Postural Tachycardia Syndrome

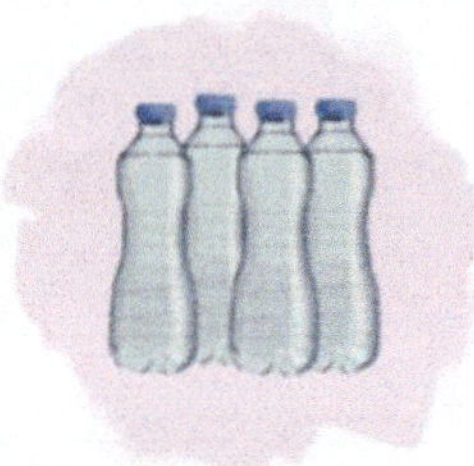

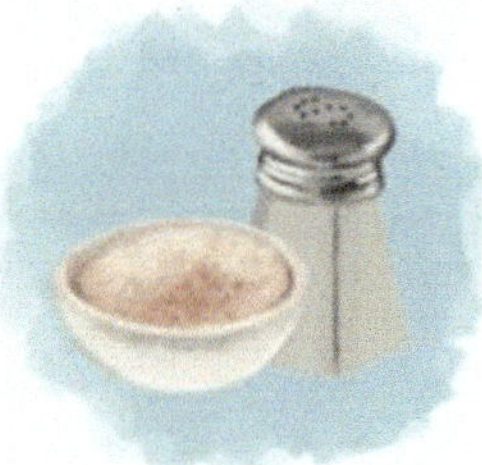

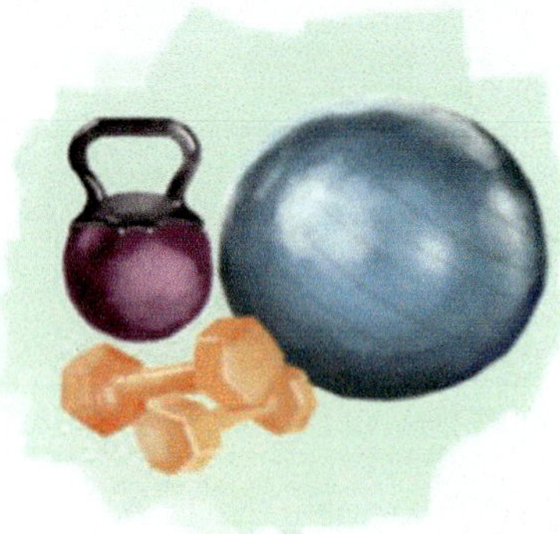

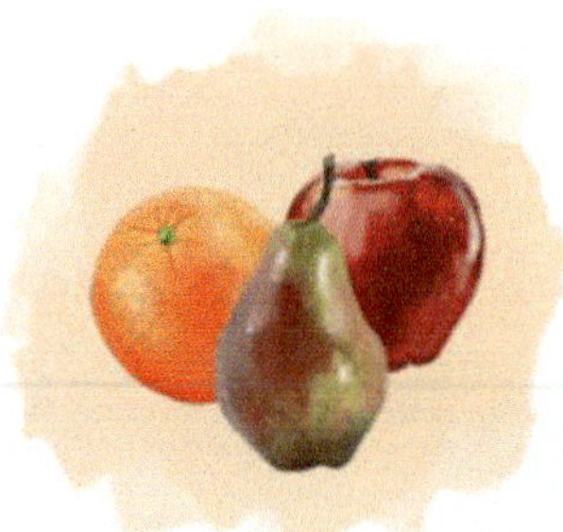

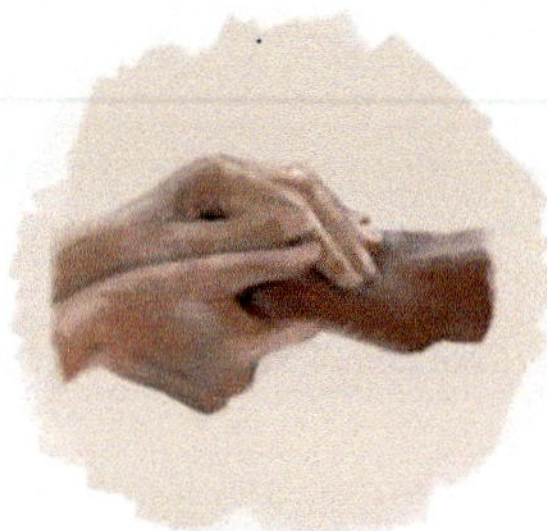

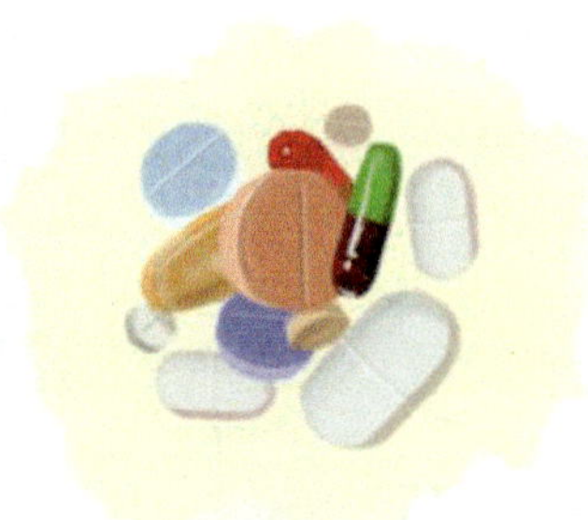

Nicholas Gall · Lesley Kavi ·
Melvin D. Lobo
Editors

Postural Tachycardia Syndrome

A Concise and Practical Guide to Management and Associated Conditions

Springer

Editors
Nicholas Gall
King's College Hospital
London, UK

Melvin D. Lobo
Barts NIHR Biomedical Research
Centre, William Harvey Research
Institute, Queen Mary
University of London
London, UK

Lesley Kavi
Faculty of Health, Education and Life
Sciences, Birmingham City University
Birmingham, UK

ISBN 978-3-030-54164-4 ISBN 978-3-030-54165-1 (eBook)
https://doi.org/10.1007/978-3-030-54165-1

This Springer imprint is published by the registered company Springer Nature Switzerland AG
The registered company address is: Gewerbestrasse 11, 6330 Cham, Switzerland

Foreword

Postural Tachycardia Syndrome is common, distressing, and has symptoms reaching far beyond simple postural tachycardia. Fortunately, we have seen recent rapid progress in studies of its origin and pathogenesis. Similarly, progress in clinical management that was slow for many years, has accelerated considerably. There are even recent consensus statements from the Heart Rhythm Society and the Canadian Cardiovascular Society. However, these statements usually provide only simple and high-level directions on what should, could, and shouldn't be done, without tools on how to actually do it.

This beautiful and comprehensive volume fills the gap, with numerous chapters providing insight, wisdom, and tools to help assessment and care. Sir William Osler once wrote that a good physician treats the disease, but a great physician treats the patient who has the disease. The authors provide an all-round approach, from the initial clinical presentation by Dr. Gall to the crucial issue of psychological support for these all too often highly distressed patients, written by Drs. Opie, Raj, and Arnold. Read it from cover to cover, or pick it up and dip in and out, then take it to help your patient. It will stand both of you in good stead for times to come.

Prof. Dr. Robert Sheldon
Cardiac Sciences, Libin Cardiovascular Institute
Cumming School of Medicine
University of Calgary
Calgary, AL, Canada
e-mail: sheldon@ucalgary.ca

Contents

Associated Conditions

Other Conditions Linked to PoTS

Therapy

POTS, An Introduction

Introduction

Nicholas Gall

Postural tachycardia syndrome (PoTS) is also known as postural orthostatic tachycardia syndrome (POTS). It is a relatively recently described condition presenting predominantly with cardiovascular symptoms and often in younger patients, predominantly female [1]. While there have been descriptions of this condition in the literature for 150 years, as will be detailed later in this book (*see Chapter2, Historical Background*), it remains poorly understood and, in some environments, controversial. Patients in their formative years are frequently significantly incapacitated by their symptoms but nevertheless are often diagnosed with a psychological or psychiatric illness rather than a physiological one [2]. While there is no true understanding of its prevalence, it does seem to be not uncommon and as time has gone on, we have become increasingly aware of large numbers of patients who have tolerated their symptoms for months and indeed years, receiving little support. While there is a clear definition, which will be detailed later in this book, whether that definition truly provides a detailed understanding of the pathophysiology remains uncertain. The condition has only been relatively recently defined and while there are now international guidelines [3], much of the guidance available comes solely from expert opinion.

Managing these patients emphasises the multidisciplinary nature of their symptom presentation, as while there may be a focus particularly on cardiovascular symptomatology, it is clear that there are many symptoms in many different organ systems, which often require the input of different clinicians in different specialties. Recent surveys undertaken both in the UK [2] and in the United States [4] have clearly highlighted the symptomatic nature of our patients, the significant length of time it can take for them to receive a diagnosis, their multiple visits to other clinicians and to other healthcare environments, such as the emergency department, where often there is a focus on whether the presentation is psychological.

While the exact aetiology of the condition remains uncertain and as a syndrome, it may well be that there are multiple aetiologies [5], as will be detailed later in this book, it is clear that symptoms affect many different organ systems in varying ways in different patients. Indeed, different symptoms may be more important to different patients, both in terms of the system affected but also this may vary with time. Anyone who has read the literature in this area will be aware of review articles which provide some understanding of the condition but often these focus on individual organs and it can often be difficult to understand the entirety of each

N. Gall (✉)
Department of Cardiology, King's College Hospital, London SE5 9RS, UK
e-mail: nickgall@doctors.org.uk

N. Gall et al. (eds.), *Postural Tachycardia Syndrome*, https://doi.org/10.1007/978-3-030-54165-1_1

patient's condition. While the definition focuses particularly on heart rate change, it is clear to those who manage patients in this territory, that focusing purely on heart rate does not lead to an overall improvement in the patient's symptoms in these multiple territories. For that reason, many experts tend to focus on a multidisciplinary management strategy; discussions with clinicians from different parts of the world often highlights a very similar management strategy, despite being developed independently.

Patients may present to varied specialities depending upon their predominant presenting symptoms and the special interest of clinicians and structure of local services. This will often be to cardiology or to blackout and syncope services but can also be to gastroenterology, immunology, rheumatology or orthopaedics amongst others. Fatigue and concerns relating to the psychological nature of the symptoms can lead patients to the chronic fatigue syndrome service or to psychology/ psychiatry. It is therefore important for any specialist to be aware of this condition as it may present in many different guises.

As knowledge of the pathophysiology of PoTS has developed in recent years, with the growing evidence of an associated small fibre neuropathy in some and the finding of increased levels of a variety of autoantibodies, neurologists, immunologists and rheumatologists are increasingly developing an interest in PoTS, providing new services for patients and exploring new potential therapeutic opportunities. On occasion, a PoTS clinic will exist within a Medicine for the Elderly clinic, even though patients are mainly younger women; such clinics have evolved as historically Medicine for the Elderly consultants have often developed the hospital's tilt table testing service.

Whilst some areas of the UK, such as London, have a number of secondary and tertiary care clinicians who express an interest in PoTS, there are other areas not so well-served and patients often experience difficulties in obtaining out-of-area referrals. Children especially find it difficult to access a knowledgeable paediatrician.

Most PoTS clinics provide similar advice in terms of self-management strategies. However, investigations and pharmaceutical management can vary depending upon the specialism and experience of the clinician and the availability of resources.

The management difficulties in this area have been discussed amongst interested clinicians and led on to plans to collect together experts in different specialties to try to provide a more coordinated, multi-specialty understanding of the problems that we face managing these patients, and to provide some understanding of what individual symptoms may indicate, how they can be assessed, by whom and how they may be managed. We have therefore tried to collect together a number of mostly UK-based specialists who see our patients, who can provide both an understanding of the current literature but also an understanding of their experience. Others have provided similar assessments in other fora; for instance, Autonomic Neuroscience produced a series of articles in 2018 to mark the 25th anniversary of the definition of PoTS [6].

We hope that this book will provide you with some understanding of the postural tachycardia syndrome and practical suggestions on how to assess and manage these complex patients and which clinicians may be able to assist. There is active research in the field although it remains limited. Our knowledge will therefore develop as time progresses and hopefully in further editions of this book, we will see the evolution of our understanding.

References

1. Bryarly M, Phillips LT, Fu Q, Vernino S, Levine BD. Postural orthostatic tachycardia syndrome. JACC. 2019;73:1207–28.
2. Kavi L, Nuttall M, Low DA, Opie M, Nicholson LM, Caldow E, Newton JL. A profile of patients with postural tachycardia syndrome and their experience of healthcare in the UK. Br J Cardiol. 2016;23:33–6.
3. Sheldon RS, Grubb BP, Olshansky B, et al. 2015 Heart Rhythm Society Expert Consensus Statement on the diagnosis and treatment of postural tachycardia syndrome, inappropriate sinus tachycardia, and vasovagal syncope. Heart Rhythm. 2015;12:e41–63.

4. Shaw BH, Stiles LE, Bourne K, et al. The face of postural tachycardia syndrome—insights from a large cross-sectional online community-based study. J Intern Med. 2019;286:438–48.
5. Mar PL, Raj SR. Neuronal and hormonal perturbations in postural tachycardia syndrome. Frontiers in Physiology. 2014;5:1–8.
6. Raj SR, Stiles LE. Special issue for the silver anniversary of Postural Tachycardia Syndrome. Autonomic Neurosci: Basic Clin. 2018;215:1–128.

Historical Background

Kelsey Klaas and Lesley Kavi

Postural tachycardia syndrome, or PoTS, is an abnormal response by the autonomic nervous system to upright posture which results in tachycardia and symptoms of orthostatic intolerance. The condition was first described in 1993 by Schondorf and Low at the Mayo Clinic in the United States, who proposed that the condition is a type of limited autonomic neuropathy. The condition is thought to be common; although the incidence is unknown, it is estimated to affect approximately 0.2% of the general population [1]. The condition is certainly not a new one, though it has gone by various names over time.

The earliest accounts of this condition were published during the American Civil War, and described exhausted soldiers who experienced tachycardia in the erect posture, with palpitations and breathlessness. Jacob M Da Costa, a physician practising in Philadelphia, first described what he called 'irritable heart' in a letter to the War Department in 1862. Da Costa was appointed to oversee the cardiac unit of a military field hospital, and there observed over 300 patients who developed symptoms of palpitations, tachycardia, chest pain, breathlessness and digestive symptoms. In 1871, after collecting follow-up data on patients where available, he published his case series in what was one of the earliest clinical cardiology studies. Importantly, Da Costa acknowledged that his was not the first description of this condition; he had found reports of what he judged to be similar cases in British reports from the Crimean War, as well as other medical military histories and discharge records. Da Costa described irritable heart as a 'functional disorder of the heart,' and excluded cases of suspected structural disease from his case series. In his patients, the onset of symptoms followed febrile or diarrhoeal illnesses, injury, or, in over a third of cases, extreme exertion, 'particularly excessive marching'. For treatment, he advocated rest and digitalis but also trialed many other medications and supplements. Some soldiers were able to return to active duty, but many were invalided or required lighter duties [2, 3].

The condition was also observed in Great Britain. W C Maclean, Professor of Military Medicine, raised concern about the high incidence of functional disorders of the heart leading to invalidity in the British Army [4]. The War Office set up a committee to investigate, and in 1867 Maclean studied 5500 soldiers who were admitted to hospital after serving overseas and he reported that almost 10% were discharged from the army with heart disease, the

K. Klaas
Mayo Clinic, 200 First St. SW, Rochester, MN 55905, USA
e-mail: klaas.kelsey@mayo.edu

L. Kavi (✉)
Solihull Healthcare Partnership, 3 Grove Road, Solihull B91 2AG, West Midlands, UK
e-mail: lesley@potsuk.org

N. Gall et al. (eds.), *Postural Tachycardia Syndrome*, https://doi.org/10.1007/978-3-030-54165-1_2

majority of which appeared to suffer from 'irritable heart'. He suggested it was caused by the combination of constrictive military uniform, excessive weight (almost 60lb) and distribution of the equipment typically carried by the foot soldiers, along with exertion.

Interest in this condition heightened shortly after the outbreak of World War 1, when soldiers returned from the front with an 'irritable heart'. Heart disease became the third leading cause of discharge from the British army, accounting for over 10%, and it was believed that many of these cases were a result of 'disordered action of the heart' [5]. In 1915, the Medical Research Committee (renamed the Medical Research Council after 1920), under the direction of Sir James Mackenzie, investigated this problem. Mackenzie advised the War Office that a hospital should be dedicated to the treatment of this condition. Mount Vernon Hospital fulfilled this role, but as numbers increased, they were moved to a larger facility in Colchester. He observed almost 400 soldiers affected by what he called 'The Soldier's Heart.' In 1916, in a lecture at the London Hospital that was also published in the BMJ, he described their symptom complex of palpitations, shortness of breath, fatigue, precordial pain, giddiness, syncope, irritability and feeling 'rotten'. They demonstrated vasomotor instability with pale fingers becoming thick and red, and swollen lower legs. Heart rate was modest at rest but increased rapidly after minimal exertion. They appeared unwell and were 'content to lie in bed and brood over their woes'. He noted the same phenomenon in the civilian population, often following severe or infective illness. Mackenzie's observations led him to conclude that the mechanism of exhaustion and syncope was the accumulation of blood in the peripheral veins of the limbs and the large abdominal veins with consequent 'anaemia' of the brain. He specified that the soldier's heart was not primarily a heart problem and would probably prove to be 'separate conditions, each with a definite cause' [6].

A secondary outcome of investigations into the soldier's heart was the foundation of Cardiology as a specialty in the United Kingdom. The Ministry of Pensions approached specialists in heart disease for assistance in assessing soldiers who claimed to have this condition. A group of physicians were appointed and met for the first time in 1921. They became known as the Cardiac Club, which subsequently became the British Cardiovascular Society. Mackenzie was an honorary member; although ironically he vehemently opposed the idea of specialism, he stated that 'a specialist is, by the nature of his calling, a man with limited experience, and therefore he can but have a limited outlook' [7].

Treatment of the soldier's heart was of paramount importance during the war. In his 1916 publication, Mackenzie advocated fresh air and judicious congenial exercise—fishing, riding, shooting and golf for the officers and bowling, quoits or skittles for lower ranks. Many of his patients improved and returned to duty [6]. Dr. Thomas Lewis, a colleague of Mackenzie appointed by the British Medical Research Committee, advocated for a graded rehabilitative program involving recreation and exercise to be conducted in hospitals, in the Lancet in 1918 [8]. In contrast, bed rest was favoured by many American physicians, who increasingly discussed a component of 'neurosis' and anxiety in cases of irritable heart [5]. The condition by the end of the First World War was widely known as 'neurocirculatory asthenia' in the United States, a term that was used over the ensuing decades, and 'effort syndrome' in the United Kingdom. The role of psychological factors continued to be a matter of debate over the next several years.

During the Second World War, in 1941, the British Medical Journal published a series of lectures by Paul Wood, an eminent British cardiologist. He declared that effort syndrome was a somatic manifestation of fear and incapacity, and tended to be exaggerated consciously or subconsciously in order to protect the individual from further painful emotional experience. He summarised that, 'a proper psychiatric diagnosis is nearly always available' [9]. Wood was an influential figure and perhaps as a result of his writings, interest in effort syndrome waned. Affected soldiers received various diagnostic labels, mostly psychiatric in nature.

However, the soldier's heart was not only a condition of soldiers. Da Costa, Mackenzie, and several others noted its existence in their civilian patients [3, 6]. In his 1871 paper, Da Costa wrote that 'much of what I am about to say could duplicate from the experience of private practice.' Dr. Selian Neuhof believed that 'the soldier's irritable heart is no new complex, but is the same syndrome as seen in civilian life, intensified and multiplied by training and war conditions' [10]. Dr. Paul White, who had trained with Lewis, published an account in 1920 commenting on the frequency of cases of effort syndrome in his civilian practice, helping to raise awareness [11]. There were further civilian studies, which suggested the condition was actually more common in women and ran in families.

The cause of the condition has long been debated, though widely believed to be heterogeneous, even from the earliest publications. Maclean had proposed that symptoms arose from soldiers' accoutrements. Others believed excesses of tobacco, alcohol and other intoxicants were to blame [7]. Fevers, excessive marching, and gastrointestinal illnesses were identified as inciting factors. White, who collaborated with several others to publish reports on neurocirculatory asthenia throughout his career, believed that no single cause was identifiable [12]. Wood found, as earlier authors had, that signs of autonomic nervous system disturbance were frequently found, but he attributed this to psychological causes [13]. A description of overlap with anxiety disorders was also widespread in civilian populations. While it has been argued that soldier's heart became shell shock, post-traumatic stress disorder and Gulf War syndrome, in the civilian population, anxiety neurosis and cardiac neurosis were described. The name assigned to the same collection of symptoms has continued to evolve. In the 1980s it was proposed that the condition was the same as 'mitral valve prolapse syndrome' [14]. Most diagnoses have focused on cardiac symptomatology, though, regardless of the name assigned, the condition is near-universally agreed to be a functional cardiac disorder. Palpitations were noted as a symptom from the earliest descriptions of soldier's heart, and tachycardia was described consistently among the constellation of symptoms [3, 13, 15].

Rosen and Cryer coined the term 'postural tachycardia syndrome' in a 1982 publication where they described a patient with postural symptoms of palpitations, lightheadedness, and headache who had an exaggerated rise in norepinephrine on standing [16]. There were reports of diabetic patients also with an exaggerated heart rate increase on standing [17]. These reports inspired Schondorf and Low to investigate the cases they later published in their 1993 paper, in which they described a form of limited autonomic neuropathy that they called postural orthostatic tachycardia syndrome or POTS [18]. They highlighted that whilst people with presyncope/syncope and orthostatic hypotention were often recognised, patients who experienced these symptoms without a drop in blood pressure were not. They undertook a retrospective analysis of records of 188 patients between the ages of 20 and 51 who presented to their autonomic laboratory during a 32 month period and reviewed in detail the 16 patients who exhibited orthostatic tachycardia on head-up tilt testing. The majority were women who experienced sudden onset of fatigue and lightheadness, often following a recent viral illness. They concluded that many patients with POTS had idiopathic hypovolaemia, some evidence of small fibre neuropathy, mild abnormalities of arteriolar or venomotor tone and a more hyperadrenergic response to standing compared to controls. Only 2 of 11 patients followed up 6–24 months later reported resolution of their symptoms. Only patients with no assignable cause for their postural tachycardia were labeled as having POTS. This contrasts with current diagnostic criteria [1] where PoTS can be considered present in the presence of other co-existing and potentially causative conditions such as connective tissue disorders.

Since the Schondorf and Low paper in 1993 there has been growing interest in the postural

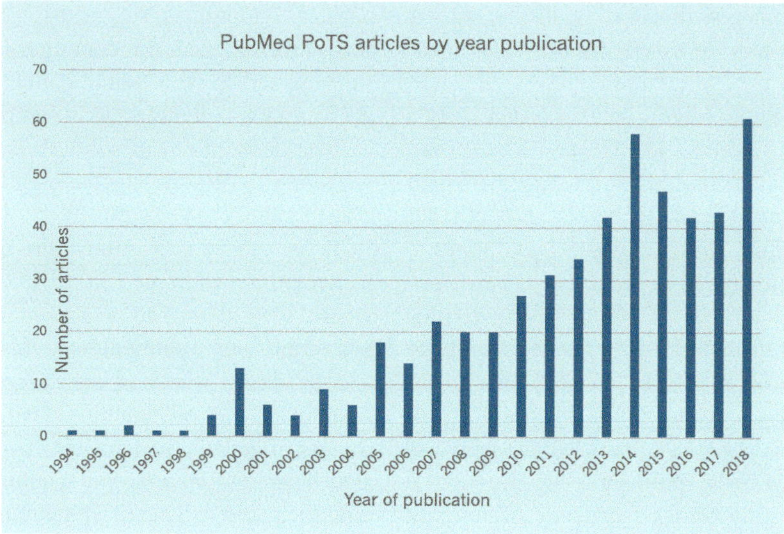

Fig. 1 Number of journal articles by year of publication (PubMed) - search terms postural tachycardia syndrome

tachycardia syndrome. A PubMed search for journal articles using the term 'postural tachycardia syndrome' revealed 1 article in 1994, steadily growing to 61 articles (both research papers and reviews) published in 2018 (see Fig. 1). Whilst there is better understanding of the symptom profile, pathophysiology, associated medical conditions, and management of PoTS, there remains much work to be done in order to fully understand this challenging condition.

References

1. Sheldon RS, Grubb BP, 2nd, Olshansky B, Shen WK, Calkins H, Brignole M, et al. 2015 heart rhythm society expert consensus statement on the diagnosis and treatment of postural tachycardia syndrome, inappropriate sinus tachycardia, and vasovagal syncope. Heart Rhythm. 2015;12(6):e41–63.
2. DaCosta JM. Medical diagnosis: with special reference to practical medicine: a guide to the knowledge and discrimination of diseases. Philadelphia, PA: J.B. Lippincott & Co.; 1864.
3. DaCosta JM. On irritable heart; a clinical study of a form of functional cardiac disorder and its consequences. Am J Med Sci. 1871;61.
4. Maclean WC. Diseases of the heart in the British army: the cause and the remedy. Br Med J. 1867:161–4.
5. Cohn AE. The cardiac phase of the war neurosis. Am J Med Sci. 1919;158:453–70.
6. Mackenzie J. The soldier's heart. BMJ. 1916;1(2873):117–9.
7. Howell JD. "Soldier's heart": the redefinition of heart disease and specialty formation in early twentieth-century Great Britain. Med Hist Suppl. 1985(5):34–52.
8. Lewis T. Observations upon prognosis, with special reference to the condition described as the "irritable heart of soldiers.". Lancet. 1918:181–3.
9. Wood P. Da Costa's syndrome: aetiology. Lecture III. Br Med J. 1941;1(4196):845–51.
10. Neuhof S. The irritable heart in general practice: a comparison between it and the irritable heart of soldiers. Arch Intern Med. 1919:51–64.
11. White PD. The diagnosis of heart disease in young people. JAMA. 1920;74(9):580–2.
12. Cohen ME, White PD. Neurocirculatory asthenia: 1972 concept. Mil Med. 1972;137(4):142–4.
13. Wood P. Da Costa's syndrome (or effort syndrome). Lecture I. Br Med J. 1941;1(4194):767–72.
14. Wooley CF. Where are the diseases of yesteryear? DaCosta's syndrome, soldiers heart, the effort syndrome, neurocirculatory asthenia–and the mitral valve prolapse syndrome. Circulation. 1976;53(5):749–51.
15. Paul O. Da Costa's syndrome or neurocirculatory asthenia. Br Heart J. 1987;58(4):306–15.
16. Rosen SG, Cryer PE. Postural tachycardia syndrome. Reversal of sympathetic hyperresponsiveness and clinical improvement during sodium loading. Am J Med. 1982;72(5):847–50.
17. Hoeldtke RD, Davis KM. The orthostatic tachycardia syndrome: evaluation of autonomic function and treatment with octreotide and ergot alkaloids. J Clin Endocrinol Metab. 1991;73(1):132–9.
18. Schondorf R, Low PA. Idiopathic postural orthostatic tachycardia syndrome: an attenuated form of acute pandysautonomia? Neurology. 1993;43(1):132–7.

Clinical Presentation

Nicholas Gall

Postural tachycardia syndrome, as a *syndrome*, is defined as a collection of symptoms present for at least six months associated with cardiovascular abnormalities on standing, where the heart rate increases inappropriately and remains persistently raised without significant orthostatic hypotension [1–3]. The details of securing the diagnosis are to be found in other chapters of this text. While the clinical definition relies on a significant heart rate change, that heart rate change can vary both with the time of day [4, 5], whether the patient has eaten recently and in women with relation to the menstrual cycle [6]. There are no other specific laboratory / imaging markers for this condition and indeed it is described as a syndrome and therefore, as detailed elsewhere, it may well represent a number of different pathophysiologies. In light of that, the diagnosis should rest not only on suggestive physiological findings but also on the clinical presentation of the patient. Review articles have been published in the field, detailing the clinical presentation in major centres [7] and other organisations have also assessed patients with the condition in an effort to understand their symptoms [8, 9].

There is no true understanding of the prevalence of the condition, although 170/100,000 population is often quoted although that is an estimate based on an assumption that 40% of patients with chronic fatigue syndrome have PoTS [10]. This may mean that from 500,000 to 3,000,000 Americans are affected [2]. No UK study to date has assessed the incidence or prevalence in any formalised manner but many clinicians believe that it is likely to be more common than is often perceived. The condition is particularly common in younger women and usually presents between the ages of 15 and 25 although patients will often describe that their symptoms began earlier and indeed a recent review of patient symptoms suggests that the modal age of onset is 14 [8]. It seems to be at least three times more common in women for which there are potential explanations, detailed elsewhere. It is important to recognise this demographic as clearly, while other patients may present with PoTS-like symptoms, the more different the patient is from this classical demographic the more one needs to be concerned that there may be an alternative explanation, perhaps a more significant underlying autonomic disturbance. In some cases, patients will describe their cardiovascular symptoms as being present for as long as they can remember and from personal experience, this may be more likely in those with hypermobility. One quarter may have a family history of similar complaints [11].

In many other cases, there is a sudden onset to the symptoms, in association with another

N. Gall (✉)
Department of Cardiology, King's College Hospital, London SE5 9RS, UK
e-mail: nickgall@doctors.org.uk

N. Gall et al. (eds.), *Postural Tachycardia Syndrome*, https://doi.org/10.1007/978-3-030-54165-1_3

illness [10]. Often this may be a viral illness, for instance glandular fever (Epstein Barr virus); however many other precipitants can be associated, for instance a road traffic accident, during a pregnancy or after a complicated labour, after an operation or a vaccination. Stressful events may also be noted as a precipitant although, as detailed elsewhere, this should not be taken to suggest that the condition is purely psychological. In the end, it does not appear that one particular event precipitates PoTS, it is often a significant event potentially putting strain on the system which produces the changes. While deconditioning may be relevant to many symptoms, as will be detailed elsewhere, the sudden onset in many cases would suggest that deconditioning is not the specific driver in most cases, more often a contributor, albeit important.

PoTS tends to present with a multitude of symptoms affecting many different organ systems but is particularly focused on the cardiovascular system and it is for that reason that many patients with this condition will be seen in cardiology clinics. The table below details the frequency of these symptoms in two reviews (Table 1).

The most frequently quoted study of patient symptoms originates from the Mayo clinic. Thieban and colleagues [7] documented their experience over an 11-year period. They included patients with the classical definition of PoTS and excluded patients with orthostatic hypotension, pregnancy, other causes of autonomic failure and those with systemic illness. They identified 152 patients, 87% being female, with symptoms predating the diagnosis by an average of four years. One in eight had a family history of orthostatic intolerance and 40% had a prior history to some degree. 13% had symptoms beginning acutely within one month, 14% between one and three months and 6% with a more gradual onset over three months or more, although in two thirds the onset was not defined. In their series, one quarter felt that there was a precipitant, often a viral illness but the majority did not recognise a clear cause. They noted a wide range of symptoms, many relating to cardiovascular symptoms but other, non-orthostatic symptoms and more general symptoms were also notable. Symptoms were noted to worsen in over half of patients with exercise or heat, a quarter noted worsening around a meal and 15% around the time of their period.

Shaw and colleagues [8] have more recently summarised the characteristics of PoTS patients with a large, cross-sectional, online community-based survey, conducted between academic institutions and Dysautonomia International, a USA-based patient advocacy organisation. There will clearly be some limitation as the data originates from self-reported diagnosis and symptoms but is a much larger sample, involving 4835 participants. The mean age of symptom onset in their cohort was 21 (±12) years with a median of 17 and a modal age of onset at 14. Nearly 50% noted their symptoms began after the age of 18. 41% of patients reported that their symptoms had started within three months of a particular event, in particular an infection in 41%, after surgery in 12%, with a pregnancy in 9%, after a vaccination in 6%, after an accident in 6%, with puberty in 5%, after a concussion in 4% or with an emotional stress/trauma in 3%. In this self-selected group, 94% of patients were female. A median of 24 months for diagnosis from symptom onset was notable. 16% of patients had some form of autoimmune disease.

A survey of PoTS patients based in the UK derived from the Newcastle PoTS clinic and subscribing to the PoTS-UK charity [9], assessed 136 patients with a mean age of 33, 10% of whom were male. On average, their symptoms began at 24 years of age but were diagnosed at 31 suggesting that diagnosis may take up to 7 years in many cases. They noted significant associated conditions including 21% diagnosed with chronic fatigue syndrome, 18% diagnosed with EDS/hypermobility, 10% with irritable bowel syndrome, 10% with thyroid problems and 7% with fibromyalgia. They also noted that 43% of PoTS patients who had not been diagnosed with chronic fatigue syndrome would in fact have fulfilled criteria for that condition.

Table 1 The symptoms associated with PoTS have been studied in a number of series; detailed here is a summary of findings from the Mayo clinic and a more recent patient questionnaire

	Symptom	Thieben et al. [7] (%)	Shaw et al. [8] (%)
Orthostatic	Lightheadedness /dizzy	77	99
	Pre-syncope	61	9
	Weakness	50	
	Palpitations	75	87
	Tremor	38	78
	Shortness of breath	28	88
	Chest pain	24	7
	Loss of sweating	5	
	Excessive sweating	9	
	Syncope		36
Non-orthostatic	Bloating	24	79
	Nausea	39	90
	Vomiting	9	
	Abdominal pain	15	83
	Constipation	15	71
	Diarrhoea	18	69
	Bladder problems	9	68
General symptoms	Fatigue	48	
	Sleep disturbance	32	
	Migraines	28	94
	Myofascial pain	16	84
	Neuropathic pain	2	
	Difficulty concentrating		94
	Memory problems		87
	Dry mouth		66
	Dry eyes		60
	Muscle weakness		83
	Skin flushing		69

The most common symptoms relate to a sense of faintness, particularly associated with standing, not only when patients stand initially (initial orthostatic hypotension), but also when patients stand for any length of time. Patients will often feel that they have a sense that they need to sit or lie down in those situations to avoid losing consciousness. As will be detailed later, there is also an association with more vertiginous dizziness where patients may fear that they will fall from being off-balance which does need to be differentiated from these feelings of faintness. While PoTS patients are at risk of losing consciousness with a vasovagal mechanism, this is perhaps less common than might be assumed, perhaps 30% [6]. There is also a distinct association with dissociative syncope in this condition. From personal experience, although the exact reasons for that remain uncertain, this will also produce an apparent loss of consciousness. However, these two forms of collapse can be differentiated. Vasovagal syncope is usually associated with autonomic symptoms and a rapid recovery of consciousness albeit with patients feeling generally unwell and washed out afterwards, whereas dissociative syncope [12] may happen more frequently (many times a day), may be more prolonged (minutes and even longer), may be associated with atypical seizure-like movements and may be associated with eye closure which is not something that occurs with vasovagal syncope.

Many PoTS patients complain of chest pain although there is very little understanding of the exact aetiology [6]. It can take a number of different forms including sharp, stabbing pains which may be more musculoskeletal, and may potentially link in with hypermobility. There can be associations with gastrointestinal disturbance, as will be detailed later, which can also precipitate chest pain of a more oesophageal quality. A number of patients describe angina-like chest tightness, which may associate with their sinus tachycardia. ECG changes in the inferior leads may occur [6]. The exact aetiology is uncertain, but this may also associate with dysfunctional breathing which is recognised to associate with PoTS (*see Chapter 39 and Physiotherapy intervention for Patients with PoTS Presenting with Breathlessness*). Dysfunctional breathing will also produce breathlessness on exertion, where patients will feel that their exercise abilities are limited. However, it may not associate with other respiratory symptoms, may be described as 'air hunger' and may associate with either gasping or yawning respiration, potentially with hand or facial paraesthesiae. This can also occur when patients are lying flat in bed but is different to orthopnoea in character. Patients may note some ankle swelling, but often they also tend to report red or purple discolouration of their legs when dependent (acrocyanosis), which is often described as pooling, although this may represent skin ischaemia [2, 13].

Patients often describe palpitation, some of which will relate to sensing ectopic beats as flutters, pauses, missed or extra beats. However, it does not appear that PoTS patients suffer any more ectopic beats than any other patient, although they do seem to be more aware of those symptoms. Their sinus rate is often inappropriately fast and therefore much of the palpitation will relate to a sense that their heart is beating harder, more strongly and faster than is required for the circumstances. It may be that this is noted suddenly. However usually this form of palpitation passes off gradually, therefore differentiating it from other arrhythmias such as supraventricular tachycardia (SVT).

Differing forms of PoTS have been recognised by some, for instance neuropathic and hyperadrenergic. They may present with differing symptoms; hyperadrenergic PoTS may be more likely to present with palpitation, anxiety, tachycardia and tremor [10]. Kanjwal in the Cardiology Journal in 2011 [14] also describe their experience with this form. They felt that in their series, these patients had a more gradual onset of symptoms in comparison to others. They also note complaints of feeling cold and sweaty when upright and also note migraine in more than half. They also found that one third of their patients had high blood pressure. Differentiating these two distinct forms, if they exist, may however be not so clear-cut from personal experience.

With the associated features and conditions, which are detailed elsewhere in this text, it is well-recognised that PoTS patients also describe symptoms in other organ territories although these can vary from patient to patient. They may present with gastrointestinal symptoms, urological symptoms, migraines, joint symptoms perhaps associating with hypermobility [15] and allergic symptoms associating with potential mast cell activation. In many patients, more vertiginous dizziness is often described which seems in many to link in with vestibular migraine. There can be a significant association with fatigue although there is little true understanding as to the exact causes of fatigue and it is for that reason that there is an overlap with chronic fatigue syndrome. Garland et al. [2] note that chronic fatigue may affect 48–77% of PoTS patients with 17–23% of patients being diagnosed formally with chronic fatigue syndrome.

Many patients complain of cold hands and feet, often with features of Raynaud's and poor temperature control, that is persistently feeling the wrong temperature for the environment; again, the reasons for these symptoms remain uncertain. Grubb and colleagues [16] note in addition significant functional impairment similar to patients with chronic obstructive pulmonary disease or heart failure.

In light of the widespread and disparate symptoms associated with this condition, many patients will present to a number of different physicians, potentially over a number of months and even years and indeed studies would suggest that many patients may take years prior to their receiving a diagnosis, having seen multiple different physicians in the interim [8, 9]. In many cases, the large number of symptoms associated can cause confusion in clinicians who are not aware of this problem and may consider that there can be little physiological basis to these multitudinous symptoms. Abnormalities in the autonomic nervous system, of course, can provide a clear explanation for the widespread issues.

The diagnosis of PoTS therefore rests not only on the suggestive findings of a significant heart rate change on a stand test but also the presentation in a patient of the correct age, beginning in a classical manner, without an alternative explanation. The response to medications, which will be detailed elsewhere and indeed lifestyle change, will also provide support for the diagnosis. Clinicians in the field no longer focus to such an extent on the absolute heart rate change, an acknowledgment of the complexity of the presentation which is reflected in the Canadian Cardiac Society guidance [17].

References

1. 2015 Heart rhythm society expert consensus statement on the diagnosis and treatment of postural Tachycardia syndrome, inappropriate sinus Tachycardia, and Vasovagal syncope. Heart Rhythm Soc [Internet] [cited 2019 Nov 27]. https://www.hrsonline.org/clinical-resources/2015-heart-rhythm-society-expert-consensus-statement-diagnosis-and-treatment-postural-tachycardia.
2. Garland EM, Celedonio JE, Raj SR. Postural Tachycardia syndrome: beyond orthostatic intolerance. In: Current neurology and neuroscience reports, vol. 15. Current Medicine Group LLC 1; 2015.
3. Carew S, Connor MO, Cooke J, Conway R, Sheehy C, Costelloe A, et al. A review of postural orthostatic tachycardia syndrome. Europace. 2009;11:18–25.
4. Plash WB, Diedrich A, Biaggioni I, Garland EM, Paranjape SY, Black BK, et al. Diagnosing postural tachycardia syndrome: Comparison of tilt testing compared with standing haemodynamics. Clin Sci [Internet]. 2013 [cited 2020 Jan 12];124(2):109–14. https://www.ncbi.nlm.nih.gov/pubmed/22931296.
5. Nwazue VC, Arnold AC, Raj V, Black BK, Biaggioni I, Paranjape SY, et al. Understanding the placebo effect in clinical trials for postural tachycardia syndrome. Clin Exp Pharmacol Physiol. 2014;41(5):325–30.
6. Raj SR. Postural tachycardia syndrome (POTS). Circulation. 2013;127(23):2336–42.
7. Thieben MJ, Sandroni P, Sletten DM, Benrud-Larson LM, Fealey RD, Vernino S, et al. Postural orthostatic tachycardia syndrome: the Mayo clinic experience. Mayo Clin Proc [Internet]. 2007 [cited 2020 Jan 12];82(3):308–13. https://www.ncbi.nlm.nih.gov/pubmed/17352367.
8. Shaw BH, Stiles LE, Bourne K, Green EA, Shibao CA, Okamoto LE, et al. The face of postural tachycardia syndrome—insights from a large cross-sectional online community-based survey. J Intern Med. 2019;286(4):438–48.
9. McDonald C, Koshi S, Busner L, Kavi L, Newton JL. Postural tachycardia syndrome is associated with significant symptoms and functional impairment predominantly affecting young women: a UK perspective. BMJ Open. 2014;4(6).
10. Low PA, Sandroni P, Joyner M, Shen WK. Postural tachycardia syndrome (POTS): clinical review. J Cardiovasc Electrophysiol. 2009;20:352–8.
11. Benarroch EE. Postural tachycardia syndrome: a heterogeneous and multifactorial disorder. In: Mayo clinic proceedings, vol. 87. Elsevier Ltd; 2012. p. 1214–25.
12. Blad H, Lamberts RJ, Dijk JG Van, Thijs RD. Tilt-induced vasovagal syncope and psychogenic pseudosyncope. Neurology. 2015;85(23):2006–10.
13. Medow MS, Stewart JM. The postural tachycardia syndrome. Cardiol Rev. 2007;15:67–75.
14. Kanjwal K, Saeed B, Karabin B, Kanjwal Y, Grubb BP. Clinical presentation and management of patients with hyperadrenergic postural orthostatic tachycardia syndrome. A single center experience. Cardiol J [Internet]. 2011 [cited 2020 Jan

12];18(5):527–31. https://www.ncbi.nlm.nih.gov/pubmed/21947988.
15. Mathias CJ, Low DA, Iodice V, Owens AP, Kirbis M, Grahame R. Postural tachycardia syndrome—current experience and concepts. Nat Rev Neurol. 2012;8:22–34.
16. Grubb BP, Kanjwal Y, Kosinski DJ. The postural tachycardia syndrome: a concise guide to diagnosis and management. J Cardiovasc Electrophysiol. 2006;17(1):108–12.
17. Raj SR, Guzman JC, Harvey P, et al. Canadian Cardiovascular Society Position Statement on Postural Orthostatic Tachycardia Syndrome (POTS) and Related Disorders of Chronic Orthostatic Intolerance. Can J Cardiol. 2020; 36(3):357–72. https://doi.org/10.1016/j.cjca.2019.12.024.

Specialty Assessment

Diagnostic Criteria for Postural Tachycardia Syndrome: Consideration of the Clinical Features Differentiating PoTS from Other Disorders of Orthostatic Intolerance

Kate M. Bourne, Matthew G. Lloyd and Satish R. Raj

Abbreviations

ADHD	Attention deficit hyperactivity disorder
HR	Heart Rate
IOH	Initial Orthostatic Hypotension
IST	Inappropriate Sinus Tachycardia
OH	Orthostatic Hypotension
PoTS	Postural Tachycardia Syndrome
NET	Norepinephrine transporter
SNRI	Serotonin-norepinephrine reuptake inhibitor

Background

The current definition of Postural Tachycardia Syndrome (PoTS) was developed in 1993 by Ron Schondorf and Phillip Low in an effort to provide a standardized profile for this disorder [1]. Prior to this, accounts of PoTS in the literature only referred to small or single sample cases [1]. Through reviewing a set of patients age 20–51 years who demonstrated orthostatic tachycardia during testing at the Mayo Autonomic Reflex Laboratory, a PoTS diagnosis was made if the heart rate (HR) increase was 2 standard deviations above the mean increase for a sex-matched control population [1]. Importantly, these data excluded children and adolescents.

Diagnostic Criteria

PoTS is a chronic form of orthostatic intolerance marked by excessive orthostatic tachycardia and associated symptoms. Specifically, a PoTS diagnosis is made when, upon assumption of upright posture, a sustained HR increase of 30 beats per minute (bpm) or more is observed in association with symptoms of orthostatic intolerance [2, 3]. In youth under 19 years of age, this HR increase should be 40 bpm or more. Diagnosing PoTS in pediatric patients will be discussed later in this chapter. The duration of the increased HR should be sustained – in other words, seen on at least 2 consecutive recordings. This orthostatic tachycardia should develop within 10 minutes of upright posture [2]. It is not unusual, but not necessary for diagnosis, for the HR to exceed 120 bpm [2, 3]. Orthostatic symptoms should improve with recumbence, and may include lightheadedness, blurry vision, tremulousness, and weakness [2, 3]. The observed postural tachycardia should also be in the absence of orthostatic hypotension (>20/10 mmHg decrease in blood pressure [BP]) [3], and symptoms should

K. M. Bourne · M. G. Lloyd · S. R. Raj (✉)
University of Calgary, Calgary, AB, Canada
e-mail: Satish.raj@ucalgary.ca

S. R. Raj
Vanderbilt University Medical Center, Nashville, TN, USA

N. Gall et al. (eds.), *Postural Tachycardia Syndrome*, https://doi.org/10.1007/978-3-030-54165-1_4

be chronic (lasting at least 3–6 months) [4]. The critical concern is that PoTS patients must have both excessive orthostatic tachycardia and symptoms of orthostatic intolerance in order to meet the criteria for this disorder. The diagnostic criteria are summarized in Table 1.

Clinical Evaluation of a Patient with Suspected PoTS

While seemingly simple, there are many caveats to the PoTS diagnosis that are important when differentiating between this disorder and other causes of orthostatic intolerance. All diagnostic criteria must be fulfilled for a diagnosis of PoTS. A more in-depth look at each of the diagnostic criteria is discussed below:

Orthostatic Tachycardia Must Occur Within 10 minutes

The orthostatic HR increase of 30 bpm or more (or 40 bpm or more in youth 12–19 years of age) should occur within 10 minutes of standing [2]. In a study investigating tilt table testing and PoTS, 15 PoTS patients and 15 healthy controls underwent 30 minutes tilt table and active stand tests [5]. Orthostatic HR changes were evaluated at the 10 and 30 minutes tilt and stand time points. During head up tilt, if the 30 minutes time point and 30 bpm increase were used for diagnosis, 80% of the healthy controls would have met the HR criterion for PoTS diagnosis [5]. This is compared to only 60% within 10 minutes [5]. The increased orthostatic tachycardia in healthy controls during the longer tilt tests corresponds to physiological changes in the body that occur over a long period of orthostasis [5]. Blood return to the heart is decreased, as plasma is filtered through the microvasculature into the interstitial spaces, reducing blood volume [5, 6]. However, with the active stand testing, the excessive tachycardia in healthy controls was less pronounced, with only 47% of control participants meeting the PoTS HR criterion at the 30 minutes time point [5]. In the PoTS group, 14 of the 15 participants met the PoTS HR criterion during the 10 minutes tilt [5]. While the majority of PoTS patients met the HR criterion within the first 10 minutes, the majority of healthy control participants met the HR criterion by the 30 min time point. The 10 min duration for the head-up tilt serves to capture patients with PoTS, while limiting

Table 1 PoTS diagnostic criteria

Clinical feature	Diagnostic criterion	Assessment
Excessive Orthostatic Tachycardia	HR increase >30 bpm (>40 bpm in <19 years of age) within 10 minutes of upright posture [4] Duration of tachycardia $\geq$30 seconds [5]	Active stand or head up tilt table test [5, 7]
Symptoms of Orthostatic Intolerance	Orthostatic symptoms which improve with recumbence [4]	Clinical evaluation and history [5]
Absence of Orthostatic Hypotension	No decrease in BP>20/10 mmHg through the duration of orthostasis [5]	Active stand or head up tilt table test [5, 7]
Chronicity	Orthostatic symptoms have been present for a period of 3–6 months [6, 21]	Clinical evaluation and history [5]
Absence of other causes	Other conditions causing orthostatic tachycardia and symptoms have been ruled out [8]	Clinical evaluation and history [5]

inadvertent diagnosis of healthy individuals (false positives).

Symptoms of Orthostatic Intolerance and Symptoms Independent of Orthostasis

Symptoms of orthostatic intolerance must be present in addition to orthostatic tachycardia (Table 2). If a patient has orthostatic tachycardia, but no (or minimal) orthostatic symptoms, they do not meet the requirements for a PoTS diagnosis. There must be clinical history of postural symptoms, but they are not required to be present at the time of orthostatic assessment. Clinical history may also reveal symptoms independent of orthostasis including gastrointestinal disturbances, fatigue, sleep problems [3] and difficulty concentrating [2].

Patients may also have symptoms related to comorbid disorders including, but not limited to, Ehlers-Danlos Syndrome, mast cell activation syndrome, and autoimmune disorders [7]. About 20–30% of patients may also experience syncope [8]. The mechanistic relationships between these disorders are not fully understood at this time.

PoTS is a Chronic Disorder

For a formal diagnosis of PoTS, the orthostatic intolerance should be chronic, and present for a period of 6 months or longer [4]. Some centers use a minimum of 3 months. Realistically, it is unusual for PoTS symptoms to disappear between 3 and 6 months, so these likely represent the same populations. Many people will develop orthostatic intolerance with acute infectious illnesses that can mimic PoTS. Unlike in PoTS patients, when seen with the "flu", these symptoms will usually resolve after a few days [8]. Generally, if signs and symptoms of orthostatic intolerance are present for a prolonged period of time, clinical investigation and treatment should not be withheld, even if the time frame of symptom onset is less than 6 months.

Other Causes of Tachycardia

A detailed clinical history should rule out other disorders or physiological conditions that may have a similar clinical presentation to PoTS [3]. If a patient has another overt cause for their sinus tachycardia, a diagnosis of PoTS should NOT be made. A summary of these causes is provided in Table 3.

Dehydration and Acute Blood Volume Loss

Dehydration leads to reduced circulating plasma volume, and compensatory tachycardia will result from the body's attempts to compensate for the reduced fluid volume [4]. For example, patients with acute gastrointestinal bleeding may present with orthostatic tachycardia ($\geq$30 bpm increase), indicating a plasma volume loss of 50% or more [9].

Table 2 PoTS symptoms

Symptoms dependent upon orthostasis [3, 18]	Symptoms independent of orthostasis [3, 18]
Lightheadedness	Fatigue
Shortness of breath	Sleep difficulties
Sensation of rapid heart rate/palpitation	Difficulty concentrating
Chest pain or discomfort	Gastrointestinal disturbances including nausea, vomiting, diarrhea, bloating and abdominal pain
Weakness	Migraine headache
Tremulousness	

Deconditioning

Severe deconditioning and prolonged bed rest can lead to orthostatic intolerance and PoTS-like symptoms. A deconditioned patient may present with physiological findings including hypovolemia [10], cardiac atrophy [10] and/or reduced stroke volume [11]. It is important to determine if a patient is deconditioned secondary to PoTS, or if it is the primary pathogenic mechanism of their orthostatic intolerance [11]. This will help to guide treatment, from basic reconditioning in a deconditioned patient, to treatment of a patient with pathogenic mechanisms. Deconditioning is common in patients with PoTS. In a study of patients with PoTS or orthostatic intolerance but not PoTS, 93% of participants were found to be deconditioned [11]. However, whether deconditioning is cause or consequence is still under investigation. Some patients seen in clinic report periods of bedrest for 16 or more hours per day. While they are supine, their symptoms are improved, but the situation is self-perpetuating and deconditioning worsens. In cases of extreme bedrest and deconditioning, a PoTS diagnosis should not be made. Prolonged bedrest produces orthostatic intolerance similar to PoTS [12]. The physiological findings in individuals who have undergone prolonged bedrest are similar to the physiological findings in PoTS [12]. Similarly, research into spaceflight and microgravity has shown the presence of orthostatic intolerance in astronauts who have returned to earth. Prolonged exposure to low-zero gravity conditions alters the body's physiological responses to standing. Cardiovascular autonomic regulatory mechanisms are disrupted, leading to a presentation of orthostatic intolerance comparable to individuals with PoTS [13].

A study of orthostatic intolerance and space flight involved astronauts engaging in a cardiovascular conditioning program for the duration of their space travel [14]. Astronauts who participated in this study were found to have reduced left ventricular mass as well as reduced plasma and red cell volume [14]. However, despite these physiological changes, the astronauts did not have significant orthostatic tachycardia suitable for PoTS diagnosis [14]. The authors suggest that the conditioning program while in space, helped to counter the effects of deconditioning experienced upon return to earth [14]. A separate study of 12 astronauts (n = 4 female) studied orthostatic hypotension and showed a similar result [15]. Throughout the 6 months the astronauts were in space, they participated in a resistance and endurance conditioning program. Upon return to earth, they were infused with 500–1000 mL of IV saline. No astronauts developed orthostatic hypotension upon return to earth, demonstrating that a regular conditioning program and acute volume loading were sufficient to prevent orthostatic intolerance [15].

Table 3 Other causes of tachycardia to consider when diagnosing PoTS

Medications	Some medications may exacerbate tachycardia. Caffeine and alcohol use can also exacerbate tachycardia. A clinical review of medications is required. See Table 3.
Dehydration	Dehydration will exacerbate tachycardia. Decreased plasma volume decreases venous return, leading to decreased stroke volume. Heart rate is increased to maintain cardiac output.
Physical deconditioning	Physical deconditioning may cause orthostatic tachycardia. Clinical review is important to ascertain what lead to the deconditioning. For example, onset of PoTS symptoms leading to deconditioning as a consequence could warrant a PoTS diagnosis. A prolonged period of bedrest leading to symptoms of orthostatic intolerance may not be a PoTS mechanism.
Medical conditions	Some medical conditions including anemia, hyperthyroidism and pheochromocytoma can lead to orthostatic tachycardia. Lab investigation and clinical history should rule out these disorders.

Medications

Medications including vasodilators, diuretics, stimulants, as well as some antidepressant, antipsychotic, and anxiolytic medications may cause tachycardia [7, 16]. Medications that inhibit norepinephrine reuptake (via the norepinephrine transporter [NET]), can cause tachycardia due to increased stimulation of norepinephrine receptors. NET-inhibitor medications including atomoxetine and reboxetine [4], and serotonin-norepinephrine reuptake inhibitor (SNRI) agents including duloxetine and venlafaxine [8] are examples of these medications. Attention deficit hyperactivity disorder (ADHD) medication including methylphenidate has sympathomimetic effects, and stimulates adrenergic receptors, leading to tachycardia [12]. Drospirenone, a spironolactone-analog containing oral contraceptive may also promote a sinus tachycardia due to diuretic effects [16]. Caffeine and alcohol can also contribute to orthostatic tachycardia [7]. A summary of these medications and their effects are listed in Table 4.

Other Medical Conditions

Some medical conditions cause tachycardia that can be confused with PoTS. Anemia [16] can lead to tachycardia, as the body works to maintain adequate tissue oxygenation [17]. Clinical evaluation of the anemic patient may reveal pale skin, a history of heavy menstrual periods, and/or a vegetarian diet [12]. Hyperthyroidism [7, 16] can also cause tachycardia. Increased thyroid hormone (T_3) alters the renin–angiotensin–aldosterone axis, with an end result of increased HR, and excessively increased cardiac output (50–300% larger) [18]. Patients may present with warm and moist skin, tremor, pretibial myxedema [12], weight loss and/or thyroid bruit [19]. A neuroendocrine tumour called pheochromocytoma [7, 12] presents with tachycardia independent of orthostasis [12]. Plasma metanephrine levels are often, and non-positionally, elevated in the presence of this condition [12]. Other medical conditions including pulmonary embolism, acute coronary syndrome, and arrhythmic disorders [12] should also be ruled out before making a diagnosis of PoTS. Acute infectious illness will also often present with transient symptoms of orthostatic intolerance, which should resolve within a few days [8].

Diurnal Variability in Orthostatic Tachycardia

PoTS patients experience variability of symptoms, and most often symptoms are worse in the morning [12]. Consideration of the time of testing should be given when diagnosing PoTS, as orthostatic tachycardia and symptoms may be lessened later in the day. A study of 54 PoTS patients found a significantly greater proportion of patients meeting PoTS diagnostic criteria in the morning than with testing in the evening (60 vs. 42%, $p=0.008$) [20]. Another important finding in this study is the percentage of healthy

Table 4 Medications that can cause PoTS-like tachycardia

Medication type	Effect	Examples
Vasodilators	Vasodilation, reduced blood return	Nitroglycerin
Diuretics	Decreased fluid volume	Drospirenone Oral Contraceptive
Norepinephrine transporter (NET) inhibitors	Reduced norepinephrine reuptake	Atomoxetine, reboxetine
Selective-norepinephrine reuptake inhibitors	Reduced norepinephrine reuptake	Duloxetine, venlafaxine
Tricyclic Antidepressants	Reduced norepinephrine reuptake	Nortriptyline
Attention Deficit Hyperactivity Disorder Medications	Sympathomimetic	Methylphenidate, Amphetamine
Beta-adrenergic Receptor Agonists	Direct ionotropic effects. Vasodilation	Salbutamol

controls who met the PoTS HR criterion in the morning but not in the afternoon (31 vs. 4%). Again, the presence of chronic orthostatic symptoms are important in the diagnosis of this clinical syndrome.

Similarly, women may experience fluctuations in symptom severity during different phases of the menstrual cycle. Estradiol and progesterone regulate fluids and sodium in the body [21]. A study of women with PoTS investigated the function of the renin–angiotensin–aldosterone system at different phases of the menstrual cycle [22]. Prolonged standing tests (up to 2 hours), were conducted to compare participants responses during the early follicular phase (EFP; low estrogen and progesterone) and mid-luteal phase (MLP; high estrogen and progesterone) phases of the menstrual cycle [22]. Plasma renin activity and aldosterone levels with a 2 hours standing test were higher during MLP than during EFP in PoTS patients [22]. The authors conclude that the increased estrogen and progesterone in the MLP are associated with increased renal hormones and exaggerated volume retention, leading to improved standing tolerance [22]. In a separate study, participants reported an increase in lightheadedness in the late-luteal and menstrual phases of their cycle [23]. These research findings demonstrate that menstrual cycle phase should be a consideration in the evaluation of PoTS.

Common Misconceptions Regarding the Diagnosis of PoTS

Tilt Table Testing

PoTS can be diagnosed with either a tilt table test or active stand testing [5]. Orthostatic tachycardia is likely to be more pronounced with tilt due to the passive standing mechanisms and lack of engagement of the skeletal muscle pump [5]. However, a tilt table test is not required for PoTS diagnosis [12]. A simple "free stand" for 10 minutes with repeated measurements of HR and blood pressure is a valid diagnostic test [5]. Further information comparing active stand and tilt testing in the diagnosis of PoTS is included in chapter "Autonomic Testing: Active Stand and Tilt Table Test" of this book.

Specialist Referral

A PoTS diagnosis can be made by a general clinician using an in office active stand test in combination with clinical assessment and ECG [3].

Syncope

A common misconception is that patients must faint in order to meet the criteria for PoTS. In reality, only about 20–30% of patients with PoTS will experience syncope [8]. A patient with PoTS could also have a syncope diagnosis, but syncope is not a requirement for a PoTS diagnosis. Prolonged pre-syncope is extremely common, and patients frequently report they are "going to faint", but most often "frank syncope" does not occur. PoTS is primarily a disorder of "feeling faint" rather than a "fainting" disorder.

Distinguishing PoTS from Other Types of Orthostatic Intolerance

There are several different causes of orthostatic tachycardia, and it is important to rule out these other types of orthostatic intolerance to ensure an accurate diagnosis of PoTS.

Orthostatic Tachycardia Without Orthostatic Symptoms

Some patients may present with excessive orthostatic tachycardia in the absence of orthostatic symptoms. The recent increase in consumer HR monitoring devices may be contributing to this increased presentation in clinic as patients are able to readily monitor their own data. However, without orthostatic symptoms, PoTS should not be diagnosed. The mechanistic differences behind orthostatic tachycardia with and without symptoms are not well understood.

An increase in HR with exercise is not PoTS (even if perceived to be excessive), and should not be diagnosed as such. PoTS is a clinical syndrome and requires the presence of symptoms [8].

Orthostatic Symptoms Without Orthostatic Tachycardia

Some patients may present with symptoms of orthostatic intolerance without meeting the corresponding HR criterion. Both criteria are required for PoTS diagnosis. These patients may be diagnosed with orthostatic intolerance, but not PoTS. It is important to note that orthostatic intolerance without orthostatic tachycardia is a legitimate diagnosis and warrants appropriate treatment. Some patients may seek out an incorrect PoTS diagnosis in order to validate their illness. A representative diagram is shown in Fig. 1.

Inappropriate Sinus Tachycardia (IST)

IST is a disorder where excessive sinus tachycardia is present independent of position. HR is sustained >100 bpm at rest in association with symptoms of palpitation [3]. IST presents in the absence of a clear causative medical condition, physiological process, or medication effect [24]. Similar to PoTS, IST primarily presents in adolescent and young adult females [24]. Mechanistic similarities between IST and PoTS have been proposed, however, PoTS is distinct in that the development of tachycardia only occurs with orthostasis [24]. If patients continue to have tachycardia independent of orthostasis, a PoTS diagnosis would not be appropriate.

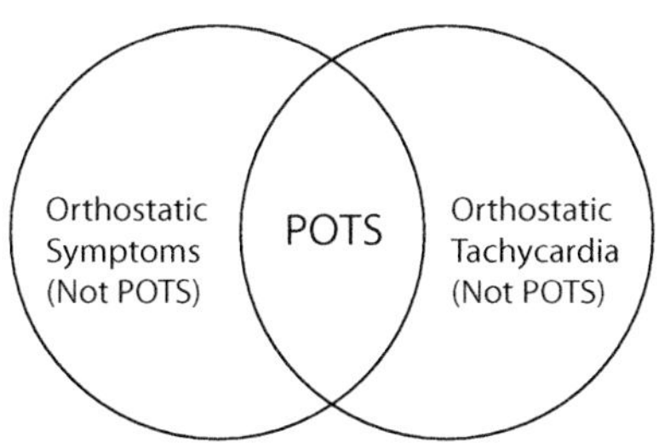

Fig. 1 For a diagnosis of PoTS, both orthostatic tachycardia and orthostatic symptoms are required

Orthostatic Hypotension (OH) and Initial Orthostatic Hypotension (IOH)

OH is defined as a decrease in BP >20/10 mmHg within 3 minutes of standing [25]. PoTS patients may experience OH at times, especially if they are hypovolemic, but they must also experience an orthostatic HR increase independent of a decrease in BP (at other times) to meet PoTS diagnostic criteria [8].

IOH is defined as a transient decrease in BP >40 mmHg systolic BP or >20 mmHg diastolic BP within 15 seconds of standing [2]. IOH quickly resolves within 20–30 seconds of standing [26]. IOH occurs in seemingly young, healthy individuals and the pathophysiology has not been fully elucidated [26]. Proposed mechanisms include the role of the muscle pump, as well as sympathetic withdrawal and/or vasodilation upon standing [26]. Reflex tachycardia in response to these decreased pressure states can result as the baroreceptors detect fluid shifts due to gravity. In IOH, this tachycardia should resolve as the BP returns to normal. Although PoTS patients may also experience IOH, PoTS should not be diagnosed in such cases where tachycardia is only observed in response to the acutely decreased BP, and is not sustained when the BP returns to a normal level (Fig. 2).

Supine Bradycardia: Patients with a low resting HR may have an orthostatic HR increase that meets or exceeds PoTS criteria. However, a PoTS diagnosis may not be appropriate unless their upright HR is significantly elevated [2].

Diagnosing PoTS in the Pediatric Patient

Children and youth are more prone to physiological orthostatic tachycardia than adults [27]. With aging into later adulthood, physiological

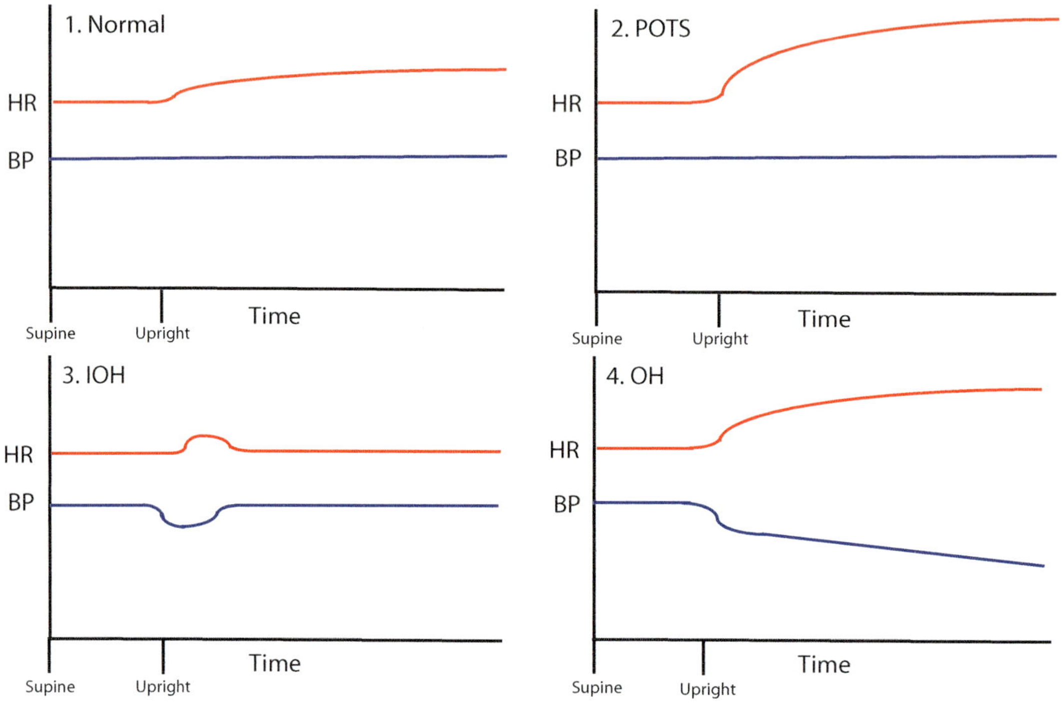

Fig. 2 Blood pressure and heart rate trends in a normal individual and in disorders orthostatic intolerance. 1. Normal blood pressure and heart rate response upright posture. A gradual heart rate increase is observed over time. Blood pressure remains unchanged. 2. Postural Tachycardia Syndrome (PoTS): Upon assumption of upright posture, excessive orthostatic tachycardia is observed. Blood pressure remains relatively unchanged. 3. Initial Orthostatic Hypotension (IOH): Upon upright posture, blood pressure transiently decreases and then recovers. A brief reflex tachycardia is observed. 4. Orthostatic Hypotension (OH): Upon upright posture, blood pressure continually declines. A reflex tachycardia is observed. Figure modified from [31]

orthostatic tachycardia decreases even further. Therefore, many youths may experience orthostatic tachycardia >30 bpm when upright, but are asymptomatic. A study established normal orthostatic HR increase in 100 healthy youth age 12–19 using active stand testing [28]. The mean HR upon upright posture was 21.5 ± 21.2 bpm (2 standard deviations above the mean) [28]. The established Schondorf and Low criteria indicate PoTS should be diagnosed when the HR is 2 standard deviations above the mean or more [1]. Based on this study, the HR target would be >42.7 bpm [28] for a diagnosis of PoTS. A separate study of 108 healthy youth found 42% increased their HR by 30 bpm or more when upright during tilt table testing [27]. To adjust for this common tachycardia in children and youth, an orthostatic HR increase of >40 bpm must be achieved for a diagnosis of PoTS in patients 12–19 years of age. A period of ≥3 months may be suitable to establish chronicity of symptoms in a pediatric population [29]. The standard test to diagnose PoTS in a pediatric population is a 10 min head-up tilt test [3, 29]. Although active stand testing is a validated diagnostic test in adults [5], it has not been validated for a pediatric population [29]. However, a research study has used standing as a diagnostic test for PoTS in 93 youth (mean age 17) while investigating appropriate duration of testing [30]. Participants stood freely with their back against a wall for 10 minutes while orthostatic vitals and symptoms were measured [30]. Notably this work found that if upright tests were conducted for only 2 or 5 minutes, 54 and 27% of participants with PoTS, respectively, would be misdiagnosed [30]. The researchers also used a 2 minutes supine post-stand measurement, to determine the value of lowest supine HR, as pre-stand supine HR was often higher than post-stand supine HR [30]. With this change, an additional 14% of adolescents met the PoTS criteria. Measurement of the lower, post-stand HR may be a more accurate value for diagnosis of PoTS [30]. Although, as mentioned, the stand test has not been validated in a pediatric population, it can be used for diagnosis. This is especially true when access to a testing center or specialist care may be limited and may be barrier to diagnosis and appropriate treatment.

Conclusions

The primary diagnostic criteria for PoTS require an excessive orthostatic tachycardia within 10 min of assuming upright posture in association with chronic symptoms of orthostatic intolerance. This must occur chronically and in the absence orthostatic hypotension, and other disorders or medications which could independently cause orthostatic tachycardia. A thorough clinical review and consideration of related disorders is critical to ensure the accurate diagnosis of PoTS and appropriate clinical treatment plan.

Acknowledgments The authors would like to acknowledge the many patients that have volunteered their time to contribute to this body of work. Their participation is critical to the ongoing investigation of PoTS.

Funding Dr. Raj has a research grant related to Postural Tachycardia Syndrome from the Canadian Institutes of Health Research, Ottawa, Canada (grant number MOP142426). Dr. Lloyd has a post-doctoral scholarship through the Cumming School of Medicine. Kate Bourne holds a Canadian Institutes of Health Research Canada Graduate Scholarship.

Disclosures Dr. Raj is a network investigator of the Cardiac Arrhythmia Network of Canada (CANet; London, Ontario, Canada). Dr. Raj serves on the Medical Advisory Board of Dysautonomia International and PoTS UK, both without financial compensation. Dr. Lloyd has reported that he has no relationships relevant to the contents of this chapter to disclose. Kate Bourne has also reported that she has no relationships relevant to the contents of this chapter to disclose.

References

1. Schondorf R, Low PA. Idiopathic postural orthostatic tachycardia syndrome: an attenuated form of acute pandysautonomia? Neurology. 1993;43:132–7.
2. Freeman R, Wieling W, Axelrod FB, Benditt DG, Benarroch E, Biaggioni I, et al. Autonomic Neuroscience : Basic and Clinical Consensus statement on the definition of orthostatic hypotension, neurally mediated syncope and the postural tachycardia syndrome. Auton Neurosci Basic Clin [Internet]. Elsevier B.V.; 2011;161:46–8.
3. Sheldon RS, Grubb BP, Olshansky B, Shen W-K, Calkins H, Brignole M, et al. 2015 heart rhythm society expert consensus statement on the diagnosis and treatment of postural tachycardia syndrome, inappropriate sinus tachycardia, and vasovagal syncope. Hear Rhythm. 2015;12:e41.
4. Raj SR. The Postural Tachycardia Syndrome (PoTS): pathophysiology, diagnosis & management. Raj SR, editor. Indian Pacing Electrophysiol J. 2006;6:84–99.
5. Plash WB, Diedrich A, Biaggioni I, Garland EM, Paranjape SY, Black BK, et al. Diagnosing postural tachycardia syndrome: comparison of tilt testing compared with standing haemodynamics. Clin Sci (Lond) [Internet]. 2013;124:109–14.
6. Fawcett JK, Wynn V. Effects of posture on plasma volume and some blood constituents. J Clin Pathol. 1960;13:304–10.
7. Lei LY, Chew DS, Sheldon RS, Raj SR. Evaluating and managing postural tachycardia syndrome. Cleve Clin J Med. United States; 2019;86:333–44Lei LY, Chew DS, Sheldon RS, Raj SR. Evaluating and managing postural tachycardia syndrome. Cleve Clin J Med. 2019;86:333–44.
8. Arnold AC, Ng J, Raj SR. Postural tachycardia syndrome—diagnosis, physiology, and prognosis. Auton Neurosci Basic Clin [Internet]. 2018;215:3–11.
9. Prasad Kerlin M, Tokar JL, Cotton D, Taichman D, Williams S. Acute gastrointestinal bleeding. Ann Intern Med. 2013;159:ITC2.2.
10. Fu Q, Vangundy TB, Galbreath MM, Shibata S, Jain M, Hastings JL, et al. Cardiac origins of the postural orthostatic Tachycardia syndrome. J Am Coll Cardiol. 2010;55:2858–68.
11. Parsaik A, Allison T, Singer W, Sletten D, Joyner M, Benarroch EE, et al. Deconditioning in patients with orthostatic intolerance. Neurology. 2012;79:1435–9.

12. Bryarly M, Phillips LT, Fu Q, Vernino S, Levine BD. Postural orthostatic Tachycardia syndrome. 2019;73.
13. Robertson D, Shannon JR, Biaggioni I, Ertl AC, Diedrich A, Carson R, et al. Orthostatic intolerance and the postural tachycardia syndrome: genetic and environment pathophysiologies. Neurolab Autonomic Team. Pflugers Arch. 2000;441:R48.
14. Tank J, Baevsky R, Funtova I, Diedrich A, Slepchenkova I, Jordan J. Orthostatic heart rate responses after prolonged space flights. An Int J Fast Commun Res Treat Relat to Auton Funct Dysfunct. 2011;21:121–4.
15. Fu Q, Shibata S, Hastings JL, Platts SH, Hamilton DM, Bungo MW, et al. Impact of prolonged spaceflight on orthostatic tolerance during ambulation, and blood pressure profiles in astronauts. Circulation; 2019.
16. Raj SR. Postural Tachycardia Syndrome (PoTS). Circulation. 2013;127:2336–42.
17. Porter WB, James GW 3rd. The heart in anemia. Circulation. 1953;8:111–6.
18. Klein I, Danzi S. Thyroid disease and the heart. Circulation. 2007;116:1725–35.
19. Pavlik D, Agnew D, Stiles L, Ditoro R. Recognizing postural orthostatic tachycardia syndrome. J Am Acad Physician Assist. 2016;29:17–23
20. Brewster JA, Garland EM, Biaggioni I, Black BK, Ling JF, Shibao CA, et al. Diurnal variability in orthostatic tachycardia: implications for the postural tachycardia syndrome. Clin Sci (Lond). 2012;122:25–31.
21. Stachenfeld NS. Sex hormone effects on body fluid regulation. Exerc Sport Sci Rev. 2008;36:152–9.
22. Fu Q, Vangundy TB, Shibata S, Auchus RJ, Williams GH, Levine BD. Menstrual cycle affects renal-adrenal and hemodynamic responses during prolonged standing in the postural orthostatic tachycardia syndrome. Hypertension. 2010;56:82–90.
23. Peggs KJ, Nguyen H, Enayat D, Keller NR, Al-Hendy A, Raj SR. Gynecologic disorders and menstrual cycle lightheadedness in postural tachycardia syndrome. Int J Gynecol Obstet. 2012;118:242–6.
24. Peyrol M, Levy S. Clinical presentation of inappropriate sinus tachycardia and differential diagnosis. J Interv Card Electrophysiol. 2016;46:33–41.
25. Neurology TCC of the AAS and the AA of. Consensus statement on the definition of orthostatic hypotension, pure autonomic failure, and multiple system atrophy. Neurology. 1996;46:1470.
26. Wieling W, Krediet CTP, van Dijk N, Linzer M, Tschakovsky ME. Initial orthostatic hypotension: review of a forgotten condition. Clin Sci (Lond). 2007;112:157–65.
27. Singer W, Sletten DM, Opfer-gehrking TL, Brands CK, Fischer PR, Low PA. Postural tachycardia in children and adolescents: what is abnormal? J Pediatr. 2019;160:222–6.
28. Horam WJ, Roscelli JD. Establishing standards of orthostatic measurements in normovolemic adolescents. Am J Dis Child. 1992;146.
29. Stewart JM, Boris JR, Chelimsky G, Fischer PR, Fortunato JE, Grubb BP, et al. Pediatric Disorders of Orthostatic Intolerance. Pediatrics. 2018;141.
30. Roma M, Marden CL, Rowe PC. Passive standing tests for the office diagnosis of postural tachycardia syndrome: New methodological considerations. Fatigue Biomed Heal Behav. 2018;6:179–92.
31. Arnold AC, Ng J, Lei L, Raj SR. Autonomic Dysfunction in Cardiology : Pathophysiology , Investigation , and Management. Can J Cardiol. 2017;33:1524–34.

Pathophysiology and Classification of PoTS

Matthew G. Lloyd and Satish R. Raj

Abbreviations

PoTS	Postural Tachycardia Syndrome
NET	Norepinephrine transporter
QSART	Quantitative sudomotor axon reflex testing
BP	Blood pressure
QDIRT	Quantitative direct and indirect reflex testing
IENFD	Intra-epidermal nerve fiber density
QST	Quantitative sensory testing
RAAS	Renin–Angiotensin–Aldosterone system
MCAS	Mast Cell Activation Syndrome
CBF	Cerebral Blood Flow

Introduction

The central clinical sign in PoTS, orthostatic tachycardia, appears to be due to the convergence of multiple heterogeneous pathophysiological processes. A comprehensive etiology, including a precise description of how these various processes interact, is not yet understood. PoTS subtypes (or endophenotypes) have been developed in an effort to better understand the pathology of PoTS (Fig. 1). The primary problem with this paradigm is the implied exclusivity of each subtype. PoTS patients often have overlapping clinical features involving more than one subtype. A secondary problem of subtyping is that the definitions for each subtype are not standard, which may lead to confusion in the literature, and may also negatively impact patient care. In our clinical experience, these subtypes are often not clinically helpful. A third problem is that a PoTS subtype provides limited information about the pathophysiology that underlies the phenotype. For instance, several mechanisms, including (but not limited to) hypovolemia, norepinephrine transport deficiency, or mast cell activation, may underlie the "hyperadrenergic" phenotype. While the last 20 years of research has added several novel mechanisms that contribute to PoTS (Fig. 2), we still do not fully understand the degree to which these mechanisms overlap, and how they might interact and contribute to the clinical presentation of a given PoTS patients.

M. G. Lloyd · S. R. Raj (✉)
Libin Cardiovascular Institute of Alberta, Cumming School of Medicine, University of Calgary, Calgary, Canada
e-mail: satish.raj@ucalgary.ca

Partial Sympathetic Neuropathy

In 1988, Streeten et al. observed that during orthostasis, PoTS patients exhibited excessive venous pooling in the legs [1]. They concluded that reduced venoconstriction was indicative of sympathetic denervation of the legs. The same group later observed that PoTS patients have

N. Gall et al. (eds.), *Postural Tachycardia Syndrome*, https://doi.org/10.1007/978-3-030-54165-1_5

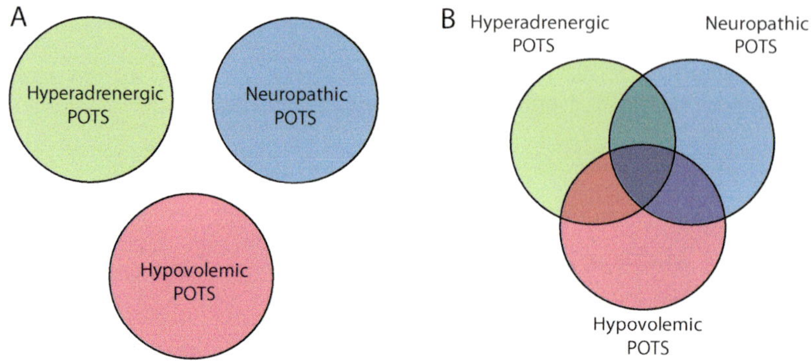

Fig. 1 The issue with POTS subtype labels is that they imply exclusivity from one another (**a**). In reality, subtypes often overlap (**b**) and patients may present with features consistent with all three POTS subtypes. Figure recreated with permission from [80]

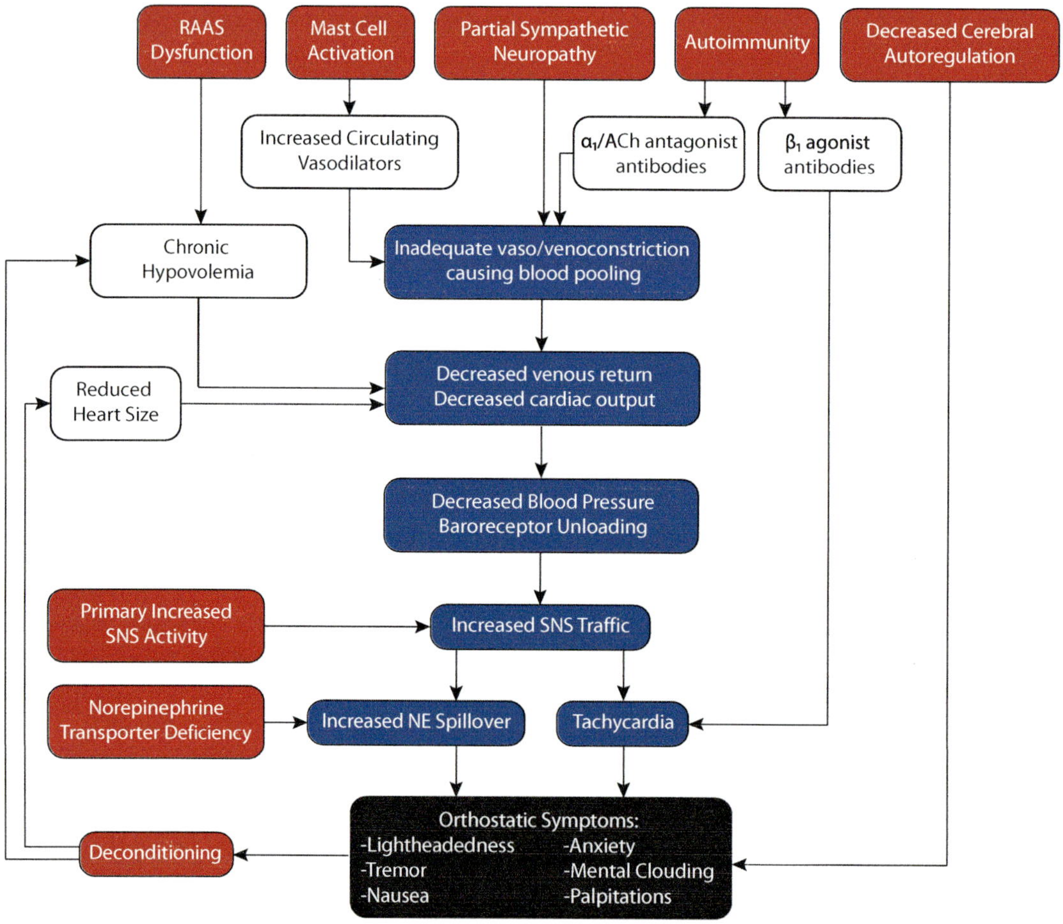

Fig. 2 Schematic diagram of the possible pathophysiological processes involved in POTS. Note that many processes converge to common physiological pathways. RAAS: renin–angiotensin–aldosterone system, Ach: Acetylcholine, SNS: sympathetic nervous system, NE: norepinephrine. Figure modified with permission from [80]

hypersensitive responses to infusion of the sympathetic agonist norepinephrine (the main sympathetic neurotransmitter in the cardiovascular system) in the lower limb [2], so-called "denervation hypersensitivity." One of the first *direct* observations of autonomic neuropathy in PoTS appeared in a 1993 publication by Ron Schondorf and Phillip Low in the journal Neurology [3]. They assessed postganglionic sympathetic nerve function using quantitative sudomotor axon reflex testing (QSART), and thermoregulatory sweat testing in patients with PoTS. Abnormal sweat responses (patchy anhidrosis) were found in 5/10 patients, and abnormal QSART results in 4/16 patients. They also noted that in many patients, the acute onset of orthostatic symptoms were preceded by a viral-like prodrome. Given the remarkable similarities in medical history to patients with Guillain-Barré (the acute onset of symptoms preceded by a viral-like prodrome), Schondorf and Low concluded that many instances of PoTS may be due to an attenuated form of acute autonomic neuropathy.

In 2000, a seminal paper by Giris Jacob and colleagues in the New England Journal of Medicine coined the term "neuropathic PoTS [4]." This thorough investigation of sympathetic nerve function conclusively demonstrated that a subset of PoTS patients have peripheral sympathetic neuropathy. However, the time-consuming and specialized methods used are inappropriate for routine clinical diagnoses, and identification of these patients remains difficult.

The putative mechanism underlying PoTS in patients with autonomic neuropathy is excessive venous pooling due to inadequate venoconstriction in the legs [1], and perhaps the splanchnic vasculature [5], which causes reduced cardiac output. A larger sympathetic outflow is required in order to maintain blood pressure (BP), and causes excessive orthostatic tachycardia.

Unfortunately, there is no gold standard method of diagnosing peripheral sympathetic neuropathy in PoTS. A variety of assessments of the sympathetic nerves have been used, including: (1) QSART [6], (2) thermoregulatory sweat testing [7], (3) quantitative direct and indirect reflex testing (QDIRT) [8], (4) local assessment of norepinephrine spillover [4], and (5) intra-epidermal nerve fiber density (IENFD) from skin biopsies [8, 9]. This has made it difficult to precisely describe the prevalence, etiology, and physiological consequences, particularly as concordance between the tests in PoTS patients is poor [8]. Estimates of peripheral sympathetic neuropathy in PoTS vary with the diagnostic test, but appear to converge to a prevalence of approximately 50% in PoTS patients [4, 6–9] (Table 1).

The most comprehensive investigation of neurological function in PoTS patients was performed by Gibbons and colleagues in 2013 [8]. They performed quantitative sensory testing (QST), QDIRT, and IENFD testing in 24 PoTS patients. They defined neuropathic PoTS as those patients with IENFD scores below the

Table 1 Studies describing peripheral sympathetic neuropathy in POTS. IENFD, intra-epidermal nerve fiber density; QSART, quantitative sudomotor axon reflex test; QST, quantitative sensory testing; QDIRT, quantitative direct and indirect sudomotor testing; NE, norepinephrine

Paper	Method	Participants (n)	Findings (% abnormal)
Haensch et al. [9]	Skin biopsy (IENFD)	84	45%
Gibbons et al. [8]	Skin biopsy (IENFD)	24	38%
	QST		50%
	QDIRT		33%
Peltier et al. [6]	QSART	30	57%
Thieben et al. [7]	Thermoregulatory sweat test	78	54%
Jacob et al. [4]	NE spillover	10	Not reported

5th percentile, *and* at least one of the other tests (QDIRT/QST) below the 5th percentile. This study revealed several important insights into PoTS neuropathies: (1) the remarkable lack of concordance between the various nerve function tests observed in this study implies distinct pathophysiological mechanisms, (2) the clinical presentation of neuropathic PoTS is distinct from non-neuropathic PoTS in several ways (Table 2), and (3) neuropathic PoTS patients do not generally report symptoms of a painful small-fiber neuropathy, and (4) neuropathic PoTS patients exhibited a smaller phase IV overshoot during the Valsalva maneuver than the non-neuropathic group.

Chronic Hypovolemia and Renin–Angiotensin–Aldosterone System

Chronic hypovolemia, including deficits in red blood cell and plasma volume, is a common finding in PoTS [10–14]. The magnitude of deficit appears to be approximately 11–13% [10, 12], but may range as high as 22% in a subset of patients [11]. This hypovolemic state contributes to reduced venous return and subsequent cardiac output, requiring a heightened sympathetic activation (with resultant tachycardia) to maintain BP via the baroreflex. Methods of blood volume assessment [15] used in PoTS include direct assessments of plasma volume with ^{131}I-labeled human serum albumin [10] or dye-dilution [11], and direct assessments of red cell volume with chromium-labelled red blood cells or carbon monoxide rebreathing [12].

In healthy people, blood volume is typically maintained by the Renin–Angiotensin–Aldosterone system (RAAS), via increased renal sodium and water reabsorption. In PoTS patients, despite hypovolemia, the RAAS fails to rectify blood volume. The specific underlying deficit in the RAAS pathway is unclear—PoTS patients have been observed to have reduced [16], similar [10, 17] and increased [12] circulating renin, similar [11, 12] and increased [11] circulating angiotensin II, and reduced [10], similar [11, 12, 16] and increased [17] circulating aldosterone compared to healthy controls. RAAS function appears to be dependant on menstrual phase and body position [12], which may underlie these different findings as not all studies tracked menstrual phase.

What is clearly demonstrated over all studies is a disparity between blood volume and expected RAAS function, with two studies reporting a reduced aldosterone:renin ratio, termed the "renin-aldosterone paradox" [10]. Several mechanisms have been proposed to explain the paradox, including deconditioning[12], low blood vessel capacitance, and reduced activity of angiotensin-converting enzyme 2 [10]. The adrenal and kidney responses to infused angiotensin II appear to be intact in PoTS patients [18], however the pressor response to angiotensin II infusion is blunted in PoTS patients.

Recently, autoantibodies to the angiotensin II receptor were discovered in 12/17 PoTS patients [19]. Presence of these autoantibodies has previously been shown to inhibit angiotensin II mediated vasoconstriction in a rabbit model [20], which likely underlies the reduced pressor response to infused angiotensin II observed in PoTS [18].

The importance of hypovolemia to orthostatic intolerance and orthostatic tachycardia in PoTS is illustrated by the observation that expansion of blood volume via intravenous saline or desmopressin (a vasopressin analog) attenuates standing heart rate and improves orthostatic symptoms [13, 21–23].

Hyperadrenergic State

Approximately 50% of PoTS patients exhibit a hyperadrenergic phenotype, which can be characterized by standing plasma norepinephrine ≥600 pg/mL, an orthostatic increase in systolic arterial pressure ≥ 10 mmHg, or symptoms of sympathetic activation during orthostasis (e.g. palpitations, tremulousness, anxiety) [24]. These patients display increased systolic BP at the end of phase II, and exaggerated phase IV systolic BP overshoot during the Valsalva maneuver.

Table 2 Clinical markers that differ between neuropathic POTS and non-neuropathic POTS

Characteristics of neuropathic POTS versus non-neuropathic POTS
Lower resting and tilted heart rate
Lower measures of parasympathetic function
Lower phase 4 Valsalva overshoot
Lower anxiety and depression
Greater ability to carry out usual activities
Greater self-perceived overall health-related quality of life

In most cases, this hyperadrenergic state is likely secondary to reduced vasoconstriction capacity due to peripheral neuropathy, or excessive sympathetic activation to maintain BP during hypovolemia. Thus, these patients may display an otherwise normal autonomic response to other primary physiological deficits. However, high sympathetic activation may also relate to increased levels of interleukin-6 [25], which may in turn cause increased sympathetic activation [26] and cause a positive feedback cycle. A small subset of hyperadrenergic patients (<10%) exhibit standing norepinephrine in excess of 1000 pg/mL, and large increases in BP upon standing. This disproportionate orthostatic response may indicate excessive central sympathetic discharge, and/or an absence of baroreflex buffering of BP [27]. Some purists would consider this latter subgroup the only true form of "hyperadrenergic PoTS".

Hyperadrenergic State: Norepinephrine Transporter Deficiency

While we often think of a hyperadrenergic state as one with increased sympathetic nerve traffic and increase norepinephrine release, another mechanism of increasing synaptic norepinephrine levels is to decrease clearance of the norepinephrine once it is has been released into the synapse. A key physiological contributor to the hyperadrenergic phenotype that has emerged in the last 20 years is reduced function/expression of the norepinephrine transporter (NET). The NET is a $Na^+/Cl-$ dependant transmembrane protein responsible for re-uptake of norepinephrine from the synapse into the pre-synaptic, noradrenergic neuron. It therefore plays a key role in the physiological outcomes of sympathetic activation [28].

In PoTS, the central hypothesis is that in a subset of the hyperadrenergic phenotype, reduced NET activity (via reduced expression or impaired function) leads to diminished norepinephrine clearance, and consequentially high orthostatic heart rates. One family with orthostatic tachycardia has been identified to have a loss-of-function mutation in the NET gene SLC6A2 [29]. However, subsequent sequence analysis of the SLC6A2 gene in other PoTS patients has revealed no additional genetic polymorphisms that could account for reduced NET expression/function, indicating that this genetic mutation is rare and is unlikely to account for the majority of NET dysfunction in PoTS [30, 31]. Nevertheless, reduced expression of NET in vein biopsies [30], and reduced SLC6A2 gene expression in cultured leukocytes [31], have been observed in PoTS patients in the absence of gene mutation. Pharmacological NET inhibition can increase synaptic norepinephrine levels, causing a PoTS-like phenotype in healthy controls [32, 33].

The underlying pathophysiology behind reduced NET function in PoTS is poorly understood. Bayles and colleagues identified epigenetic modulation of NET expression via histone acetylation modification and binding of a repressive regulatory complex (methyl-CpG binding protein 2) to the SLC6A2 gene [34]. NET expression in PoTS (and other conditions) may also be partly explained by modulation by microRNAs [31]. Given the well-documented RAAS dysfunction in PoTS, it is notable that angiotensin II regulates NET expression and function via multiple pathways [28]. This presents an interesting (but unexplored) avenue of investigation.

The pharmacological treatment of neuropsychiatric disorders involves a host of drugs that inhibit NET function, including tricyclic antidepressants, NET inhibitors such as atomoxetine or reboxetine, and serotonin-norepinephrine reuptake inhibitors such as duloxetine and venlafaxine. Indeed, NET inhibition has been used previously for PoTS in an attempt to enhance orthostatic vasoconstriction [35]. However, a double-blind, placebo-controlled trial demonstrated that acute NET inhibition with atomoxetine in PoTS patients worsened orthostatic tachycardia and symptoms in PoTS [36]. This is not surprising, as neuronal reuptake of norepinephrine is relatively higher in the heart than the general circulation [37, 38], and NET inhibitors may therefore have a relatively larger effect on synaptic norepinephrine levels in the heart than the peripheral vasculature. Medications inhibiting NET should therefore be used with caution in PoTS patients [24].

Immune-Mediated

The immune system is implicated in the pathophysiology of PoTS patients for several reasons. POTS patients often report that the onset of their disorder follows an acute viral illness or vaccination [3, 39], which is reminiscent of autoimmune neurological disorders such as Guillain–Barre syndrome. There are a spectrum of common symptoms in PoTS, including myalgias, fatigue, gastrointestinal complaints, and nausea, that are similar to those seen in chronic viral syndromes or autoimmune disorders. There is also considerable clinical overlap between PoTS and Sjögren's Syndrome, a common chronic autoimmune disorder that primarily affects exocrine glands, resulting in dry eyes and dry mouth [40]. A recent case series of 13 patients with Sjögren's Syndrome that were referred to the Mayo Clinic Arizona autonomic clinic found that 8 (62%) presented with PoTS [40]. A diagnosis of Sjögren's Syndrome may be considered in PoTS patients presenting with dry eyes, dry mouth, and/or gastrointestinal symptoms.

The earliest findings of an autoimmune role in PoTS was published in the New England Journal of Medicine in 2000 by Steven Vernino and colleagues [41]. They found ganglionic acetylcholine receptor antibodies in one PoTS patient (out of 16). Subsequent studies have reported low titer of ganglionic acetylcholine receptor antibodies in 5–29% PoTS patients [7, 42, 43]. There is some debate about the clinical relevance of these findings, as low titers of acetylcholine receptor autoantibodies are also found in healthy controls [39].

Circulating antibodies to several G-protein coupled receptors have also been found in PoTS patients. Antibodies to alpha-1 adrenergic receptors appear to have a partial antagonistic effect, which may reduce sympathetically-mediated vasoconstriction in PoTS patients, and necessitate high sympathetic outflow to maintain BP [44, 45]. Sympathetically-mediated vasoconstriction may also be reduced by the presence of β_2 adrenergic receptor antibodies, which appear to have an agonist effect to the vasodilatory function of the receptor [44, 45]. Agonist antibodies to the β_1 adrenergic receptor have also been found in PoTS, providing a direct mechanism for orthostatic tachycardia in these patients [44, 45].

A number of additional antibodies have been found in PoTS patients, including cardiac lipid raft-associated proteins [46], muscarinic receptors 1 and 2 [39], and the angiotensin II type 1 receptor [19]. Further research is needed to understand the clinical significance of these findings. This topic is covered more in chapter "Inherited Metabolic Diseases", Is PoTS an autoimmune condition?

Mast Cell Activation

A subset of the wide symptomatology of PoTS includes "allergic-like" reactions to food, odors, and medications [47]. This observation has led to the examination of a connection between mast cell disorders and PoTS. Mast cells are white blood cells that reside in close proximity to blood vessels and peripheral nerves [48]. They are involved in a variety of immune responses, such as neuro-immune responses, autoimmunity, and allergic reactions [49]. Mast cell activation disorders refer to a set of diseases including (but not limited to) monoclonal mast cell activation syndrome, chronic autoimmune urticaria, and mast cell activation syndrome (MCAS)[50]. In particular, MCAS has been implicated in the pathophysiology of PoTS [48, 51].

MCAS is characterized by the following criteria: (1) typical symptoms (flushing, lightheadedness, chest pain, rapid heart rate, muscle and bone pain, diarrhea, dizziness/vertigo, etc.); (2) a substantial increase (>20%) in a mast-cell-derived mediator (e.g. serum total tryptase, urinary methylhistamine, urinary prostaglandin D_2, etc.), during or shortly after a symptomatic event, and (3) a response of clinical symptoms to H1- and H2-histamine receptor blockers, high dose aspirin, cromolyn-based agents, or other mast cell targeting agents [49].

The evidence supporting a connection between PoTS and MCAS is scant, with only one study directly examining the prevalence of MCAS in PoTS [51]. Shibao et al. evaluated patients with orthostatic intolerance referred to the autonomic dysfunction clinic at Vanderbilt. Out of 24 PoTS patients, eight women had concurrent MCAS, defined as a history of facial or upper trunk flushing, and urine methylhistamine>230 μg/g. These patients presented as "hyperadrenergic," with an exaggerated sympathetic pressor response during phase II_{Late} and phase IV of the Valsalva maneuver, compared to PoTS patients without MCAS. The purported mechanism linking mast cell activation with PoTS is via increased histamine release from mast cells, which causes systemic vasodilation, an excessive baroreflex-mediated increase in sympathetic activity to maintain BP, and associated tachycardia [51]. This raises the question: is PoTS a common finding among patients with MCAS?

While the prevalence of PoTS within patients with mast cell disorders has not been officially examined, one study found that 71% of patients with mastocytosis/MCAS report light-headedness daily or occasionally [52]. Many additional symptoms reported by MCAS patients overlap significantly with POTS patients: brain fog, anxiety, diarrhea, headache, bloating, joint pain, etc. To our knowledge, no other studies have examined mast cell activation in PoTS patients with hypertryptasemia. However, Lyons and colleagues [53] performed a survey of 96 patients, and found 46% presented with autonomic dysfunction, defined as an elevated composite autonomic symptom score (COMPASS 31) [54].

Despite the paucity of evidence linking PoTS with MCAS, the bi-directional interaction between mast cells and neurons provide a strong basis of plausibility for a pathophysiological link. Many symptoms associated with allergic reactions (itchy eyes, bronchospasm, and mucous production) are mediated to a large degree by neuronal activity [55]. Neurons can activate mast cells via the release of substance P and calcitonin gene-related peptide [56, 57]. Mast cells can also affect neuronal activity via a number of chemical messengers, including tryptase, cysteinyl leukotrienes, prostaglandins, tumor necrosis factor α, neurotrophin, and nerve growth factor [58].

This topic is covered in more detail in chapter "Mast Cell Activation Syndrome (MCAS)", "Mast Cell Activation Syndrome."

Deconditioning

PoTS patients commonly present with poor cardiovascular fitness and low activity levels, even those who were very active and athletic before they became ill. Most PoTS patients have reduced quality of life and exhibit functional disability [59, 60]. Their recurrent, and often incessant, orthostatic intolerance likely leads to reduced physical activity. The physiological response to orthostasis in PoTS patients is reminiscent of deconditioned patients following prolonged bed rest (orthostatic tachycardia, exercise intolerance, reduced left ventricular mass, reduced stroke volume, reduced blood volume) [61–64]. PoTS patients also have reduced blood volume and left ventricular mass [65], characteristics also commonly seen with prolonged bed rest [62, 66]. Reduced cardiac size produces a less "distensible" heart, and reduced stroke volume during orthostasis via the Frank-Starling mechanism. Therefore, heart rate must increase to maintain cardiac output, providing a direct mechanistic link between deconditioning and PoTS. Supervised, PoTS-specific exercise programs have been shown to increase blood volume and left ventricular mass in PoTS patients [65], and improve orthostatic tachycardia, orthostatic symptoms, and quality of life [67]. Exercise treatment is covered in more detail in chapter "Exercise Guidelines for Postural Tachycardia Syndrome".

Impaired Cerebral Autoregulation

Symptoms of orthostatic intolerance are a major cause of reduced quality of life in PoTS patients [60, 68]. The presence of these symptoms during normal BP while upright implies a reduced ability for the cerebral vasculature to maintain constant cerebral blood flow (CBF) over a range of perfusion pressures, a phenomenon known as cerebral autoregulation. Cerebral autoregulation can be modeled as "static," referring to the absolute cerebral blood flow at a given BP, or "dynamic," which refers to the acute cerebral blood flow responses to fluctuations in BP [69].

The issue of static cerebral autoregulation in PoTS is controversial. Several studies have shown excessive reduction in middle cerebral artery blood flow velocity during head-up tilt [70–73], implying impaired static cerebral autoregulation. This may be due to hyperpneic hypocapnia [73] (hyperventilation with deep breathing), but has also been observed under normocapnic conditions [74]. Reduced orthostatic CBF may be due to a sympathetically-mediated increase in cerebrovascular resistance [72], but has also been observed in PoTS patients prior to an orthostatic increase in sympathetic outflow [75]. Other studies have observed normal static cerebral autoregulation [71, 76–78]. The reasons behind these disparate findings are unclear, as there are no significant methodological differences to explain the divergent results. While orthostatic hyperpneic hypocapnia is present in approximately 25% of PoTS patients [79], many patients remain normocapnic during tilt. Sympathetically-mediated cerebral vasoconstriction would be expected to be enhanced in hyperadrenergic PoTS patients. However, in part due to a lack of standardized definitions, these subgroup comparisons have not been performed, which may underpin the controversy in the literature. The role of static cerebral autoregulation remains a point of debate [80].

Cerebral autoregulation can also be modeled as a dynamic process. BP oscillates with breathing at around 0.3 Hz, but also oscillates at ~0.1 Hz, so-called "Mayer waves [81]." The buffering of these oscillations by the cerebral circulation, among other processes, is termed dynamic cerebral autoregulation [69]. The integrity of dynamic cerebral autoregulation in PoTS is also controversial. Schondorf et al. examined this in PoTS patients, and found no difference between PoTS patients and controls in the transfer function coherence between BP and CBF, and concluded that dynamic cerebral autoregulation is intact in PoTS patients [76].

However, several subsequent publications from Dr. Julian Stewart's group at New York Medical College have demonstrated increased BP-CBF coherence [71, 74, 82] in PoTS patients. While this may be indicative of reduced dynamic cerebral autoregulation, it may also be that larger BP oscillations in PoTS exceed the autoregulatory range [71]. Both BP and CBF variability increase in magnitude with head-up tilt angle in a dose-dependent manner [71]. The central consequences of these large CBF oscillations may be reduced cognitive function and functional cerebral hyperemia [71]. This provides a potential mechanistic underpinning the "brain fog" commonly reported in PoTS patients. One might argue that this relationship is purely co-incident (and not causal), however inducing large oscillations in BP in healthy controls also reduces working memory [83] and functional hyperemia [84]. This literature would be enhanced by further confirmatory publications from other groups.

Conclusion

The physiology behind PoTS is complex and incompletely understood. As we expand our understanding of the separate mechanisms that can contribute to the PoTS phenotype, the development of standardized clinical tests and definitions is needed to allow us to examine whether treatment should be tailored to the underlying pathology. A necessary step to this tailored approach is a description of the interplay between pathophysiological mechanisms, as many PoTS patients present with characteristics of several PoTS subtypes. Understanding the interaction of pathologies in a given PoTS patient is critical to individualized treatment.

Acknowledgments The authors would like to acknowledge the many patients that have volunteered their time to contribute to this body of work. Their participation is critical to the ongoing investigation of POTS.

Funding Dr. Raj has a research grant related to Postural Tachycardia Syndrome from the Canadian Institutes of Health Research, Ottawa, Canada (grant number MOP142426). Dr. Lloyd has a post-doctoral scholarship through the Cummings School of Medicine.

Disclosures Dr. Raj is a network investigator of the Cardiac Arrhythmia Network of Canada (CANet; London, Ontario, Canada). Dr. Raj serves on the Medical Advisory Board of Dysautonomia International and PoTS UK, both without financial compensation. Dr. Lloyd has reported that he has no relationships relevant to the contents of this chapter to disclose.

References

1. Streeten DH, Anderson GH, Richardson R, Thomas FD. Abnormal orthostatic changes in blood pressure and heart rate in subjects with intact sympathetic nervous function: evidence for excessive venous pooling. J Lab Clin Med. 1988 [cited 2019 Jun 2];111:326–35. https://www.ncbi.nlm.nih.gov/pubmed/3343547.
2. Streeten DHP. Pathogenesis of hyperadrenergic orthostatic hypotension. Evidence of disordered venous innervation exclusively in the lower limbs. J Clin Invest. 1990;86:1582–8.
3. Schondorf R, Low PA. Idiopathic postural orthostatic tachycardia syndrome: an attenuated form of acute pandysautonomia? Neurology. 1993 [cited 2019 Apr 27];43:132–7. https://www.ncbi.nlm.nih.gov/pubmed/8423877.
4. Jacob G, Costa F, Shannon J, Robertson RM, Wathen M, Stein M, et al. The neuropathic postural tachycardia syndrome. N Engl J Med. 2000;343:1008–14.
5. Stewart JM, Medow MS, Glover JL, Montgomery LD. Persistent splanchnic hyperemia during upright tilt in postural tachycardia syndrome. Am J Physiol Circ Physiol. 2006;290:H665–73.
6. Peltier AC, Garland E, Raj SR, Sato K, Black B, Song Y, et al. Distal sudomotor findings in postural tachycardia syndrome. Clin Auton Res. 2010;20:93–9.
7. Thieben MJ, Sandroni P, Sletten DM, Benrud-Larson LM, Fealey RD, Vernino S, et al. Postural orthostatic tachycardia syndrome: the mayo clinic experience. Mayo Clin Proc. 2007;82:308–13.
8. Gibbons CH, Bonyhay I, Benson A, Wang N, Freeman R. Structural and functional small fiber abnormalities in the neuropathic postural tachycardia syndrome. PLoS ONE. 2013;8:1–8.
9. Haensch CA, Tosch M, Katona I, Weis J, Isenmann S. Small-fiber neuropathy with cardiac denervation in postural tachycardia syndrome. Muscle Nerve. 2014;50:956–61.
10. Raj SR, Biaggioni I, Yamhure PC, Black BK, Paranjape SY, Byrne DW, et al. Renin-aldosterone paradox and perturbed blood volume regulation underlying postural tachycardia syndrome. Circulation. 2005;111:1574–82.
11. Stewart JM, Glover JL, Medow MS. Increased plasma angiotensin II in postural tachycardia syndrome (POTS) is related to reduced blood flow and blood volume. Clin Sci. 2006;110:255–63.
12. Fu Q, Vangundy TB, Shibata S, Auchus RJ, Williams GH, Levine BD. Menstrual cycle affects renal-adrenal and hemodynamic responses during prolonged standing in the postural orthostatic tachycardia syndrome. Hypertension. 2010;56:82–90.
13. Jacob G, Shannon JR, Black B, Biaggioni I, Mosqueda-Garcia R, Robertson RM, et al. Effects of volume loading and pressor agents in idiopathic orthostatic tachycardia. Circulation. 1997 [cited 2019 May 9];96:575–80. https://www.ncbi.nlm.nih.gov/pubmed/9244228.
14. Hoeldtke RD, Horvath GG, Bryner KD. Treatment of orthostatic tachycardia with erythropoietin. Am J Med. 1995;99:525–9.
15. Ertl AC, Diedrich A, Raj SR. Techniques used for the determination of blood volume. Am J Med Sci. 2007;334:32–6.
16. Jacob G, Robertson D, Mosqueda-Garcia R, Ertl AC, Robertson RM, Biaggioni I. Hypovolemia in syncope and orthostatic intolerance role

of the renin-angiotensin system. Am J Med. 1997;103:128–33.
17. Garland EM, Raj SR, Black BK, Harris PA, Robertson D. The hemodynamic and neurohumoral phenotype of postural tachycardia syndrome. Neurology. 2007;69:790–8.
18. Mustafa HI, Raj SR, Diedrich A, Black BK, Paranjape SY, Dupont WD, et al. Altered systemic hemodynamic and baroreflex response to angiotensin II in postural tachycardia syndrome. Circ Arrhythmia Electrophysiol. 2012;5:173–80.
19. Yu X, Li H, Murphy TA, Nuss Z, Liles J, Liles C, et al. Angiotensin II type 1 receptor autoantibodies in postural tachycardia syndrome. J Am Heart Assoc. 2018;7:1–7.
20. Li H, Kem DC, Zhang L, Huang B, Liles C, Benbrook A, et al. Novel Retro-Inverso Peptide Inhibitor Reverses Angiotensin Receptor Autoantibody-Induced Hypertension in the Rabbit. Hyptertension. 2015;65:793–9.
21. Coffin ST, Black BK, Biaggioni I, Paranjape SY, Orozco C, Black PW, et al. Desmopressin acutely decreases tachycardia and improves symptoms in the postural tachycardia syndrome. Hear Rhythm. 2012;9:1484–90. https://doi.org/10.1016/j.hrthm.2012.05.002.
22. Ruzieh M, Baugh A, Dasa O, Parker RL, Perrault JT, Renno A, et al. Effects of intermittent intravenous saline infusions in patients with medication—refractory postural tachycardia syndrome. J Interv Card Electrophysiol. 2017;48:255–60.
23. Victor M G, Tonette L O-G, Novak V, Low PA. Hemodynamic and symptomatic effects of acute interventions on tilt in patients with postural tachycardia syndrome. Clin Auton Res. 2000;10:29–33. https://www.embase.com/search/results?subaction=viewrecord&from=export&id=L32250283.
24. Sheldon RS, Grubb BP, Olshansky B, Shen WK, Calkins H, Brignole M, et al. 2015 Heart rhythm society expert consensus statement on the diagnosis and treatment of postural tachycardia syndrome, inappropriate sinus tachycardia, and vasovagal syncope. Hear Rhythm. 2015;12:e41–63. https://doi.org/10.1016/j.hrthm.2015.03.029.
25. Okamoto LE, Raj SR, Gamboa A, Shibao CA, Arnold AC, Garland EM, et al. Sympathetic activation is associated with increased IL-6, but not CRP in the absence of obesity: lessons from postural tachycardia syndrome and obesity. Am J Physiol Circ Physiol. 2015;309:H2098–107. https://www.physiology.org/doi/10.1152/ajpheart.00409.2015.
26. Torpy DJ, Papanicolaou DA, Lotsikas AJ, Wilder RL, Chrousos GP, Pillemer SR. Responses of the sympathetic nervous system and the hypothalamic-pituitary-adrenal axis to interleukin-6: a pilot study in fibromyalgia. Arthritis Rheum. 2000;43:872–80.
27. Raj SR. The postural tachycardia syndrome (POTS) pathophysiology, diagnosis & management. Indian Pacing Electrophysiol J. 2006;6:84–99.
28. Mandela P, Ordway GA. The norepinephrine transporter and its regulation. J Neurochem. 2006;97:310–33.
29. Shannon JR, Flattem NL, Jordan J, Jacob G, Black BK, Biaggioni I, et al. Orthostatic intolerance and tachycardia associated with norepinephrine-transporter deficiency. N Engl J Med. 2000;342:541–9.
30. Lambert E, Eikelis N, Esler M, Dawood T, Schlaich M, Bayles R, et al. Altered sympathetic nervous reactivity and norepinephrine transporter expression in patients with postural tachycardia syndrome. Circ Arrhythm Electrophysiol. 2008;1:103–9.
31. Marques FZ, Eikelis N, Bayles RG, Lambert EA, Straznicky NE, Hering D, et al. A polymorphism in the norepinephrine transporter gene is associated with affective and cardiovascular disease through a microRNA mechanism. Mol Psychiatry; 2017;22:134–41. https://doi.org/10.1038/mp.2016.40.
32. Vincent S, Bieck PR, Garland EM, Loghin C, Bymaster FP, Black BK, et al. Clinical assessment of norepinephrine transporter blockade through biochemical and pharmacological profiles. 2004;3202–7.
33. Schroeder C, Tank J, Boschmann M, Diedrich A, Sharma AM, Biaggioni I, et al. Selective norepinephrine reuptake inhibition as a human model of orthostatic intolerance. Circulation. 2002;105:347–53.
34. Bayles R, Kn H, Lambert E, Baker EK, Agrotis A, Guo L, et al. Epigenetic modification of the norepinephrine transporter gene in postural tachycardia syndrome. Arterioscler Thromb Vasc Biol. 2012;32:1910–6.
35. Grubb BP. Postural tachycardia syndrome. Circulation. 2008;117:2814–7.
36. Green EA, Raj V, Shibao CA, Biaggioni I, Black BK, Dupont WD, et al. Effects of norepinephrine reuptake inhibition on postural tachycardia syndrome. J Am Heart Assoc. 2013;2:1–9.
37. Kopin IJ, Rundqvist B, Friberg P, Lenders J, Goldstein DS, Eisenhofer G. Different relationships of spillover to release of norepinephrine in human heart, kidneys, and forearm. Am J Physiol—Regul Integr Comp Physiol. 1998;275:R165–73.
38. Goldstein DS, Brush JE, Eisenhofer G, Stull R, Esler M. In vivo measurement of neuronal uptake of norepinephrine in the human heart. Circulation. 1988;78:41–8.
39. Vernino S, Stiles LE. Autoimmunity in postural orthostatic tachycardia syndrome: current understanding. Auton Neurosci Basic Clin. 2018;215:78–82. https://doi.org/10.1016/j.autneu.2018.04.005.

40. Goodman BP, Crepeau A, Dhawan PS, Khoury JA, Harris LA. Spectrum of autonomic nervous system impairment in Sjögren syndrome. Neurologist. 2017;22:127–30.
41. Vernino S, Low PA, Fealey RD, Stewart JD, Farrugia G, Lennon VA. Autoantibodies to ganglionic acetylcholine receptors in autoimmune autonomic neuropathies. N Engl J Med. 2000;343:847–55.
42. Vernino S, Hopkins S, Okamoto L, Black B, Paranjape SY, Raj SR. Prevalence of ganglionic AChR antibodies in postural tachycardia syndrome (POTS). Clin Auton Res. 2016;26:328.
43. Watari M, Nakane S, Mukaino A, Nakajima M, Mori Y, Maeda Y, et al. Autoimmune postural orthostatic tachycardia syndrome. Ann Clin Transl Neurol. 2018;5:486–92.
44. Li H, Yu X, Liles C, Khan M, Vanderlinde-Wood M, Galloway A, et al. Autoimmune basis for postural tachycardia syndrome. J Am Heart Assoc. 2014;3:1–10.
45. Fedorowski A, Li H, Yu X, Koelsch KA, Harris VM, Liles C, et al. Antiadrenergic autoimmunity in postural tachycardia syndrome. Europace. 2017;19:1211–9.
46. Wang XL, Ling TY, Charlesworth MC, Figueroa JJ, Low P, Shen WK, et al. Autoimmunoreactive IgGs against cardiac lipid raft-associated proteins in patients with postural orthostatic tachycardia syndrome. Transl Res. 2013;162:34–44. https://doi.org/10.1016/j.trsl.2013.03.002
47. Doherty TA, White AA. Postural orthostatic tachycardia syndrome and the potential role of mast cell activation. Auton Neurosci Basic Clin. 2018;215:83–8. https://doi.org/10.1016/j.autneu.2018.05.001.
48. Frieri M. Mast cell activation syndrome. J Allergy Clin Immunol. 2018;54:353–65.
49. Valent P, Akin C, Arock M, Brockow K, Butterfield JH, Carter MC, et al. Definitions, criteria and global classification of mast cell disorders with special reference to mast cell activation syndromes: a consensus proposal. Int Arch Allergy Immunol. 2012;157:215–25.
50. Akin C, Valent P, Metcalfe DD. Mast Cell Activation Syndrome: Proposed Diagnostic Criteria. J Allergy Clin Immunol. 2010;126(1099–1104):e4.
51. Shibao C, Arzubiaga C, Roberts LJ, Raj S, Black B, Harris P, et al. Hyperadrenergic postural tachycardia syndrome in mast cell activation disorders. Hypertension. 2005;45:385–90.
52. Jennings S, Russell N, Jennings B, Slee V, Sterling L, Castells M, et al. The mastocytosis society survey on mast cell disorders: patient experiences and perceptions. J Allergy Clin Immunol Pract. 2014;2:70–6. https://doi.org/10.1016/j.jaip.2013.09.004.
53. Lyons JJ, Yu X, Hughes JD, Le QT, Jamil A, Bai Y, et al. Elevated basal serum tryptase identifies a multisystem disorder associated with increased TPSAB1 copy number. Nat Genet. 2016;48:1564–9.
54. Sletten DM, Suarez GA, Low PA, Mandrekar J, Singer W. COMPASS 31: A refined and abbreviated composite autonomic symptom score. Mayo Clin Proc. 2012;87:1196–201. https://doi.org/10.1016/j.mayocp.2012.10.013.
55. Undem BJ, Taylor-Clark T. Mechanisms underlying the neuronal-based symptoms of allergy. J Allergy Clin Immunol. 2014;133:1521–34. https://doi.org/10.1016/j.jaci.2013.11.027.
56. Keller JT, Marfurt CF. Peptidergic and serotoninergic innervation of the rat dura mater. J Comp Neurol. 1991;309:515–34.
57. Stead RH, Tomioka M, Quinonez G, Simon GT, Felten SY, Bienenstock J. Intestinal mucosal mast cells in normal and nematode-infected rat intestines are in intimate contact with peptidergic nerves. Proc Natl Acad Sci. 1987;84:2975–9.
58. Mittal A, Sagi V, Gupta M, Gupta K. Mast cell neural interactions in health and disease. Front Cell Neurosci. 2019;13:1–6.
59. Benrud-Larson LM, Sandroni P, Haythornthwaite JA, Rummans TA, Low PA. Correlates of functional disability in patients with postural tachycardia syndrome: preliminary cross-sectional findings. Heal Psychol. 2003;22:643–8.
60. Benrud-Larson LM, Dewar MS, Sandroni P, Rummans TA, Haythornthwaite JA, Low PA. Quality of life in patients with postural tachycardia syndrome. Mayo Clin Proc. 2002 [cited 2019 May 9];77:531–7. https://linkinghub.elsevier.com/retrieve/pii/S0025619611619952.
61. Fu Q, VanGundy TB, Galbreath MM, Shibata S, Jain M, Hastings JL, et al. Cardiac origins of the postural orthostatic tachycardia syndrome. J Am Coll Cardiol. 2010;55:2858–68. https://doi.org/10.1016/j.jacc.2010.02.043.
62. Levine BD, Zuckerman JH, Pawelczyk JA. Cardiac atrophy after bed-rest deconditioning: a nonneural mechanism for orthostatic intolerance. Circulation. 1997 [cited 2019 May 9];96:517–25. https://www.ncbi.nlm.nih.gov/pubmed/9244220.
63. Tank J, Baevsky RM, Funtova II, Diedrich A, Slepchenkova IN, Jordan J. Orthostatic heart rate responses after prolonged space flights. Clin Auton Res. 2011;21:121–4.
64. Joyner MJ, Masuki S. POTS versus deconditioning: the same or different? Clin Auton Res. 2008;18:300–7.
65. Fu Q, Vangundy TB, Galbreath MM, Shibata S, Jain M, Hastings JL, et al. Cardiac origins of the postural orthostatic tachycardia syndrome. J Am Coll Cardiol. 2010 [cited 2014 Apr 13];55:2858–68. https://www.pubmedcentral.nih.gov/articlerender.fcgi?artid=2914315&tool=pmcentrez&rendertype=abstract.
66. Dorfman TA, Levine BD, Tillery T, Peshock RM, Hastings JL, Schneider SM, et al. Cardiac atrophy

in women following bed rest. J Appl Physiol. 2007;103:8–16.
67. Fu Q, Levine BD. Exercise and non-pharmacological treatment of POTS. Auton Neurosci Basic Clin. 2018;215:20–7.
68. Bagai K, Song Y, Ling JF, Malow B, Black BK, Biaggioni I, et al. Sleep disturbances and diminished quality of life in postural tachycardia syndrome. J Clin Sleep Med. 2011;7:204–10.
69. Tan CO, Taylor JA. Integrative physiological and computational approaches to understand autonomic control of cerebral autoregulation. Exp Physiol. 2014;99:3–15.
70. Ocon AJ, Kulesa J, Clarke D, Taneja I, Medow MS, Stewart JM. Increased phase synchronization and decreased cerebral autoregulation during fainting in the young. Am J Physiol Heart Circ Physiol. 2009;297:H2084–95.
71. Medow MS, Del Pozzi AT, Messer ZR, Terilli C, Stewart JM. Altered oscillatory cerebral blood flow velocity and autoregulation in postural tachycardia syndrome. Front Physiol. 2014 [cited 2019 May 9];5. https://journal.frontiersin.org/article/10.3389/fphys.2014.00234/abstract.
72. Jordan J, Shannon JR, Black BK, Paranjape SY, Barwise J, Robertson D. Raised cerebrovascular resistance in idiopathic orthostatic intolerance: evidence for sympathetic vasoconstriction. Hypertension. 1998;32:699–704.
73. Novak V, Spies JM, Novak P, McPhee BR, Rummans T, Low PA. Hypocapnia and cerebral hypoperfusion in orthostatic intolerance. Stroke. 1998;29:1876–81. https://www.embase.com/search/results?subaction=viewrecord&from=export&id=L28399981.
74. Ocon AJ, Medow MS, Taneja I, Clarke D, Stewart JM. Decreased upright cerebral blood flow and cerebral autoregulation in normocapnic postural tachycardia syndrome. Am J Physiol Circ Physiol. 2009;297:H664–73.
75. Del Pozzi AT, Schwartz CE, Tewari D, Medow MS, Stewart JM. Reduced cerebral blood flow with orthostasis precedes hypocapnic hyperpnea, sympathetic activation, and postural tachycardia syndrome. Hypertension. 2014;63:1302–8.
76. Schondorf R, Benoit J, Stein R, Benoit J, Cerebral RS. Cerebral autoregulation is preserved in postural tachycardia syndrome. Am J Physiol-Heart Circ Physiol. 2005;99:828–35.
77. Hermosillo AG, Jauregui-Renaud K, Kostine A, Marquez MF, Lara JL, Cardenas M. Comparative study of cerebral blood flow between postural tachycardia and neurocardiogenic syncope, during head-up tilt test. Europace. 2002;4:369–74.
78. Endo A, Fujita Y, Fuchigami T, Takahashi S, Mugishima H, Skatani K. Changes in cerebral blood oxygenation induced by active standing test in children with POTS and NMS. Adv Exp Med Biol. 2014 [cited 2019 May 30];812:253–61. https://link.springer.com/10.1007/978-1-4939-0620-8_34.
79. Stewart JM, Pianosi P, Shaban MA, Terilli C, Svistunova M, Visintainer P, et al. Postural hyperventilation as a cause of postural tachycardia syndrome: increased systemic vascular resistance and decreased cardiac output when upright in all postural tachycardia syndrome variants. J Am Heart Assoc. 2018;7:1–11.
80. Arnold AC, Ng J, Raj SR. Postural tachycardia syndrome—diagnosis, physiology, and prognosis. Auton Neurosci Basic Clin. 2018;215:3–11. https://doi.org/10.1016/j.autneu.2018.02.005.
81. Killip T. Oscillation of blood flow and vascular resistance during Mayer waves. Circ Res. 1962 [cited 2019 May 31];11:987–93. https://www.ncbi.nlm.nih.gov/pubmed/14032613.
82. Stewart JM, Del Pozzi AT, Pandey A, Messer ZR, Terilli C, Medow MS. Oscillatory cerebral blood flow is associated with impaired neurocognition and functional hyperemia in postural tachycardia syndrome during graded tilt. Hypertension. 2015;65:636–43.
83. Merchant S, Medow MS, Visintainer P, Terilli C, Stewart JM. Oscillatory lower body negative pressure impairs working memory task-related functional hyperemia in healthy volunteers. Am J Physiol Circ Physiol. 2017;312:H672–80.
84. Stewart JM, Balakrishnan K, Visintainer P, Del Pozzi AT, Messer ZR, Terilli C, et al. Oscillatory lower body negative pressure impairs task related functional hyperemia in healthy volunteers. Am J Physiol Circ Physiol. 2016;310:H775–84.

Cardiological Considerations: Tests to Consider, Are They Useful and What Do They Show?

Tushar V. Salukhe

History taking is fundamental to the diagnosis of PoTS. Careful symptom assessment and physical examination will, in most patients, raise sufficient suspicion towards diagnosis and avoid a shotgun approach to further investigation. Important aspects of history and examination are covered elsewhere.

The premise of performing cardiac investigations in patients suspected of PoTS is to exclude other diagnoses, to describe cardiovascular physiology and to plan treatment. Patients attending specialist clinics for presyncope or transient loss of consciousness should routinely have a 12-lead ECG. The patient's history, physical examination and 12 lead ECG will uncover most red flag signs to warrant further investigation. These red flags signs are covered later. In the context of a suggestive history and a normal 12 lead ECG the yield of further cardiac investigation is very low.

Echocardiography

Documentation of normal structure and function of cardiac chambers and valves may be useful in a selection of PoTS patients. This is particularly so when dizziness and palpitations occur in the context of comorbidities such as known coronary disease, known structural heart disease, concomitant symptoms of heart failure, a family history of early, unexpected death or an abnormal 12 lead ECG. In the absence of these red flag signs, the added diagnostic value of echocardiography is diminished.

Palpitations with symptoms suggestive of cardiovascular compromise such as dizziness or transient loss of consciousness may have a more sinister connotation when associated with structural heart disease. Structural and functional abnormalities such as ventricular dilatation, hypertrophy, wall motion abnormalities or impaired function should prompt specific effort to exclude malignant explanations for such symptoms and early referral to a cardiologist.

In the absence of red flag signs, echocardiography should not be considered routine investigation in the majority of young (under 40 years old) PoTS patients.

Holter Electrocardiography

The Holter ECG is an invaluable tool for the cardiologist to achieve an arrhythmic diagnosis, assess arrhythmia burden and heart rate variability, yet it is often used ineffectively. Skilled and productive use of Holter ECG relies on careful evaluation of palpitations, with particular

T. V. Salukhe (✉)
Royal Brompton Hospital and Imperial College, London, UK
e-mail: t.salukhe@imperial.ac.uk

N. Gall et al. (eds.), *Postural Tachycardia Syndrome*, https://doi.org/10.1007/978-3-030-54165-1_6

attention to symptom frequency, duration, onset/offset and triggers.

Palpitations in PoTS are typically associated with upright posture. Capturing symptoms on pulse palpation or ECG may be readily achieved with an in-clinic stand test or tilt testing. Thus, the sinus tachycardia associated with postural symptoms is easy to document. Holter monitoring is not required for PoTS diagnosis but may have some value to exclude pathological arrhythmia, assessing sinus tachycardia burden and assist in differentiating adrenergic subtypes of PoTS or the often-overlapping inappropriate sinus tachycardia [1]. Such differences may be assessed with mean heart rates and the shape of heart rate histograms on Holter analysis. However, such sub-classification may have little impact on management.

Cardiopulmonary Exercise Testing

Orthostatic symptoms are often presented as exercise intolerance by PoTS patients. The mechanisms of reduced exercise tolerance are likely to be multifactorial and not simply confined to lower body pooling and venodilatation. Deconditioning and cognitive misperception of effort also have a role.

There is evidence that VO_{2max} is reduced in patients with PoTS. This has largely been documented with upright exercise on treadmill, a position in which PoTS patients are particularly vulnerable [2, 3]. The VO_2 deficit does not reflect a deficit in cardiovascular reserve but is rather a function of deconditioning, the hallmark of which is an excessive heart rate response to exercise and slow recovery.

The argument for postural decondition is further supported by the observation that there is no measurable difference in maximum heart rate and VO_{2max} in patients with PoTS when compared to age-matched normal controls in *recumbent* bicycle exercise VO_{2max} [4]. Moreover, in patients with the oft-compared chronic fatigue syndrome, there is a clear difference in the *perceived effort* made by patients with chronic fatigue, who subjectively reported a greater level of effort than controls to achieve the same levels of activity. Although there is ample data to show that deconditioning in PoTS is reversible with exercise training, this is readily assessed with clinical symptoms and does not require the use of routing exercise testing.

In summary, the demonstration of a sinus tachycardia within 10 minutes of assuming upright posture (typically by 30 bpm in adults) defines postural orthostatic tachycardia. The diagnosis of the *syndrome* requires the presence of several of the varied constellation of symptoms associated with this exaggerated physiological response. The uses of ancillary cardiac investigations, however simple or non-intrusive, are used to exclude other pathologies if suspected clinically and are rarely helpful for diagnosis or monitoring treatment in PoTS patients.

References

1. Garland EM, Celedonio JE, Raj SR. Postural Tachycardia syndrome: beyond orthostatic intolerance XE "Orthostatic intolerance." Curr Neurol Neurosci Rep. 2015;15(9):60.
2. Parsaik A1, Allison TG, Singer W, Sletten DM, Joyner MJ, Benarroch EE, Low PA, Sandroni P. Deconditioning in patients with orthostatic intolerance. Neurology. 2012;79(14):1435–9.
3. Shibata S, Perhonen M, Levine BD. Supine cycling plus volume loading prevent cardiovascular XE "Cardiovascular" deconditioning during bed rest. J Appl Physiol. 2010;108:1177–86.
4. Arnold AC, Okamoto LE, Diedrich A, Paranjape SY, Raj SR, Biaggioni I, Gamboa A. Low-dose propranolol and exercise capacity in postural tachycardia syndrome: a randomized study. Neurology. 2013; 80(21): 1927–33.

Neurological Investigations

Robert Shane Delamont

Neurological Investigations in PoTS

An Approach to Neurological Investigations in PoTS

For those outside in the non-specialised world, PoTS has come to mean any condition which is associated with non-specific symptoms. These symptoms can relate to the cardiovascular, neurological, respiratory, gastroenterological, genitourinary, skin, sleep as well as neuro-cognitive and psychological components of bodily function. The nervous system innervates all aspects of the body, so, at first presentation and initial assessment, it can be difficult to know where to start. In fact, as in most areas in medicine, the initial and most important step is to take a detailed history and establish which symptoms are most troubling for the patient. This guides subsequent assessments, including neurological investigations.

After the initial history is taken, the clinician has to decide how many and in which order to undertake their investigations. This relates to all investigations and not just to neurological ones. Neurological investigations should support and complement non-neurological investigations. This may be best delivered by taking a multi-disciplinary team approach to managing investigations in this group of patients. Managing the complexities of modern testing is also helped by taking a tiered approach to investigations as is already used in other areas of medicine such as in oncology and various surgery meetings, such as for undertaking epilepsy surgery. For patients with PoTS, the challenge is to combine relevant investigations outside the cardiovascular system, so that they usefully contribute to diagnosing and stratifying the disorder.

Finally, one has to take into account the health system in which the doctor and patient operate. Judicious and timely investigation is always our goal in clinical medicine, but the practicalities of delivering that can be quite challenging. Within the UK, and its popular NHS, health care is delivered across networks, some with a hub and spoke structure, such that some of the neurological tests are delivered within primary care, some within District General Hospitals and some within Tertiary centres with a greater collection of specialists in PoTS, both within neurology and outside the specialty.

R. S. Delamont (✉)
Departments of Neurology and Clinical Neurophysiology, King's College Hospital, Denmark Hill, London 5 9RS, UK
e-mail: robert.delamont@nhs.net

R. S. Delamont
Department of Neurology, Darent Valley Hospital, Dartford, Kent D2 8DA, UK

N. Gall et al. (eds.), *Postural Tachycardia Syndrome*, https://doi.org/10.1007/978-3-030-54165-1_7

Neurological Investigations Within Primary Care

The role of primary care is to ensure that any issues related to the general medical state of the patient have been assessed. This includes basic haematology including FBC, biochemistry including renal function, electrolytes, liver function tests, calcium and bone minerals, a fasting blood sugar and an HbA1c. Knowing whether there is an abnormality in these basic parameters is essential because of their significant impact on neurological function both acutely and in the longer term. Given the increasing incidence of diabetes and pre-diabetes in communities around the world, this must be any baseline testing. Serum B12 and folate available as a baseline are important because of their impact on neurological function and because many patients with PoTS may have gastro-intestinal disorders with secondary effects on absorption of nutrients including B12 and folate.

A 12 lead ECG should also be available. While it can be seen as relating to the heart, the frequent presentation with dizziness and possible pre-syncope often coming through neurology clinics, an ECG should be regarded as essential. This gives us an idea if there are cardiological issues requiring their input and may also flag up conduction abnormalities which may be markers of channelopathies which themselves can be associated with neurological disorders such as epilepsy which can co-exist with syncope and pre-syncope.

Whether to image and which modality to use depends on what is available in primary care and the initial set of symptoms leading to further assessment. Imaging may be more widely available in the secondary sector or in investigational centres for PoTS. Where the initial presentation relates to experiential symptoms, early cerebral imaging with adequate anatomical detail is recommended. This is largely by MRI of the head including the cranio-cervical junction. Imaging at this level in the health service will usually deliver reports often by general radiologists and not the images to review by the referring clinician. Careful wording in the referral is useful to ensure that the reporting radiologist has included the cranio-cervical junction in their assessment.

CT is sometimes more widely available and can be used in lieu of MRI. This can have implications for patients with PoTS as they are often young women and it is arguable whether they should have CT as a first line investigation at all in this situation. Subsequently, MRI in Investigational Centres may be necessary to ensure that alternative diagnoses have been effectively eliminated. Where fatigue has been a dominant symptom and if subtle neurological abnormalities are identified on examination, identifying other conditions is important. Within the central nervous system, multiple sclerosis would be important to have considered and eliminated.

Neurological Investigations Within Secondary/Tertiary Care

Diagnosing a PoTS response can be achieved by a simple 10 minutes prolonged stand. While this enables labelling, it does not confirm that there is no evidence of autonomic failure contributing to the disorder and for this reason autonomic function testing is one of the initial investigations undertaken.

Autonomic Function testing frequently shows evidence of exaggerated HR responses to standing but they may not reach the criteria of a sustained 30 bpm increase in the first 10 minutes of standing (see also Chapter 8: The active stand/tilt tests). This can lead to a lack of clarity for patients. It should be remembered that there is a diurnal variation in postural HR responses [1], that circumstances of testing can vary despite the best attempts to standardise testing conditions, patient hydration state, room temperature and anxiety are all important considerations.

Ancillary features to note in addition to crude heart rate changes include the presence of Mayer type waves which can be seen pre-syncopally, but may be seen during a prolonged stand when the patient complains of difficulty focusing and brain fog [2]. On standing there can be an exaggerated rise in blood pressure which is sustained for the 10 minutes. During Valsalva manoeuvres, elevated phase II late and phase IV blood pressures can be seen.

Syncopal events can be triggered and this should be interpreted in light of the history.

Further neurophysiology of peripheral nerve function will be influenced by the results of autonomic function testing (see chapters "Additional Autonomic Tests" and "PoTS from a Patient's Perspective"). If there is evidence of autonomic failure, it is essential to undertake large fibre neurophysiology to identify evidence for a large fibre neuropathy.

Up to 50% of PoTS patients evaluated at tertiary centres have evidence of partial sympathetic denervation of the lower limbs. This is assessed by thermoregulatory sweat test (TST), quantitative sudomotor axon reflex testing, intra-epidermal nerve fibre density [3] and with meta-iodobenzylguanidine (MIBG) scans, though this last feature remains subject to on-going debate.

Undertaking small fibre studies, remains a specialised test, but promises to illuminate more about the pathophysiology of the disorder and may enable sub-grouping in the future. Consistent abnormalities in different parameters of C-fibre function in a large proportion of PoTS patients have been demonstrated. Specifically, the relative time occurrence of the supernormal and the refractory period of excitability of sympathetic axons indicates depolarised axonal membrane potentials [4]. Also, some PoTS patients with comorbid chronic pain have signs of spontaneous activity in C-nociceptors.

For patients with evidence of a small fibre neuropathy, more detailed history should be undertaken as the list for causes of small fibre neuropathies is long and is outlined in Table 1 [5]. Such a list is not complete and is always subject to updating. This is particularly true for drugs and toxins which are, an ever expanding cause of small fibre disease. The other area which is being increasingly recognised is that of paraneoplastic causes. Both should be looked for very carefully.

Table 1 Causes of small fibre neuropathy

Impaired glucose control	Diabetes mellitus
	Rapid glycaemic control
Vitamin B12 deficiency	
Dyslipidaemia	
Hypothyroidism	
Chronic kidney disease	
Hereditary/genetic	Nav1.7 mutations
	Nav 1.8 mutations
	Familial amyloid polyneuropathy
	Fabry's disease
	Tangier's disease
Infections	HIV
	Hepatitis C
	Influenza
Toxins and Drugs	Anti-retroviral
Antibiotics	Metronidazole
	Nitrofurantoin
	Linezolid
Chemotherapy: Proteasome Inhibitor	Bortezomib
Anti-arrhythmic agents	Flecainide
Statins	
Alcohol	
Vitamin B6 toxicity	
Immune disorders	Coeliac disease
	Sarcoidosis
	Sjögren's syndrome
	Rheumatoid disease
	Systemic lupus erythematosus
	Vasculitis
	Inflammatory bowel disease
Paraneoplastic disorders	
Monoclonal gammopathy/amyloid	

Once detailed clinical history and examination have been undertaken, targeted laboratory testing can be undertaken. However, not all of these potential investigations will be available as clinical tests. Some are very specialized and will be available only in specialized hospitals or Units including National Centres. There is little evidence to suggest that routine testing for ganglionic acetylcholine receptor antibodies is useful as a routine practice. The role for identifying α1-adrenergic or β-adrenergic antibodies in routine clinical practice remains subject to debate and discussion [6].

Where experiential phenomena are a prominent component of the history, thought should be given to capturing an attack. This can be during autonomic function testing where continuous heart rate and blood pressure records are available. All patients should ideally have their testing done under video surveillance to be able to carefully review any phenomena that occur at the time.

The true incidence of syncope in patients with PoTS remains unclear. Experiential symptoms such as brain fog, detachment, light headedness, blurred vision, nausea, headache and tremor are well described and on occasion may raise the question of whether epilepsy may be relevant. Careful history taking usually enables the treating clinician to delineate between the two types of experiential disorder, but it is not always easy. This group of patients also have a high prevalence of migraine which can confuse the treating clinician (see also Chapter 15: Headache). An electroencephalogram (EEG) is needed on occasion and sometimes an attempt to activate the attacks may be needed. This should be undertaken in a laboratory which is familiar with this procedure and is able to interpret EEGs [7]. It also enables differentiation between syncope and non-syncopal and non-epileptic attacks [8]. Dissociative attacks are well recognised in the epilepsy field. Hypokinetic dissociative attacks are less well recognised and often associated with delayed diagnosis [9]. They can be misdiagnosed as epilepsy and increasingly syncope.

In Summary

The key to deciding on the neurological investigations needed in patients with PoTS lies in the history. This requires sufficient time for the clinician to establish the time course, progression, relapsing features and the predominant bodily systems involved. This enables the clinician to take a tiered approach to investigations. This particularly applies to any neurologist who sees patients with PoTS.

References

1. Brewster JA, Garland EM, Biaggioni I, Black BK, Ling JF, Shibao CA, Robertson D, Raj SR. Diurnal variability in orthostatic tachycardia: implications for the postural tachycardia syndrome. Clin. Sci. (Lond.). 2012;122:25–31.
2. Delamont S. "Syncope" 0029 Oxford textbook of clinical neurophysiology Ed: K Mills; Chap. 29 OUP; 2016. Print ISBN-13. https://doi.org/10.1093/med/9780199608997.003.0029.
3. Haensch CA, Tosch M, Katona I, Weis J, Isenmann S. Small-fiber neuropathy with cardiac denervation in postural tachycardia syndrome. Muscle Nerve. 2014;50:956–61.
4. Z'Graggen WJ, Solà R, Graf NE, Serra J, Bostock H. Sensitivity to ischaemia of single sympathetic nerve fibres innervating the dorsum of the human foot. J Physiol. 2017;595(13):4467–73.
5. Themistocleous AC, Ramirez JD, Serra J, Bennett DLH. The clinical approach to small fibre neuropathy and painful channelopathy. Pract Neurol. 2014;14:368–79. https://doi.org/10.1136/practneurol-2013-000758.
6. Vernino S, Stiles LE. Autoimmunity in postural tachycardia syndrome: current understanding. Auton Neurosci. 2018;215:78–82.
7. Whitehead K, Kane N, Wardrope A, Kandler R, Reuber M. Proposal for best practice in the use of video-EEG when psychogenic non-epileptic seizures are a possible diagnosis. Clin Neurophysiol Pract. 2017;2:130–9.
8. LaRoche S, Taylor D, Walter P. Tilt table testing with video EEG monitoring in the evaluation of patients with unexplained loss of consciousness. Clin EEG Neuro Sci. 2011;42(3):202–5.
9. Goldstein LH, Robinson EJ, Reuber M, Chalder T, Callaghan H, Eastwood C, Landau S, McCrone P, Medford N, Metters JDC, Moore M, Mosweu I, Murray J, Perdue I, Pilecka I, Richardson MP, Carson A, Stone J; on behalf of the CODES Study Group. Characteristics of 698 patients with dissociative seizures: a UK multicentre study. Epilepsia. 2019;60(11):2182–93.

The Active Stand and Tilt Tests

Matthew G. Lloyd, Kate Bourne and Satish R. Raj

Abbreviations

PoTS	Postural Tachycardia Syndrome
HR	Heart rate
AST	Active stand testing
HUT	Head-up tilt
VOSS	Vanderbilt Orthostatic Symptom Score

Assessment of Orthostatic Tachycardia

Clinical evaluation of orthostatic tachycardia is critical to the diagnostic assessment of postural tachycardia syndrome (PoTS). A key diagnostic criterion for PoTS is a heart rate (HR) increase of ≥30BPM within 10 minutes of positional change from supine to standing, and without orthostatic hypotension (>20/10 mmHg reduction) [1]. Active stand testing (AST) and head up tilt table testing (HUT) can both be used to evaluate the presence of this tachycardia. While there are methodological differences between the two tests, the commonalities of assessing orthostatic tachycardia in PoTS will be discussed first.

M. G. Lloyd · K. Bourne · S. R. Raj (✉)
Cumming School of Medicine, Libin Cardiovascular Institute of Alberta, University of Calgary, Calgary, Canada
e-mail: satish.raj@ucalgary.ca

Continuous measurement of beat-to-beat blood pressure (BP) and heart rate (HR) are preferable during both AST and HUT. If continuous monitoring is not available, HR and BP readings should be recorded at regular time intervals [2]. HR measurements using pulse oximetry, non-invasive brachial blood pressure cuff measurements or manual palpation are acceptable in the clinical diagnostic setting, but do not allow for detection of non-sinus rhythm. Incremental blood pressure readings using a non-invasive brachial arm cuff are sufficient to rule out orthostatic hypotension in the setting of a diagnosis of PoTS.

For a diagnosis of PoTS, orthostatic tachycardia must be accompanied by a history of consistent orthostatic symptoms in daily life, which lessen with recumbence. Orthostatic symptoms often occur during an orthostatic test, and can be measured at the end of orthostasis using a symptom scale such as the Vanderbilt Orthostatic Symptom Score (VOSS) [3]. This scale rates nine common orthostatic symptoms from a scale of 0–10. The presence of orthostatic symptoms during the clinical exam is not necessary for a PoTS diagnosis.

The HR increment of 30 bpm that is the key diagnostic sign for PoTS is typically calculated relative to the baseline, pre-orthostasis supine period. However, Roma et al. have argued that the pretest HR may not reflect the participants' true resting HR, due to pre-test anxiety [4]. They propose

N. Gall et al. (eds.), *Postural Tachycardia Syndrome*, https://doi.org/10.1007/978-3-030-54165-1_8

that two minutes of supine recovery from orthostasis should also be considered when assessing the patients' maximum HR increment. The addition of this period increased the number of PoTS patients reaching diagnostic threshold by 10–30%, however the impact on specificity is unknown.

As the diagnostic criterion for PoTS is orthostatic tachycardia within 10 minutes of orthostasis from a supine posture, the optimal duration for the orthostatic test is 10–11 minutes [5]. This allows the patient to be evaluated for orthostatic tachycardia within the timeframe for PoTS diagnosis. Although orthostatic tachycardia before 10 minutes can occur, an abbreviated test could miss the requisite orthostatic tachycardia in some patients [6, 7]. Conversely, longer tests may allow for detection of some PoTS patients (so-called "late PoTS [8]"), but reduces specificity significantly (20% for HUT, 53% for AST).

Patients should be instructed to not move or voluntarily contract their leg muscles throughout the duration of the test in order to limit the contribution of the skeletal muscle pump to venous return [4]. Prior to orthostasis, the patient should lie supine for at least 5 minutes to allow heart rate and blood pressure to stabilize [9]. During HUT, the tilt table should be raised from supine to at least 60° [9] in one movement, and not in incremental angles over a certain time period. Due to the passive nature of the HUT, patients may experience vasovagal syncope, despite no medical history of syncope.

Sustained orthostatic tachycardia with a ≥30BPM increase in the absence of a blood pressure decrease>20/10 mmHg confirms orthostatic tachycardia [10]. The addition of chronic orthostatic symptoms (≥3 months) confirms PoTS. It is expected that heart rate will increase upon initial active standing due to unloading of the baroreceptors, and brief initial orthostatic hypotension (reduction in blood pressure>40/20 mmHg immediately upon standing) may also be present [11]. If the HR increases transiently in response to the initial BP decrease, and then returns to baseline levels in the following minutes of tilt, a diagnosis of PoTS is not be appropriate. The AST shows a greater initial blood pressure decrease, and HR increase than HUT [12].

General Considerations

Diurnal Variability: Orthostatic heart rate changes and baroreflex sensitivity fluctuate throughout the day [13]. Orthostatic tachycardia has been shown to be worse in PoTS patients in the morning than later in the day [14]. Symptoms of orthostatic intolerance are also more often experienced during morning testing versus later in the day [15]. Therefore, consideration into timing should be given when interpreting results of the AST and HUT. Patients should be tested in the morning when they are likely to have a more pronounced orthostatic heart rate increase, and may be more likely to demonstrate associated symptoms. Afternoon tests that are borderline for PoTS may be repeated in the morning.

Influence of Menstrual Cycle: Phase of the menstrual cycle during testing may affect the patient's results. Worsening orthostatic intolerance is associated with the early follicular or luteal (premenstrual) phases [1, 16–18]. Menstrual cycle phase should be recorded, and repeat testing should be considered in patients who are suspicious for PoTS, but do not have a positive testing result.

Medications: Drugs that affect heart rate, sympathetic nervous activity, or blood volume should be withheld prior to the orthostatic test.

Pediatric Considerations: The AST for the diagnosis of PoTS has not been validated in a pediatric population [19]. A 10 minute HUT is considered the standard diagnostic tool [19]. As orthostatic tachycardia in more common in children than adults, pediatric patients should demonstrate an orthostatic HR increase of ≥40BPM in addition to symptoms of orthostatic intolerance for a diagnosis of PoTS. As well, symptoms of orthostatic intolerance may not occur during HUT. A study of 22 pediatric patients, found that 7 did not experience symptoms on HUT, despite being diagnosed with PoTS [20].

Additional Considerations: Patients should be tested in a fasted state or at least 2 hours postprandial to avoid acute fluid shifts and vasodilation that can occur in response to eating and cause postprandial hypotension [21].

Patients should refrain from alcohol for 24 hours prior to the test to avoid its diuretic effects, and the consequential reduction in plasma volume. The testing room should be kept at a comfortable temperature (20–22 °C) to mitigate the well-known effects of heat stress on exacerbating orthostatic intolerance [22]. Lastly, excitatory stimuli (bright lights, loud noises) should be minimized since they can directly alter blood pressure and heart rate.

Advantages and Disadvantages of Active Stand Testing and the Head up Tilt Test

Both AST and HUT present various advantages and disadvantages in the clinical diagnosis of PoTS. In the Heart Rhythm Society 2015 consensus statement on the diagnosis and management of PoTS, AST was rated as a class I diagnostic recommendation, and HUT as a class IIb recommendation [10]. AST is convenient, cost-effective and can be performed in the primary care physician office. The AST can therefore help to make a diagnosis of PoTS without the need for specialist referral or a specialized testing centre, which could lead to a delay in diagnosis and treatment. Passive standing testing may be utilized in patients unable to stand unsupported, as the patient stands against a wall [4]. Active standing mimics standing in everyday life, which may help to recreate specific symptomology or experiences for diagnostic purposes [5]. However, it may be difficult to standardize this testing, as muscle tensing is more difficult to control.

Orthostasis with HUT allows evaluation over a longer duration of time than AST [10], and elicits higher heart rates than AST [23]. The HUT is useful in situations where the patient is unable to stand, or has a high fall risk or risk of syncope. However, HUT requires expensive, specialized equipment and the test may not be covered by insurance. Both HUT and AST may provoke orthostatic tachycardia in patients who do not have PoTS [7], which must be carefully considered in making a diagnosis (Fig. 1).

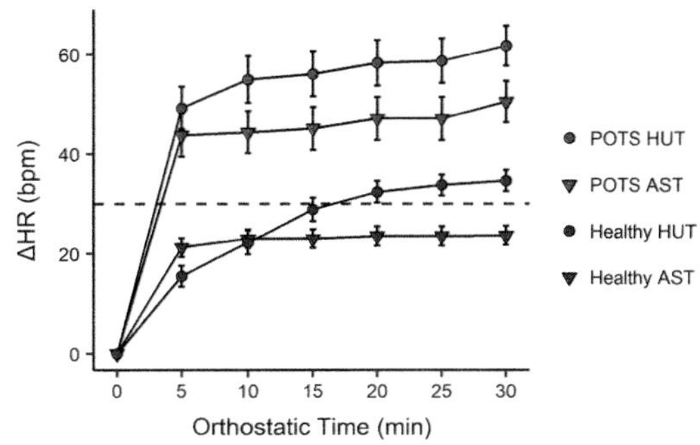

Fig. 1 The cardiac response to head-up tilt (HUT) and active stand test (AST) in patients with postural tachycardia syndrome (PoTS) and healthy controls. Note that the heart rate response to HUT is larger for both PoTS patients and healthy controls. The dashed horizontal line is the 30 bpm ΔHR criterion currently in use for the diagnosis of PoTS. Figure recreated with permission from [23]

Conclusion

Should one type of test be selected over the other for the diagnosis of PoTS? Different physiological findings may be evident in AST versus HUT, due to the role of the skeletal muscle pump [23]. A study of PoTS patients and healthy controls found a significantly higher orthostatic heart rate increase on HUT versus AST [23]. In this study, HUT and AST had similar sensitivities (93% and 87%, respectively), but specificity was lower for HUT (40% vs. 67% for AST). A different study of patients with orthostatic intolerance as well as healthy controls found similar HR measurements between AST and HUT [2]. Reflex tachycardia specific to initial orthostatic hypotension may be greater in the initial minutes of AST, compared to HUT, and this should be considered in the evaluation of early AST HR responses [12]. A summary of the comparisons between AST and HUT are found in Table 1.

Overall, the AST should be used as a first line tool in the diagnostic assessment of PoTS. Referral to a specialist centre with HUT and other autonomic testing may be considered if the patient does not experience symptom improvement with initial treatment [10], is limited in their ability to complete the AST, or another

Table 1 Summary of active stand and head up tilt testing

	Active stand testing	Head up tilt testing
Heart rate evaluation	First line diagnostic tool for PoTS	Elicits greater orthostatic tachycardia
Blood pressure evaluation	May elicit initial orthostatic hypotension	
Usage	May be performed in the physician's office	Requires specialized equipment
Sensitivity (%)	87	93
Specificity	67	40

diagnosis requiring prolonged passive standing for diagnosis (e.g. delayed orthostatic hypotension or vasovagal syncope) is being considered.

Acknowledgements The authors would like to acknowledge the many patients that have volunteered their time to contribute to this body of work. Their participation is critical to the ongoing investigation of PoTS.

Funding Dr. Raj has a research grant related to Postural Tachycardia Syndrome from the Canadian Institutes of Health Research, Ottawa, Canada (grant number MOP142426). Dr. Lloyd has a post-doctoral scholarship through the Cummings School of Medicine. Kate Bourne has a Canadian Institute of Health Research Graduate Scholarship.

Disclosures Dr. Raj is a network investigator of the Cardiac Arrhythmia Network of Canada (CANet; London, Ontario, Canada). Dr. Raj serves on the Medical Advisory Board of Dysautonomia International and PoTS UK, both without financial compensation. Dr. Lloyd has reported that he has no relationships relevant to the contents of this chapter to disclose. Kate Bourne has also reported that she has no relationships relevant to the contents of this chapter to disclose.

References

1. Raj SR. The Postural Tachycardia Syndrome (PoTS) pathophysiology, diagnosis & management. Indian Pacing Electrophysiol J. 2006;6:84–99.
2. Kirbiš M, Grad A, Meglič B, Bajrović FF. Comparison of active standing test, head-up tilt test and 24-h ambulatory heart rate and blood pressure monitoring in diagnosing postural tachycardia. Funct Neurol. 2013;28:39–45.
3. Raj SR, Black BK, Biaggioni I, Harris PA, Robertson D. Acetylcholinesterase inhibition improves tachycardia in postural tachycardia syndrome. Circulation. 2005;111:2734–40.
4. Roma M, Marden CL, Rowe PC. Passive standing tests for the office diagnosis of postural tachycardia syndrome: new methodological considerations. Fatigue Biomed Heal Behav. 2018;6:179–92 (Taylor & Francis).
5. Finucane C, van Wijnen VK, Fan CW, Soraghan C, Byrne L, Westerhof BE, et al. A practical guide to active stand testing and analysis using continuous beat-to-beat non-invasive blood pressure monitoring. Clin Auton Res. 2019.
6. Carew S, Cooke J, O'Connor M, Donnelly T, Costelloe A, Sheehy C, et al. What is the optimal duration of tilt testing for the assessment of patients with suspected postural tachycardia syndrome? Europace. 2009;11:635–7.
7. van Campen C (Linda) MC, Rowe PC, Visser FC. Low sensitivity of abbreviated tilt table testing for diagnosing postural tachycardia syndrome in adults with ME/CFS. Front Pediatr. 2018;6:1–6.
8. Mayuga KA, Butters KB, Fouad-Tarazi F. Early versus late postural tachycardia: a re-evaluation of a syndrome. Clin Auton Res. 2008;18:155–7.
9. Arnold AC, Ng J, Raj SR. Postural tachycardia syndrome—diagnosis, physiology, and prognosis. Auton Neurosci Basic Clin. 2018;215:3–11. https://doi.org/10.1016/j.autneu.2018.02.005 (Elsevier).
10. Sheldon RS, Grubb BP, Olshansky B, Shen WK, Calkins H, Brignole M, et al. 2015 Heart rhythm society expert consensus statement on the diagnosis and treatment of postural tachycardia syndrome, inappropriate sinus tachycardia, and vasovagal syncope. Hear Rhythm. 2015;12:e41–63. https://doi.org/10.1016/j.hrthm.2015.03.029 (Elsevier).
11. Wieling W, Krediet CTP, van Dijk N, Linzer M, Tschakovsky ME. Initial orthostatic hypotension: review of a forgotten condition. Clin Sci. 2007;112:157–65.
12. Tanaka H, Sjöberg BJ, Thulesius O. Cardiac output and blood pressure during active and passive standing. Clin Physiol. 1996;16:157–70.
13. Cooper V, Elliott MW, Pearson SB, Taylor CM, Hainsworth R. Daytime variability in carotid

baroreflex function in healthy human subjects. Clin Auton Res. 2007 [cited 2013 Aug 24];17:26–32. https://www.ncbi.nlm.nih.gov/pubmed/17264980.
14. Brewster JA, Garland EM, Biaggioni I, Black BK, Ling JF, Shibao CA, et al. Diurnal variability in orthostatic tachycardia: implications for the postural tachycardia syndrome. Clin Sci (Lond). 2012;122:25–31.
15. Moon J, Lee HS, Byun JI, Sunwoo JS, Shin JW, Lim JA, et al. The complexity of diagnosing postural orthostatic tachycardia syndrome: Influence of the diurnal variability. J Am Soc Hypertens. 2016;10:263–70 (Elsevier Ltd.).
16. Stickford ASL, Vangundy TB, Levine BD, Fu Q. Menstrual cycle phase does not affect sympathetic neural activity in women with postural orthostatic tachycardia syndrome. J Physiol. 2015;593:2131–43.
17. Peggs KJ, Nguyen H, Enayat D, Keller NR, Al-Hendy A, Raj SR. Gynecologic disorders and menstrual cycle lightheadedness in postural tachycardia syndrome. Int J Gynecol Obstet. 2012;118:242–6.
18. Fu Q, Vangundy TB, Shibata S, Auchus RJ, Williams GH, Levine BD. Menstrual cycle affects renal-adrenal and hemodynamic responses during prolonged standing in the postural orthostatic tachycardia syndrome. Hypertension. 2010;56:82–90.
19. Stewart JM, Boris JR, Chelimsky G, Fischer PR, Fortunato JE, Grubb BP, et al. Pediatric disorders of orthostatic intolerance. Pediatrics. 2018 [cited 2018 Jun 17];141:e20171673. https://pediatrics.aappublications.org/lookup/doi/10.1542/peds.2017-1673
20. Huh TE, Yeom JS, Kim YS, Woo HO, Park JS, Park ES, et al. Orthostatic symptoms does not always manifest during tilt-table test in pediatric postural orthostatic tachycardia syndrome patients. Korean J Pediatr. 2013;56:32–6.
21. Luciano GL, Brennan MJ, Rothberg MB. Postprandial hypotension. Am J Med. 2010;123:281.e1–6. https://doi.org/10.1016/j.amjmed.2009.06.026 (Elsevier Inc.)
22. Schlader ZJ, Wilson TE, Crandall CG. Mechanisms of orthostatic intolerance during heat stress. Auton Neurosci Basic Clin. 2016;196:37–46. https://doi.org/10.1016/j.autneu.2015.12.005 (Elsevier B.V.)
23. Plash WB, Diedrich A, Biaggioni I, Garland EM, Paranjape SY, Black BK, et al. Diagnosing postural tachycardia syndrome: comparison of tilt testing compared with standing haemodynamics. Clin Sci (Lond). 2013;124:109–14.

Additional Autonomic Tests

Peter Oketa-Onyut Julu and Melvin D. Lobo

Introduction

The physiology of postural tachycardia syndrome or PoTS is complex and is poorly understood. The magnitude of tachycardia depends on natural and normal compensatory requirement in response to orthostatic challenges. Other contributions come from the inotropic function of the heart, windkessel vascular resistance and venous vascular capacitance. It would be desirable to quantify all of these four contributions during clinical investigation of PoTS. Laboratory standardised surrogate measures of all the four cardiovascular compensatory factors and their autonomic controls are now available. Some are described here as autonomic target-organs neurophysiological tests and may be offered as an adjunct to active stand/tilt testing in some centres in order to better define PoTS phenotypes/subgroups. In addition, other forms of autonomic testing as undertaken in the National Hospital for Neurology & Neurosurgery tertiary centre are also described in chapter "A Tertiary Referral Centre for PoTS: The Autonomic Unit at the National Hospital for Neurology and Neurosurgery Experience".

P. O.-O. Julu (✉) · M. D. Lobo
Barts NIHR Cardiovascular Biomedical Research Unit, Charterhouse Square, William Harvey Research Institute, Queen Mary University London, London EC1M 6BQ, UK
e-mail: p.julu@qmul.ac.uk

M. D. Lobo
Barts BP Centre of Excellence, Barts Heart Centre, St Bartholomew's Hospital, West Smithfield, London EC17BE, UK

Autonomic Target-Organs Neurophysiological Tests (ATONT)

Definition of Autonomic Failure

The phrase "Autonomic Failure" when used as a clinical term means the inability of the autonomic nervous system to execute co-ordinated and standardised autonomic tasks that have been identified and validated for clinical examinations of the system. The autonomic tasks are set up in the form of special manoeuvres recommended for clinical tests of autonomic function by an International Committee in a consensus statement of San Antonio [1]. Diagnosis of autonomic failure cannot be based on a single abnormal test parameter because the autonomic nervous system either influences or controls the functions of all the organs in the body. It requires a set of carefully designed clinical manoeuvres aimed to examine functions of specific target-organs in order to draw conclusions whether or not such target-organs have normal functions. We have designed and validated multiple parameters described below. Some of these are derived from the internationally recommended manoeuvres

N. Gall et al. (eds.), *Postural Tachycardia Syndrome*, https://doi.org/10.1007/978-3-030-54165-1_9

mentioned above and some are improvements of the recommendations, but we have designed some entirely in our laboratory to diagnose and characterise autonomic failures according to the specific target-organs we intend to examine. We would report a failure or dysfunction of a target-organ if its function lies outside the range of our normal values. Our laboratory standards are based on 250 healthy subjects aged between 13 and 79 years.

Assessment of Central Parasympathetic Function

Resting Supine Cardiac Vagal Tone (CVT)

This is a measure of the central parasympathetic restraint of the chronotropic function of the heart regulated by the vagus nerve. It is measured continuously on a beat-to-beat basis as 'pulse-synchronised phase shifts in consecutive cardiac cycles' using the NeuroScope (Medifit Instruments Ltd, London, UK) in a quiet room at controlled room temperature of 21 ± 1 °C. It is essentially a form of jitter that is quantified continuously from the electrocardiogram (ECG) using a circuit of electronic integrators and a phase detector to convert the pulse interval jitters into voltages [2], which are then calibrated into units of the atropine-derived linear vagal scale (LVS) [3]. The least value in the units of LVS is zero, equivalent to full atropinisation of human subjects [3]. The LVS is therefore a validated clinical unit of cardiac vagal tone with an absolute zero reference point. The frequency distribution of CVT measured in units of LVS in our laboratory control population is approximately Gaussian (Fig. 1).

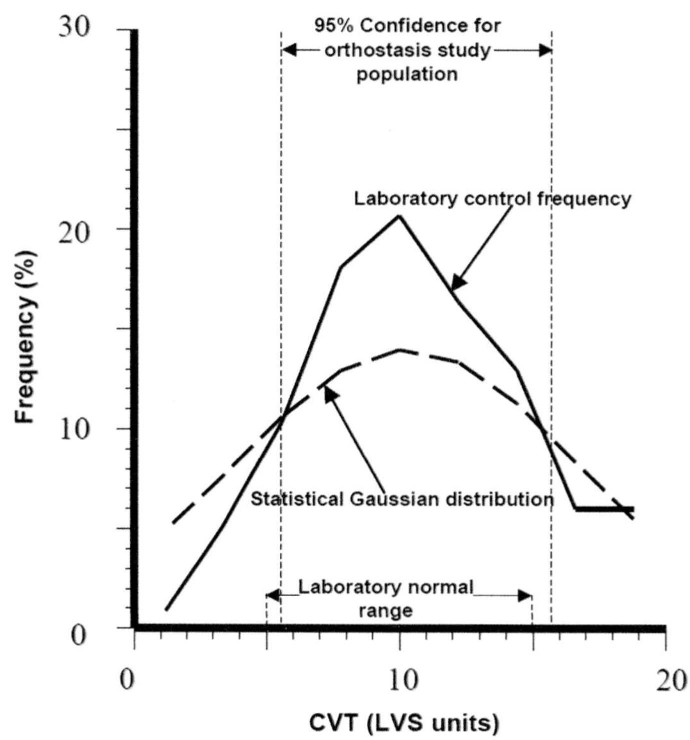

Fig. 1 A frequency distribution plot of the observed values of cardiac vagal tone (CVT) measured in units of a linear vagal scale (LVS) at rest in supine position in the laboratory control population (n = 250, see text for details). The theoretical statistical Gaussian distribution with the same population mean and standard deviation is superimposed in this plot. Chi squared test showed a normal distribution of CVT in our laboratory control population. The laboratory normal range of resting supine values of CVT is indicated in the plot together with the 95% confidence interval of baseline CVT values in a sample population used in the study of the effects of progressive orthostatic stress on autonomic regulation of the cardiovascular system (see text for details)

Respiratory Gating of Cardiac Vagal Tone (CVT) in Supine Position

The central parasympathetic tone, with inherent cardiac pulse and response to voluntary changes in breathing rhythms, is also known as cardiac vagal tone and it is generated by cardiac vagal premotor neurons (cVPN) in the nucleus ambiguus (NA) in the brainstem. The magnitude of respiratory gating of CVT at the level of cVPN in NA can be quantified and used to assess the integrity of cardiorespiratory neurons within the brainstem. This is a central cardiorespiratory cholinergic function of the brainstem at the level of cVPN [4]. Lying in supine position, the subject is asked to take a deep breath within 4 s and to breathe out forcefully to reach up to expiratory reserve volume within 6 s and repeating the exercise six times while CVT is being measured continuously using the NeuroScope (Medifit Instruments Ltd, London, UK) in a quiet room with controlled room temperature as above. Deep breathing at 0.1 Hz should increase CVT from baseline by values ranging between 5 and 15 LVS units and should show clear modulations in the continuous CVT record at the same frequency (Our laboratory standard).

Resting Supine Cardiac Sensitivity to Baroreflex (CSB)

This is a measure of the beat-to-beat baroreflex central sympathetic restraint exerted directly within the brainstem. It is a measure of the well known baroreflex restraint of sympathetic activity, mainly the vasomotor tone in the RVLM, which is coming through the NTS [5, 6]. The resting supine CSB is measured using the NeuroScope (MediFit Instruments Ltd, London) as previously described in a quiet room at controlled room temperature as described above [7]. The index is defined as the increase in pulse interval per unit increase in systolic pressure and it is measured in units of ms $mmHg-^{1}$. It is a beat-to-beat baroreflex negative feedback control of arterial blood pressure. The least value of CSB is zero representing no negative feedback cardiovascular control at all. The normal range in our laboratory population is between 6 and 12 ms $mmHg^{-1}$. The 95% confidence interval in the population sample used in a progressive orthostatic stress study described by Julu et al. [7] is between 5 and 11 ms $mmHg-^{1}$ similar to our laboratory normal range given above. The method allows the detection of rapid changes in CSB within a continuous measurement, which represents real-time engagements and disengagements of the baroreflex negative feedback cardiovascular control. Disengagement of negative feedback cardiovascular control indicates cardiovascular arousal in preparation to imminent changes in either blood pressure alone, or heart rate alone, or both heart rate and blood pressure at the same time.

Assessment of Central Baroreflex Gain

We use the isometric contraction of the skeletal muscles of the dominant hand during a sustained handgrip at 50% of the maximum sustainable force measured in Newton (N) for a target duration of three minutes to reduce and keep the baroreflex negative feedback cardiovascular restraint to its lowest level. Withdrawal of the baroreflex negative feedback control measured as CSB in the upright-seated position is achieved within one minute of sustained handgrip and stays at its least level for the remaining duration of the handgrip. This is confirmed visually on the computer screen during the test procedure. Since CSB is at its lowest level, the gradients of the concurrent rise in heart rate and arterial blood pressure during the second and third minute of sustained handgrip is regulated by the supramedullary central autonomic regulation sites (CARS). The CARS sites in the periorbital frontal lobes are the dominant bilateral supramedullary sites during the restraints of both heart rate and arterial blood pressure during isometric contraction of skeletal muscles. The gradient of concurrent changes in heart rate and arterial blood pressure is a measure of baroreflex gain and in this case it is a supramedullary central gain. We define this central baroreflex gain (BRR) as the absolute value of the ratio ΔR-R/ΔSBP, where ΔR-R is the change in the electrocardiographic (ECG) R-R interval, associated and concurrent with ΔSBP, the change in systolic BP, from baseline to the respective levels at the end of three minutes of sustained handgrip. The central baroreflex gain can be predicted from the equation BRR = $2.42 \times 10^{(3\,h-5)}$ ms mmH$-^{1}$ [8], where h is the subject's height in metres, or predicted in terms of the natural number 'e' where BRR = $6.35 \times 10^{(eh-5)}$ ms mmHg$-^{1}$ [8]. The observed value from the ratio ΔR-R/ΔSBP should be within 50% of the predicted value in the age group 15–79 years (Our laboratory standard). The ECG R-R intervals, CSB and the arterial blood pressure are monitored and measured continuously using the NeuroScope (Fig. 2) during this assessment of the central baroreflex gain.

Assessment of Peripheral Baroreflex Function

Mechanical Digital Massage of the Carotid Sinus

Carotid massage using digital pressure applied on the carotid sinus in a resting supine position at the rate of the subject's heartbeats for the duration of 15 s should cause an increase in the CVT by a range between 5 and 20 LVS units in the age group 15–79 years (Our laboratory standard). This is described as a standardised clinical measure of cardiodepressor response of

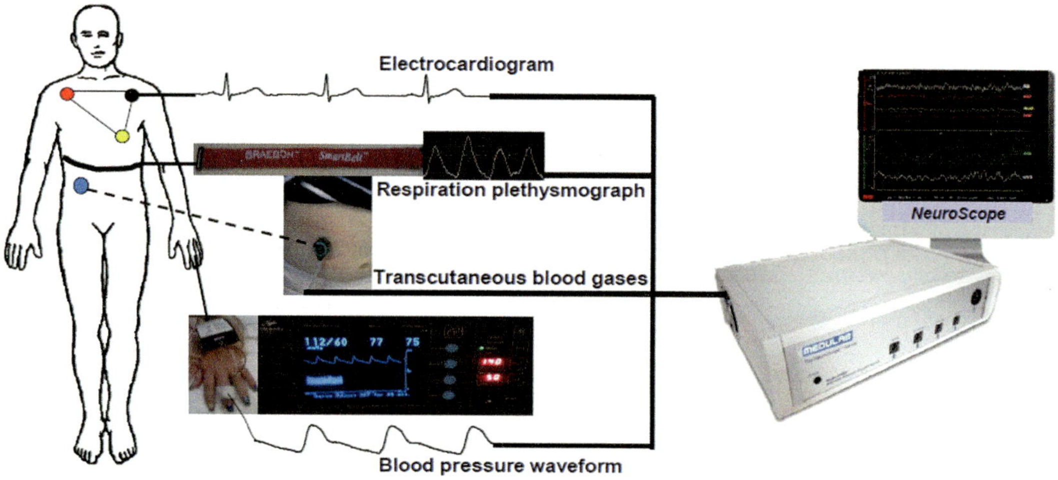

Fig. 2 A schematic representation of non-invasive continuous streams of biometrics obtained from the human body by the NeuroScope during the assessment of autonomic functions. Continuous electrocardiogram (ECG) is recorded using three chest-electrodes in a modified Einthoven's triangle, but configured within the NeuroScope as Einthoven's ECG lead II. Continuous stream of breathing movements is recorded using respiration impedance plethysmography (RIP), which is coupled within the NeuroScope to facilitate the discrimination and identification of apneusis, apnoea, Valsalva's manoeuvres and other respiratory dysrrhythmias. The respiration plethysmogram belt is applied around the chest at the xiphisternal level to capture both thoracic and upper abdominal movements. Transcutaneous blood gases are recorded continuously during autonomic assessment using the dual oxygen and carbon dioxide electrode (Radiometer, Copenhagen). The transcutaneous blood gases electrode measures tension of gases in tissues, not gas tension in the bloodstream. The tension of gases in the tissues correlates with local capillary blood flow, tissue metabolism and temperature, all of which are influenced by the autonomic nervous system and form part of autonomic functions. Tissue temperature in the surrounding of the transcutaneous blood gases sensor is kept constant using a heating element within the sensor. In our practice, the sensor is placed sub-costal in the mid clavicular line close to the liver where it is relatively warmer than other peripheral sites. Continuous stream of arterial blood pressure waveform is recorded from the finger using photoplethysmography and Penáz's principle of arterial pressure unloading through volume-clamp (Finapres Medical Systems, Enschede the Netherlands). All biometrics are synchronised to the nearest millisecond, date and time-stamped before they are used to derive cardiovascular and autonomic parameters using the VaguSoft software (Medifit Instruments Ltd, London)

peripheral baroreflex. The same carotid massage should cause a drop in systolic arterial blood pressure by not more than 30 mmHg (Our laboratory standard). This is a standardised clinical measure of the vasodepressor function of peripheral baroreflex. The CVT and the arterial blood pressure are monitored and measured continuously using the NeuroScope (Fig. 2) during this assessment of the baroreflex function.

Pharmacological Peripheral Baroreceptor Excitation

Intravenous injection of phenylephrine or other α_1-adrenergic vasoactive drugs in a resting supine position should cause a concurrent rise in both blood pressure and ECG R-R intervals and the two should be statistically associated with a gradient of R-R intervals rise per systolic blood pressure rise between 5 and 12 ms $mmHg^{-1}$ (similar to the normal range of the resting supine CSB described above) and a correlation coefficient greater than 0.9 (Our laboratory standard). The ECG R-R intervals and the arterial blood pressure are monitored and measured continuously using the NeuroScope (Fig. 2) during this assessment of peripheral baroreflex function.

Assessment of Sympathetic α_1-Adrenergic Denervation Hypersensitivity

A small intravenous bolus dose of 25 μg of phenylephrine is used to test for denervation hypersensitivity of sympathetic α_1-adrenergic nerves. This will cause systolic blood pressure rise of more than 15 mmHg in denervation hypersensitivity (Our laboratory standard). All the arterial blood pressures; SBP, DBP and MAP, including the parasympathetic restraints; CSB and CVT and the heart rate are monitored and measured continuously during this test using the NeuroScope (Fig. 2).

Assessment of Sympathetic Control of Cardioaccelerator Function

We use the isometric contraction of the skeletal muscles of the dominant hand during a sustained handgrip at 50% of the maximum sustainable force measured in Newton (N) for the duration of three minutes to reduce and keep the baroreflex negative feedback cardiovascular restraint and the central parasympathetic tone to their lowest levels. Withdrawals of both the baroreflex negative feedback control measured as CSB and the central parasympathetic activity measured as CVT in an upright-seated position are achieved within one minute of sustained handgrip and they stay at the least levels for the remaining duration of the handgrip. This is visually confirmed from the computer screen during the test procedure. We interpret the results to mean that the continual increase in heart rate during the second and third minute of sustained handgrip represents the central sympathetic drive of cardioaccelerator function with minimal parasympathetic restraint. The heart rate should increase above the resting pre-exercise value by 22–45% at the end of three minutes of sustained handgrip in subjects aged 15–79 years (Our laboratory standard). Beat-to-beat heart rate, the arterial blood pressures; SBP, DBP and MAP, including the parasympathetic restraints; CSB and CVT are monitored and measured continuously using the NeuroScope during this test (Fig. 2).

Assessment of Sympathetic Vasomotor Control of Windkessel Vascular Resistance

We use the isometric contraction of the skeletal muscles of the dominant hand during a sustained handgrip at 50% of the maximum sustainable force measured in Newton (N) for the duration of three minutes to reduce and keep the baroreflex negative feedback cardiovascular restraint and the central parasympathetic tone to their lowest levels. Withdrawals of both the baroreflex negative feedback control measured as CSB and the central parasympathetic activity measured as CVT in an upright-seated position are achieved within one minute of sustained handgrip and they stay at the least levels for the remaining duration of the handgrip. This is confirmed visually from the computer screen during the test procedure. We expect the continual increase in diastolic blood pressure (DBP) during the second and third minute of sustained handgrip to represent the central sympathetic vasomotor drive of the windkessel vascular resistance with minimal parasympathetic restraint. We use the rising DBP during sustained handgrip as a surrogate of increasing central sympathetic vasomotor drive to windkessel vascular resistance because DBP has a linear relationship with MSNA during this procedure [9]. Diastolic arterial blood pressure is a function of the windkessel vascular resistance [10]. The skeletal muscle vascular bed provides most of the windkessel vascular resistance during muscle contraction because the sympathetic drive to skin is significantly inhibited and sympathetic drive to the splanchnic vascular bed is mainly used to regulate venous vascular capacitance [11] out of the three major vascular beds used for arterial blood pressure control. The diastolic blood pressure should increase above the resting pre-exercise level by no less than 15 mmHg in all adults [12]. Our laboratory range for the age range 15–79 years is an increase above the pre-exercise level by 18–46 mmHg at the end of three minutes of sustained handgrip at 50% of the maximum sustainable force measured in Newton. All the arterial blood pressures; SBP, DBP and MAP, including the residual parasympathetic restraints; CSB and CVT and the heart rate are monitored and measured continuously during this test using the NeuroScope (Fig. 2).

Assessment of Sympathetic Control of Venous Vascular Capacitance in the Splanchnic Region

We use a positive intra-thoracic pressure of 40 mmHg lasting 15 s during Valsalva's manoeuvre to suddenly reduce venous return to the heart and provoke an auto-transfusion response [13]. The auto-transfusion is caused by a neurogenic constriction of vessels and organs in the splanchnic region. In order to optimise the assessment of venous return from the splanchnic region, the Valsalva's manoeuvre is performed in the upright-seated position with the subject stooping forwards so that the inguinal ligaments compresses the iliac veins to eliminate most of the venous return from the lower limbs. Before the auto-transfusion response, arterial blood pressure increases suddenly in a Phase I response, then it starts to fall rapidly due to lack of venous return in the early part of Phase IIe. The trough of SBP in Phase IIe should be within 25 mmHg from the pre-manoeuvre baseline level to indicate adequate and normal venous return during the positive intra-thoracic pressure (Our laboratory standard). Phase IIe is arrested at the beginning of the auto-transfusion response, which starts to restore arterial blood pressure back towards the pre-manoeuvre level during the positive intra-thoracic pressure in the late Phase IIi. This should end with SBP at or not more than 15 mmHg above the pre-manoeuvre baseline level to indicate adequate auto-transfusion response (Our laboratory standard). Abrupt end of the positive intra-thoracic pressure of Valsalva's manoeuvre reverses the pressure from positive to negative intra-thoracic creating a suction effect in Phase III, which decreases the arterial blood pressure suddenly and the SBP at the trough of Phase III should be within 25 mmHg from the pre-manoeuvre baseline level to indicate sufficient venous blood volume during negative intra-thoracic suction following the auto-transfusion response

(Our laboratory standard). All the arterial blood pressures; SBP, DBP and MAP, including the parasympathetic restraints; CSB and CVT and the heart rate are monitored and measured continuously during this test using the NeuroScope (Fig. 2).

Declaration of Interest

None

References

1. Kahn, R. Report and recommendations of the San Antonio conference on diabetic neuropathy. Ann Neurol. 1988;24(1):99–104.
2. Little CJ, Julu PO, Hansen S, Reid SW. Real-time measurement of cardiac vagal tone in conscious dogs. Am J Physiol. 1999;276(2 Pt 2):H758–65.
3. Julu PO. A linear scale for measuring vagal tone in man. J Auton Pharmacol. 1992;12(2):109–15.
4. Gilbey MP, Jordan D, Richter DW, Spyer KM. Synaptic mechanisms involved in the inspiratory modulation of vagal cardio-inhibitory neurones in the cat. J Physiol. 1984;356:65–78.
5. Dampney RA. Blood pressure regulation by C1 neurons in the rostral ventrolateral medulla: new light on the subject. J Physiol. 2009;587(Pt 23):5513.
6. Schreihofer AM, Guyenet PG. The baroreflex and beyond: control of sympathetic vasomotor tone by GABAergic neurons in the ventrolateral medulla. Clin Exp Pharmacol Physiol. 2002;29(5–6):514–21.
7. Julu PO, Cooper VL, Hansen S, Hainsworth R. Cardiovascular regulation in the period preceding vasovagal syncope in conscious humans. J Physiol. 2003;549(Pt 1):299–311.
8. Julu PO, Hansen S, Jamal GA. Is baroreflex responsiveness (BRR) a function of height during isometric muscle contraction in human volunteers? J Physiol. 1996;491.P(Suppl).
9. Halliwill JR, Taylor JA, Eckberg DL. Impaired sympathetic vascular regulation in humans after acute dynamic exercise. J Physiol. 1996;495(Pt 1):279–88.
10. Westerhof N, Lankhaar JW, Westerhof BE. The arterial Windkessel. Med Biol Eng Comput. 2009;47(2):131–41.
11. Greenway CV. Role of splanchnic venous system in overall cardiovascular homeostasis. Fed Proc. 1983;42(6):1678–84.
12. Ewing DJ, Irving JB, Kerr F, Wildsmith JA, Clarke BF. Cardiovascular responses to sustained handgrip in normal subjects and in patients with diabetes mellitus: a test of autonomic function. Clin Sci Mol Med. 1974;46(3):295–306.
13. Lundgren O. Role of splanchnic resistance vessels in overall cardiovascular homeostasis. Fed Proc. 1983;42(6):1673–7.

Cardiovascular Red Flag Symptoms in PoTS

Szablocs Nagy and P. Boon Lim

Patients with PoTS can present with a variety of cardiovascular symptoms including pre-syncope, syncope, palpitations, dizziness, shortness of breath or chest pain. It is important to consider and exclude important cardiovascular diagnoses before attributing these symptoms to PoTS. A list of these symptoms, including red-flag features are provided below.

1. Syncope

Patients with PoTS **may** have coexisting vasovagal syncope and this would be the most common cause of infrequent episodes of syncope in a patient with PoTS. Usually syncope will occur after a period of standing with **typical** symptoms of PoTS manifested prior to the syncopal event. The exuberant activation of the sympathetic nervous system often leads to the constellation of symptoms during the initial few minutes of standing, prior to the vasovagal reflex manifesting with continued standing and the eventual loss of consciousness from vasovagal syncope.

However, patients with PoTS do not usually manifest syncope unless there are other triggers such as standing for a prolonged duration, dehydration, being in a warm environment, etc. Therefore when syncope occurs frequently (every few days), an alternate diagnosis should be considered, including vasovagal syncope. If syncope occurs very frequently (a few times a day), strongly consider a diagnosis of psychogenic pseudosyncope instead. In this scenario it is worthwhile revisiting the diagnosis of PoTS by taking a full clinical history, and consider performing an active stand test, or a tilt table test. Video mobile recordings from friends or family members can be extremely helpful, or inpatient video telemetry can be diagnostic for psychogenic pseudosyncope.

Syncope is considered a "red-flag" symptom in the following circumstances and should always prompt further investigations. Syncope which is unheralded, syncope whilst supine and syncope during exercise should prompt further consideration of other diagnoses such as bradycardia, tachycardia, or structural or inherited heart disease such as hypertrophic cardiomyopathy or Brugada. In these instances, a 12 lead ECG, prolonged cardiac monitoring (Holter, 7 day event recorder or an implantable loop recorder), and imaging (echocardiogram, MRI) should be performed.

2. Palpitations

Palpitations are a common feature in PoTS patients. The robust activation of the sympathetic nervous system with postural change usually leads to an immediate sinus tachycardia

S. Nagy · P. B. Lim (✉)
Imperial Syncope Diagnostic Unit, Imperial College Healthcare NHS Trust, Hammersmith Hospital, Du Cane Road, London W12 0HS, UK
e-mail: Pblim@imperial.ac.uk

N. Gall et al. (eds.), *Postural Tachycardia Syndrome*, https://doi.org/10.1007/978-3-030-54165-1_10

and causes the heart rate rise by >30 bpm or >120 bpm, which is maintained throughout the standing period. A key, but subtle point about this heart rate rise, is that in PoTS, this rise is maintained for the duration of standing, with the inability of the heart rate to "settle". This distinction may only be seen with prolonged active standing for 10 minutes: in PoTS, the heart rate changes and symptoms will continue to manifest throughout the entirety of the standing period, but in vasovagal syncope or early orthostatic intolerance with associated appropriate reactive sinus tachycardia, the initial heart rate rise (which may be associated with PoTS-like symptoms) may gradually reduce with symptom improvement, even with prolonged standing. This subtle return to a normal heart rate and resolution of symptoms after 3–5 minutes of standing can usually help distinguish PoTS from vasovagal syncope.

Red-flag palpitations symptoms including palpitations which are sudden onset or offset, particularly if they occur without postural changes, or nocturnal palpitations which wake patients from sleep. In these instances an ECG, prolonged cardiac monitor (Holter, 7 day event recorder, implantable loop recorder) or an electrophysiological study may need to be considered to rule out primary arrhythmic diagnoses including AV nodal re-entrant tachycardia, AV re-entrant tachycardia (Wolff-Parkinson-White Syndrome), atrial fibrillation, atrial flutter, atrial or ventricular ectopy, or inappropriate sinus tachycardia.

3. Chest pain and shortness of breath

Chest pain and shortness of breath are common but ill-understood symptoms in PoTS. In these instances, the chest pain and shortness of breath usually manifests during periods of standing and is associated with the other symptoms of PoTS including palpitations, dizziness, and fatigue. One potential mechanism for this pain could be that with increasing sympathetic activation, the resulting increase in heart rate (chronotropy) and strength of contraction (inotropy) increases oxygen demand and causes a relative mismatch in supply and demand of cardiac oxygenation, resulting in chest pain. In these instances, anything that relieves sympathetic activation (such as lying down, increasing fluid and salt intake, augmenting BP with medications if low) may help improve symptoms of chest pain and shortness of breath. This understanding of the chest pain profile may help avoid unnecessary tests including CT coronary angiograms, or exercise testing (which PoTS patients may not be able to tolerate) or other forms of stress testing.

Red flag symptoms include acute chest pain at rest, or shortness of breath at rest, particularly if unresolved on lying down. In these instances, exclude a pulmonary embolus or heart rhythm abnormality such as a supraventricular tachycardia, by performing appropriate diagnostic testing such as ECG, prolonged ECG monitoring, echocardiography, or CT pulmonary angiogram.

Neurological Red Flags in Common Neurological Conditions Associated with PoTS

Evangelia Theochari

Abbreviations

MS	Multiple sclerosis
IENFD	Intra-epidermal nerve fibre density
anti-ENA	anti-extractable nuclear antigen antibodies,
nAChR	Nicotinic acetylcholine receptor
ECG	Electrocardiogram
EEG	Electroencephalogram

Introduction

The main focus of this chapter is to discuss relatively common neurological disorders that can be associated with PoTS and which red flags identified in history and examination should prompt further investigations and neurology review.

These neurological conditions are:

1. Multiple sclerosis
2. Peripheral neuropathies (autoimmune or small fibre neuropathy)
3. Epilepsy
4. Cognitive disorders
5. Headache

1. *Multiple Sclerosis associated with PoTS*

Multiple sclerosis (MS) is a chronic autoimmune demyelinating disorder that affects 2.5 million people worldwide [1]. It typically presents between the ages of 15 and 45 years. Women are affected approximately two to three times more often than men [2]. Amongst all other symptoms, autonomic dysfunction is commonly seen and usually manifests as bladder dysfunction, sleep disturbances, sweating, gastrointestinal and cardiovascular disturbances [3, 4]. The prevalence of autonomic dysfunction can vary considerably from 7 to 60% and can affect both sympathetic and parasympathetic system [5–8].

The association of MS and PoTS can be divided into two types:

(i) Causal association as MS can cause autonomic dysregulation.

The pathophysiological mechanism proposed in development of autonomic symptoms in MS is the disruption of the function of anatomical areas regulating the central autonomic system, including the insular cortex, anterior cingulate cortex, amygdala, hypothalamus, periaqueductal grey matter, parabrachial nucleus, nucleus of

E. Theochari (✉)
Department of Neurology, King's College Hospital, 1st Floor, Neurosciences Modular Building, London, UK
e-mail: Evangelia.theochari@nhs.net

N. Gall et al. (eds.), *Postural Tachycardia Syndrome*, https://doi.org/10.1007/978-3-030-54165-1_11

the solitary tract, ventrolateral reticular formation of the medulla, and medullary raphe nuclei, or their interconnections and reflex pathways due to the presence of demyelinating plaques [9, 10]. In addition the plaques can interfere with the descending autonomic nervous system pathways during their course in the brainstem or spinal cord [8]. There is a significant association between presence of autonomic dysfunction and clinical and MRI evidence of brainstem lesions [8].

One study described clinical characteristics of nine patients with a dual diagnosis of MS and PoTS, emphasizing that MS patients may manifest autonomic dysfunction by developing PoTS [11]. Another study looked at the frequency of PoTS in 112 patients with MS undergoing testing for autonomic dysfunction evaluation compared to 181 patients with orthostatic symptoms in the absence of any neurological disorder. PoTS was identified in 39 patients: 21(19%) in group 1 comparing to 18 (10%) in group 2, which suggested a close association of PoTS and MS [12]. The same authors in a later study identified the presence of PoTS as a predictor of conversion to MS in patients with clinically isolated syndrome, suggesting that PoTS seems to be associated with disease activity [13, 14]. In general, it has been suggested that parasympathetic dysfunctions are consequences of the disease itself while sympathetic dysfunction could be a trigger of new relapses [5].

(ii) Sharing common phenotypes

Shared symptoms of MS and PoTS that are common in both conditions include orthostatic intolerance, fatigue and anxiety [15, 16]. Orthostatic dizziness occurs in almost 50% of MS patients [8]. Up to 53% of patients report fatigue in MS and has a major impact of patient quality of life. The presence of fatigue is multifactorial and different underlying mechanism have been implicated, including autonomic dysregulation, although the exact mechanism remains unclear [17]. There seems to be no correlation between fatigue and disease severity [18, 19]. Although both fatigue and reduced physical activity are important consequences of MS, however, their mutual association is poorly understood. Rieteberg et al. suggested that fatigue does not seem to be related with the physical activity but it seems to represent instead a perception rather a physical tiredness following physical activity [16]. Drugs such as amantadine, affecting glutamatergic transmission, and modafinil, affecting dopaminergic transmission, have been used with variable effect as well as exercise regimes [20].

Red Flags

Therefore, when a patient presents with PoTS in clinic, it is important to ask for any typical symptoms of MS, such as previous history of visual symptoms, urinary symptoms, or other focal motor, sensory or coordination symptoms that lasted for a few days/weeks. On the other hand, it is important to ask patients with MS whether they experience any autonomic dysregulation symptoms and consider the diagnosis of PoTS depending on the symptoms. Concurrent MS and PoTS has an additive effect on morbidity and disability of these conditions. It is therefore vital for these conditions to be recognised and treatment to be offered for both early on to improve quality of life and disease burden in disability.

2. *Neuropathy and PoTS*

Neuropathic PoTS has been reported to be present in 33–50% of PoTS cases in tertiary centres [21, 22].

One of the pathophysiological mechanisms implicated in PoTS is the sympathetic denervation, particularly in the lower limbs, resulting in diminished capacity for venoconstriction [3, 22, 23]. This leads to increased venous pooling when standing and perpetuates a greater reduction in stroke volume. In neuropathic PoTS, 50% of cases have peripheral autonomic denervation. In PoTS, there also seems to be a selective involvement of autonomic C fibres; autonomic C-fibre function is impaired in a peripheral and distal distribution, whereas somatic C fibres are spared. This involvement pattern differs to the one seen in idiopathic autonomic neuropathy cases where a combined and selective distal and generalized autonomic C-fibre impairment has been observed [24].

Skin biopsy findings were compared in neuropathic versus non neuropathic cases of PoTS. Intra-epidermal nerve fibre density (IENFD) was calculated for each biopsy and as expected subjects with neuropathic PoTS (per definition) had lower IENFD than the non-neuropathic PoTS group and controls, without however the patients reporting any small fibre neuropathy symptoms [23].

Therefore although patients may not present with the typical small fibre neuropathic presentation such as painful and length dependant neuropathy, a detailed history to exclude symptoms for other system involvement, such as weight loss, joint pain, dry skins and dry eyes, and neurological examination to guide investigations for secondary causes should be performed. These may include neuronal antibodies for paraneoplastic neuropathies, serum electrophoresis, thyroid function tests, full blood count, urea and electrolytes, HbA1c, infective causes including Hepatitis and HIV, immune causes including antinuclear antibodies, anti-extractable nuclear antigen antibodies (anti-ENA) including anti-SSA (anti-Ro 52/60) and anti-SSB (anti-La), serum cryoglobulin detection and immunochemical typing, rheumatoid factor, serum immunoglobulins (IgG, IgA, IgM), and vitamin deficiencies (vitamin B12 and folate).

Rare forms of autoimmune neuropathies can also be associated with PoTS. One rare form of dysautonomia is autoimmune autonomic ganglionopathy (AAG) where antibodies against the ganglionic anti-nicotinic acetylcholine receptor (nAChR) impair transmission in autonomic ganglia causing a variety of autonomic dysregulation symptoms [25]. Antibodies against nAChR was reported in 15% of adult PoTS patients evaluated at the Mayo Clinic between 1993 and 2003 [22].

If there are symptoms suggestive of peripheral neuropathy, a careful neurological examination, neurophysiology investigations and referral to neurology should be prompted to guide towards the appropriate diagnosis and management.

3. ***Epilepsy associated with cardiac arrhythmias***

Epilepsy is one of the commonest neurological disorders globally as more than 50 million people worldwide have a diagnosis of epilepsy. Epilepsy includes a variety of clinical presentations and syndromes. Autonomic involvement due to seizures was already reported in the 1950s [26]. Cardiac arrhythmias as part of autonomic involvement in seizures, have been reported to occur before (pre-ictal), during (ictal) and immediately after (postictal) a seizure. The cardiac arrhythmias are thought to represent a direct effect of seizure activity on the autonomic central system, including its sympathetic, parasympathetic and enteric components. Anatomic areas of the brain that play an important role in the central autonomic system include insular cortex, anterior cingulate cortex, amygdala, hypothalamus, periaqueductal grey matter, parabrachial nucleus, nucleus of the solitary tract, ventrolateral reticular formation of the medulla, and medullary raphe nuclei [9, 10]. If the seizure onset zone or the seizure propagation pathway involves any of these anatomic structures or their connections then autonomic symptoms can develop by dysregulation of the central autonomic network. If the anatomic areas of sympathetic regulation are excited as part of seizure propagation, then increased sympathetic outflows will have an impact on autonomic function, whereas if cortical areas responsible for depressor responses, such as the insula, are affected, this can manifest as parasympathetic associated symptoms.

This effect of seizures on the autonomic central system regulation has been given an important emphasis in the new operational classification of Epilepsy and seizures as the term "focal autonomic seizures" has been coined for the first time to describe these clinical manifestations. As described in the new operational seizure classification, "focal autonomic seizures can present with gastrointestinal sensations, a sense of heat or cold, flushing, piloerection (goose bumps), palpitations, sexual arousal, respiratory changes, or other autonomic effects" [27]. They can represent the only seizure manifestation and may not be associated with other motor or behavioural signs and symptoms. If there are motor or behavioural manifestations following or at the same time as the autonomic symptoms, then the seizure would be classified according to the other predominant symptoms and not as a pure autonomic seizure.

Therefore, when a patient is assessed for symptomatic tachycardic symptoms, it is important to keep in mind the cardiac arrhythmias associated with seizures to make an appropriate differential diagnosis.

The cardiac arrhythmias associated with seizure activity can be divided into tachy-arrhythmias, most commonly sinus tachyarrhythmias, and bradyarrhythmias.

Tachyarrhythmias

Tachyarrhythmias can present as a pre-ictal, ictal and postictal phenomenon as already described. Their temporal association to seizures may have a localising or lateralising value, and could be of important potential diagnostic value, although further studies are needed to clarify these associations. It may be challenging to clarify the exact temporal association, as in some cases when intracranial recordings have been used, changes on the electroencephalogram (EEG) preceded changes in the electrocardiogram (ECG), but in other studies where scalp EEG was used, the ECG changes may precede the EEG or clinical manifestation of seizures [28, 29].

Ictal sinus tachycardia is the most frequently seen cardiac arrhythmia during an epileptic seizure [30]. It can be seen both in adults and in children [31, 32]. It has been reported to be present in up to 82% of seizures, and can be seen with all seizure types, focal, generalised, or focal to bilateral [33].

Ictal tachycardia may or may not be symptomatic and the patient may complain of palpitations, but it does not seem to be associated with syncope as can be seen in PoTS.

Epilepsy Localisation/Lateralisation and Tachy-Arrhythmias

Ictal tachycardia seems to be seen with a temporal lobe epileptic focus rather than in cases where the epilepsy focus is extra-temporal lobe epilepsy [33, 34]. Furthermore, it seems to present earlier when the hippocampal formation is involved rather that extra hippocampal areas of the temporal lobe [29]. A possible explanation why the temporal lobe epileptic focus seems to be more implicated with sinus tachycardia, is the anatomic proximity, especially of the hippocampus and the mesial temporal lobe, and relation of temporal lobe with cortical areas and neural circuits involved in sympathetic cardiovascular regulation [35].

Whether the lateralisation of the epileptic focus to the right or left can predict the occurrence of ictal tachycardia remains unclear. It has been speculated that seizures arising from the non-dominant hemisphere may have a stronger association with tachycardia [35–38] and this was supported by a study where stimulation of the left non-dominant insula, an area predominantly responsible for parasympathetic effects, caused bradycardia [36, 39, 40]. However, most studies produced inconsistent results and therefore a clear association of right or non-dominant hemisphere with tachycardia is not supported by most of the current literature [33, 34].

Seizure Type and Tachy-Arrhythmias

Eggleston et al. in their review of 34 articles reported ictal sinus tachycardia in 12% of subclinical seizures, 71% of focal onset seizures, 64% of generalized seizures and 76% of mixed seizure types [33]. Surges et al. in their study of 25 patients undergoing surgical evaluation for temporal lobe epilepsy, reported a significantly higher ictal heart rate and persistent postictal tachycardia in focal to bilateral tonic clonic compared to focal-only seizures [41]. However, the systematic review and metanalysis conducted by Bruno et al. concluded that the effects of seizure type remains unclear [34]. In the same systematic review and metanalysis conducted by Bruno et al. [34] the authors also concluded that "pre-ictal heart rate increase seemed to occur many seconds prior to the apparent seizure onset and more frequently in specific groups of patients with epilepsy, namely temporal lobe epilepsy adults and patients on antiepileptic medications" [34].

Cardiac Brady-Arrhythmias

Patients can also develop bradyarrhythmias including asystole. The prevalence has been reported between 1.3 and 5.5% [31, 32, 42] and can range from mild bradycardia with no associated symptoms, to more severe cases of symptomatic bradyarrhythmias including prolonged periods of asystole. The localisation seems to be in the majority of cases of temporal origin [43]. As with tachycardia, whether lateralisation of the seizure onset, right of left, is more likely to cause ictal bradyarrhythmia, the question remains unanswered within the current literature. When it comes to cases with post-ictal asystole these seem to be associated with focal to bilateral seizures and in the majority of cases reported there seem to be postictal generalised suppression on EEG.

Other Cardiac Arrhythmias

Atrial flutter/fibrillation, ventricular fibrillation in patients with epilepsy have also been described in the literature. These cases are usually associated with underlying cardiac pathology or other risk factors, including the degree of hypoxemia due to seizure, that serves as a substrate for the development of cardiac arrhythmias in a temporal association with seizures [44–48].

Red Flags

Epilepsy, especially of temporal lobe onset, can cause autonomic dysregulations that present in a similar way as symptoms due to PoTS.

Therefore, when we assess a patient presenting with tachycardic signs and symptoms it is important to take a detailed description of the events. Ask to describe the sequence of the events in detail, whether there are any triggers, or what can relieve the symptoms. PoTS symptoms typically occur when standing up from a reclining position and are relieved by sitting or lying back down. A seizure on the other hand can occur in any position. Enquire as to whether there was any loss of consciousness or altered awareness. Ask if there were any abnormal sensations such as feelings of "deja-vu" or altered awareness as, in temporal lobe epilepsy, these have been frequently implicated as localising features for autonomic seizures.

It may be worth exploring whether there are any risk factors for epilepsy such as a history of febrile convulsions, traumatic brain injury, central nervous system infections such as meningitis or encephalitis, developmental delays, or family history of epilepsy.

Neurological examination is always useful because, if any abnormalities are identified that could be localising/lateralising to a specific part of the brain, this will need further assessment with imaging and, if seizure is suspected, an EEG.

A case of a 20 year old patient has been reported where there was comorbid PoTS and right temporal lobe epilepsy [49]. Therefore, it is important to recognise the two syndromes can co-exist and require different effective treatment that involves different medications and/or other therapeutic modalities.

4. ***Cognitive issues associated with PoTS***

Cognitive symptoms are very common amongst patients with PoTS and have been reported by 77–96% of PoTS patients and are experienced by 67% on a daily basis [50].

Although patients give a vague picture of the cognitive symptoms they experience, mainly adapting the terms of "brain fog", "mental slowing" or "cognitive fatigue" to describe them, specific patterns of cognitive dysfunction in PoTS have been reported. These are typically characterized by specific deficits in working memory, [51] selective attention [52, 53], cognitive processing speed, and executive function [54]. In contrast, other measures of cognitive function including memory assessments were not impaired, implying a selective deficit rather that a generalised one.

As to what extent the posture affects the degree of the cognitive issues, the literature remains unclear. Ocon et al. showed that reductions in working memory in response to graded head-up tilt were not associated with altered cerebral blood flow in PoTS patients with comorbid chronic fatigue syndrome [54]. Stewart et al. showed the opposite effect as their study suggested that diminished cognitive performance in PoTS was indeed associated with slow oscillations in cerebral blood flow (Stewart et al. 2015). Rodriguez et al. showed that the cognitive symptoms were only present in the upright position for working memory, but were independent of attention and alertness, and went one step further to show that rapid water drinking has a positive effect on improving working memory in upright position. Furthermore, cognitive deficits in patients with comorbid PoTS and chronic fatigue syndrome seem to improve on supine position [55].

Following the contradictory results, it was suggested that these findings may indicate that the cognitive dysfunction in PoTS is not due to the increased heart rate and symptoms with standing, but rather may reflect part of the disease itself [52].

Moreover, other factors that can be present in PoTS and need to be addressed include poor sleep efficiency, mood disorders, and anxiety, either clinical or subclinical [56]. It is important to note however that PoTS patient do not seem to have an increased lifetime prevalence of psychiatric disorders.

Red Flags

As cognitive deficits are commonly present in PoTS, differentiating between subjective cognitive complaints and cognitive impairment due to neurodegenerative disorders can be difficult [57]. It is vital to take a detailed history of the specific deficits, ask for specific examples that demonstrate the nature and extent of the symptoms [58]. Once more, collateral information is vital in investigating cognitive complains. It is well recognised that patients with memory and cognitive deficits, such as in Alzheimer's Disease may underplay their symptoms, mainly due to cognitive anosognosia, whereas those with purely subjective memory complaints (the "worried well") may overemphasise difficulties. Three non-canonical signs have been shown to have diagnostic value during assessment in the cognitive clinic. These are: The "attended alone sign", "the head turning sign" and the "applause sign".

When patients attend the cognitive clinic alone, despite written and clear information to bring a close relative or friend, the so called "attended alone sign" has been strongly associated with the absence of dementia [59, 60]. As it is an indicator of subjective memory issues. When the patient is asked a question and turns his/her head towards the person accompanying them looking for the answer, is a modestly sensitive but very specific sign of cognitive impairment [61, 62]. The third one, "the applause sign" requires asking the patient to clap their hands only three times; if they do it more, this is abnormal. Although the sensitivity is poor, the specificity for cognitive impairment is good as, if negative, it can usually exclude neurodegenerative diagnosis for cognitive issues [63].

On further questioning, it is important to ask if there are any personality changes, as these can be associated with forms of dementia, such as frontotemporal dementia, which if inherited can presented in younger patients. If there is a family history of dementia in younger age as this can be associated with increased risk; specific genes have been implicated. Any abnormalities in neurological examination, for example increased tone, rigidity, abnormal gait or presence of choreiform movements, such as seen in Huntington's disease, are red flags that should prompt further investigations and evaluation by a specialist. Any signs of movement disorder should prompt further investigations. If there is previous history of strokes and headaches, then consider the possibility of CADASIL (cerebral autosomal dominant arteriopathy with subcortical infarcts and leukoencephalopathy), a rare disorder that typically presents with migraines with aura, subcortical transient ischemic attacks or strokes, or mood disorders and cognitive deficits between 35 and 55 years of age [64]. In an observational study, the cause of dementia in patients younger than 45, the neurodegenerative causes were seen in 31.1% of the cohort; Autoimmune or inflammatory causes (such as MS and autoimmune encephalopathy) accounted for 21.3%. Inborn errors of metabolism were seen more frequently in patients younger than 30 years [65].

Infective causes such as human immunodeficiency virus and treponemal associated dementia and rarer causes, prion disease or progressive multifocal leukoencephalopathy, have also been described in younger patients. If the deficits are atypical for PoTS, clinicians should have a low threshold to test for HIV and treponemal serology as these are treatable.

If the clinician remains concerned for atypical cognitive issues and/or the presence of red flags, formal cognitive testing showing the pattern of neuropsychological deficits in association with neurological signs can help establish an aetiological diagnosis.

5. ***Headaches associated with PoTS***

Migraine is a common (mis) diagnosis in patients with PoTS. Up to 2/3 of patients suffer with orthostatic headaches, especially if they are younger than 30. Orthostatic headaches may be associated with decrease in spinal venous pressure and decrease in cerebrospinal fluid volume due to absolute or orthostatic hypovolaemia [66].

Detailed history and physical examination have a pivotal role in identifying reg flags and organising further appropriate investigations and referrals. A detailed association of headaches in PoTS is described in another chapter of this book.

References

1. Leray E, Moreau T, Fromont A, Edan G. Epidemiology of multiple sclerosis. Rev Neurol (Paris). 2016;172(1):3–13.
2. Goodin DS. The epidemiology of multiple sclerosis-Chapter 11: insights to disease pathogenesis. Elsevier Health Sciences; 2014. p. 231–66.
3. Haensch CA, Tosch M, Katona I, Weis J, Isenmann S. Small-fiber neuropathy with cardiac denervation in postural tachycardia syndrome. Muscle Nerve. 2014;50(6):956–61.
4. Haensch CA, Jorg J. Autonomic dysfunction in multiple sclerosis. J Neurol. 2006;253(Suppl 1):I3-9.
5. Flachenecker P, Reiners K, Krauser M, Wolf A, Toyka KV. Autonomic dysfunction in multiple sclerosis is related to disease activity and progression of disability. Mult Scler. 2001;7(5):327–34.
6. Frontoni M, Fiorini M, Strano S, Cerutti S, Giubilei F, Urani C, et al. Power spectrum analysis contribution to the detection of cardiovascular dysautonomia in multiple sclerosis. Acta Neurol Scand. 1996;93(4):241–5.
7. Acevedo AR, Nava C, Arriada N, Violante A, Corona T. Cardiovascular dysfunction in multiple sclerosis. Acta Neurol Scand. 2000;101(2):85–8.
8. Vita G, Carolina Fazio M, Milone S, Blandino A, Salvi L, Messina C. Cardiovascular autonomic dysfunction in multiple sclerosis is likely related to brainstem lesions. J Neurol Sci. 1993;120(1):82–6.
9. Cersosimo, Benarroch MEGE. Central control of autonomic function and involvement in neurodegenerative disorders; 2013. p. 45–57.
10. Benarroch EE. The central autonomic network: functional organization, dysfunction, and perspective. Mayo Clin Proc. 1993;68(10):988–1001.
11. Khalil Kanjwal BKYKBPG. Autonomic dysfunction presenting as postural orthostatic tachycardia syndrome in patients with multiple sclerosis. Int J Med Sci. 2010;7(2):62–7.
12. Adamec I, Lovric M, Zaper D, Barusic AK, Bach I, Junakovic A, et al. Postural orthostatic tachycardia syndrome associated with multiple sclerosis. Auton Neurosci. 2013;173(1–2):65–8.
13. Adamec I, Bach I, Barusic AK, Mismas A, Habek M. Assessment of prevalence and pathological response to orthostatic provocation in patients with multiple sclerosis. J Neurol Sci. 2013;324(1–2):80–3.
14. Habek M, Krbot Skoric M, Crnosija L, Gabelic T, Barun B, Adamec I. Postural orthostatic tachycardia predicts early conversion to multiple sclerosis after clinically isolated syndrome. Eur Neurol. 2017;77(5–6):253–7.
15. Hoad A, Spickett G, Elliott J, Newton J. Postural orthostatic tachycardia syndrome is an

under-recognized condition in chronic fatigue syndrome. QJM: Int J Med. 2008;101(12):961–5.
16. Rietberg MB, van Wegen EE, Uitdehaag BM, Kwakkel G. The association between perceived fatigue and actual level of physical activity in multiple sclerosis. Mult Scler. 2011;17(10):1231–7.
17. Manjaly Z-M, Harrison N, Critchley HD, Do CT, Stefanics G, Wenderoth N, et al. Pathophysiological and cognitive mechanisms of fatigue in multiple sclerosis. 2019.
18. Tartaglia MC, Narayanan S, Francis SJ, Santos AC, De Stefano N, Lapierre Y, et al. The relationship between diffuse axonal damage and fatigue in multiple sclerosis. Arch Neurol. 2004;61(2):201–7.
19. Bakshi R, Miletich RS, Henschel K, Shaikh ZA, Janardhan V, Wasay M, et al. Fatigue in multiple sclerosis: cross-sectional correlation with brain MRI findings in 71 patients. Neurology. 1999;53(5):1151–3.
20. Heine M, van de Port I, Rietberg MB, van Wegen EE, Kwakkel G. Exercise therapy for fatigue in multiple sclerosis. Cochrane Database Syst Rev. 2015(9):Cd009956.
21. Jacob G, Costa F, Shannon JR, Robertson RM, Wathen M, Stein M, et al. The neuropathic postural tachycardia syndrome. N Engl J Med. 2000;343(14):1008–14.
22. Thieben M, Sandroni P, Benrud-Larson L, Fealey R, Vernino S, Lennon V, et al. Postural tachycardia syndrome—Mayo Clinic experience. J Neurol Sci. 2005;238:S79–S.
23. Gibbons CH, Bonyhay I, Benson A, Wang N, Freeman R, Gonzalez-Alegre P. Structural and functional small fiber abnormalities in the neuropathic postural tachycardia syndrome. PLoS One. 2013;8(12).
24. Singer W, Spies JM, McArthur J, Low J, Griffin JW, Nickander KK, et al. Prospective evaluation of somatic and autonomic small fibers in selected autonomic neuropathies. Neurology. 2004;62(4):612–8.
25. Vernino S, Hopkins S, Wang Z. Autonomic ganglia, acetylcholine receptor antibodies, and autoimmune ganglionopathy. Auto Neurosci: Basic Clin. 2009;146(1–2):3–7.
26. So-Called GH. "Psychomotor" and "temporal" epilepsy. Epilepsia. 1953;C2(1):59–76.
27. Fisher RS, Cross JH, French JA, Higurashi N, Hirsch E, Jansen FE, et al. Operational classification of seizure types by the international league against epilepsy: position paper of the ILAE commission for classification and terminology. Epilepsia. 2017;58(4):522–30.
28. Jansen K, Lagae L. Cardiac changes in epilepsy. Seizure: Eur J Epilepsy. 2010;19(8):455–60.
29. Hirsch M, Altenmüller DM, Schulze-Bonhage A. Latencies from intracranial seizure onset to ictal tachycardia: a comparison to surface EEG patterns and other clinical signs. Epilepsia. 2015;56(10):1639–47.
30. Sevcencu C, Struijk JJ. Autonomic alterations and cardiac changes in epilepsy. Oxford, UK; 2010. p. 725–37.
31. Blumhardt LD, Smith PEM, Owen L. Electrocardiographic accompaniments of temporal lobe epileptic seizures. The Lancet. 1986;327(8489):1051–6.
32. Smith PEM, Howell SJL, Owen L, Blumhardt LD. Profiles of instant heart rate during partial seizures. Electroencephalogr Clin Neurophysiol. 1989;72(3):207–17.
33. Eggleston KS, Olin BD, Fisher RS. Ictal tachycardia: the head–heart connection. Seizure: Eur J Epilepsy. 2014;23(7):496–505.
34. Bruno E, Biondi A, Richardson MP. Pre-ictal heart rate changes: a systematic review and meta-analysis. Seizure. 2018;55:48–56.
35. Di Gennaro G, Quarato PP, Sebastiano F, Esposito V, Onorati P, Grammaldo LG, et al. Ictal heart rate increase precedes EEG discharge in drug-resistant mesial temporal lobe seizures. Clin Neurophysiol. 2004;115(5):1169–77.
36. Massetani R, Strata G, Galli R, Gori S, Gneri C, Limbruno U, et al. Alteration of cardiac function in patients with temporal lobe epilepsy: different roles of EEG-ECG monitoring and spectral analysis of RR variability. Epilepsia. 1997;38(3):363–9.
37. Leutmezer F, Schernthaner C, Lurger S, Potzelberger K, Baumgartner C. Electrocardiographic changes at the onset of epileptic seizures. Epilepsia. 2003;44(3):348–54.
38. Mayer H, Benninger F, Urak L, Plattner B, Geldner J, Feucht M. EKG abnormalities in children and adolescents with symptomatic temporal lobe epilepsy. Neurology. 2004;63(2):324–8.
39. Oppenheimer SM, Kedem G, Martin WM. Left-insular cortex lesions perturb cardiac autonomic tone in humans. Clin Auton Res. 1996;6(3):131–40.
40. Oppenheimer SM, Gelb A, Girvin JP, Hachinski VC. Cardiovascular effects of human insular cortex stimulation. Neurology. 1992;42(9):1727–32.
41. Surges R, Scott CA, Walker MC. Enhanced QT shortening and persistent tachycardia after generalized seizures. Neurology. 2010;74(5):421–6.
42. Devinsky O. Effects of seizures on autonomic and cardiovascular function. Epilepsy Curr. 2004;4(2):43–6.
43. Tényi D, Gyimesi C, Kupó P, Horváth R, Bóné B, Barsi P, et al. Ictal asystole: a systematic review. Epilepsia. 2017;58(3):356–62.
44. Nei M, Ho RT, Sperling MR. EKG Abnormalities during partial seizures in refractory epilepsy. Epilepsia. 2000;41(5):542–8.
45. Keilson M, Hauser W, Magrill JP. Electrocardiographic changes during electrographic seizures. Arch Neurol. 1989;46(11):1169–70.
46. van der Lende M, Surges R, Sander JW, Thijs RD. Cardiac arrhythmias during or after

epileptic seizures. J Neurol Neurosurg Psychiatry. 2016;87(1):69–74.
47. Park KJ, Sharma G, Kennedy JD, Seyal M. Potentially high-risk cardiac arrhythmias with focal to bilateral tonic–clonic seizures and generalized tonic–clonic seizures are associated with the duration of periictal hypoxemia. Epilepsia. 2017;58(12):2164–71.
48. Britton JW, Ghearing GR, Benarroch EE, Cascino GD. The ictal bradycardia syndrome: localization and lateralization. Epilepsia. 2006;47(4):737–44.
49. Seeck M, Blanke O, Zaim S. Temporal lobe epilepsy and postural orthostatic tachycardia syndrome (POTS). Epilepsy Behav. 2002;3(3):285–8.
50. Deb A, Morgenshtern K, Culbertson CJ, Wang LB, Hohler AD. A survey-based analysis of symptoms in patients with postural orthostatic tachycardia syndrome. Proc (Bayl Univ Med Cent). 2015;28(2):157–9.
51. Anderson JW, Lambert EA, Sari CI, Dawood T, Esler MD, Vaddadi G, et al. Cognitive function, health-related quality of life, and symptoms of depression and anxiety sensitivity are impaired in patients with the postural orthostatic tachycardia syndrome (POTS). Front Physiol. 2014;5:230.
52. Arnold AC, Haman K, Garland EM, Raj V, Dupont WD, Biaggioni I, et al. Cognitive dysfunction in postural tachycardia syndrome. Clin Sci (Lond). 2015;128(1):39–45.
53. Snowden JS, Rollinson S, Thompson JC, Harris JM, Stopford CL, Richardson AM, et al. Distinct clinical and pathological characteristics of frontotemporal dementia associated with C9ORF72 mutations. Brain. 2012;135(Pt 3):693–708.
54. Ocon AJ, Messer ZR, Medow MS, Stewart JM. Increasing orthostatic stress impairs neurocognitive functioning in chronic fatigue syndrome with postural tachycardia syndrome. Clin Sci (Lond). 2012;122(5):227–38.
55. Stewart JM, Medow MS, Messer ZR, Baugham IL, Terilli C, Ocon AJ. Postural neurocognitive and neuronal activated cerebral blood flow deficits in young chronic fatigue syndrome patients with postural tachycardia syndrome. Am J Physiol Heart Circ Physiol. 2012;302(5):H1185.
56. Raj V, Opie M, Arnold AC. Cognitive and psychological issues in postural tachycardia syndrome. Auton Neurosci. 2018;215:46–55.
57. Bradford A, Kunik ME, Schulz P, Williams SP, Singh H. Missed and delayed diagnosis of dementia in primary care: prevalence and contributing factors. Alzheimer Dis Assoc Disord. 2009;23(4):306–14.
58. Al-Hameed S, Benaissa M, Christensen H, Mirheidari B, Blackburn D, Reuber M. A new diagnostic approach for the identification of patients with neurodegenerative cognitive complaints. PLoS ONE. 2019;14(5):e0217388.
59. Larner AJ. "Who came with you?" A diagnostic observation in patients with memory problems? J Neurol Neurosurg Psychiatry. 2005;76(12):1739.
60. Larner AJ. 'Attended alone' sign: validity and reliability for the exclusion of dementia. Age Ageing. 2009;38(4):476–8.
61. Larner AJ. Head turning sign: pragmatic utility in clinical diagnosis of cognitive impairment. J Neurol Neurosurg Psychiatry. 2012;83(8):852–3.
62. Ghadiri-Sani M, Larner AJ. Head turning sign for diagnosis of dementia and mild cognitive impairment: a revalidation. J Neurol Neurosurg Psychiatry. 2013;84(11):e2.
63. Bonello M, Larner AJ. Applause sign: screening utility for dementia and cognitive impairment. Postgrad Med. 2016;128(2):250–3.
64. Buffon F, Porcher R, Hernandez K, Kurtz A, Pointeau S, Vahedi K, et al. Cognitive profile in CADASIL. J Neurol Neurosurg Psychiatry. 2006;77(2):175–80.
65. Kelley BJ, Boeve BF, Josephs KA. Young-onset dementia: demographic and etiologic characteristics of 235 patients. Arch Neurol. 2008;65(11):1502–8.
66. Mokri AB, Low AP. Orthostatic headaches without CSF leak in postural tachycardia syndrome. Neurology. 2003;61(7):980–2.

Associated Conditions

Rheumatology and Postural Tachycardia Syndrome

Alan J. Hakim, Jane V. Simmonds and Arvind Kaul

PoTS and Joint Hypermobility

Alan J. Hakim

Introduction

The term joint hypermobility describes the ability to move a joint through a wider range of movement than normal. A number of factors can influence the ability to do this including age, gender, race, training, injury, and the presence of medical disorders or syndromes that cause joint tissue laxity [1]. Injury can induce laxity in a previously stable joint or lead to a reduced range of movement in a previously hypermobile joint.

Typically, children have a wide range of movement in their joints that is normal and may decrease or be lost with growth during adolescence and into adulthood. For this reason, scoring tools used to define generalised or widespread joint hypermobility have higher cut-off points for a description of generalised hypermobility in children than in adults [2].

Similarly, adults lose mobility with age. For this reason, scoring tools used to define generalised hypermobility have a lower cut-off for those after the age of 50 years.

In addition, women tend to have greater prevalence of generalised joint hypermobility than men.

The distribution of joint hypermobility can also vary between individuals. It may be:

- Mono-articular—found in just a single joint
- Pauci-articular—identified in a few joints
- Regional—such as upper or lower limb dominant, or in the small joints of the hands and feet (i.e. 'peripheral'), or
- Poly-articular or Generalised—found throughout the body.

A. J. Hakim (✉)
The Wellington Hospital, London, UK
e-mail: contact@alanhakim.com

A. J. Hakim
School of Medicine, PennState University, State College, USA

A. J. Hakim
The Ehlers-Danlos Society, Montgomery, USA

J. V. Simmonds (✉)
Great Ormond Street Institute of Child Health, University College London, London, UK
e-mail: jane.simmonds@ucl.ac.uk

J. V. Simmonds
London Hypermobility Unit, Platinum Centre, Wellington Hospital, London, UK

A. Kaul (✉)
St. George's University of London, London, UK
e-mail: akaul@sgul.ac.uk

N. Gall et al. (eds.), *Postural Tachycardia Syndrome*, https://doi.org/10.1007/978-3-030-54165-1_12

Identifying Joint Hypermobility

A general physical examination is required to identify joint hypermobility. For mono, pauci, and regional hypermobility there are no scoring systems. The findings are descriptive, having identified the joints affected. One might have hypermobility at the shoulders with joint instability and related injury and pain but have no other sites of hypermobility. One might, for example, have unstable ankles causing regional pain and changes in the biomechanics and function of the legs, pelvis and lower back.

For generalised joint hypermobility the most commonly applied scoring tool to define it is the Beighton Score (Box 1) [3], a modification of an earlier scoring system by Carter and Wilkinson [4]. The Beighton score is a set of 9 manoeuvers or points (Box 1).

Box 1: Assessing the Beighton Score

- One point if, while standing and bending forward, the individual can place their palms on the ground with the legs straight
- One point for each elbow that extends more than 10 degrees
- One point for each knee that extends more than 10 degrees
- One point for each thumb that, with the wrist flexed and arm straight, can be manipulated to touch the forearm
- One point for each fifth finger that extends beyond 90 degrees.

Children are considered to have generalised joint hypermobility if their Beighton score is 7 or more; adolescents and adults under the age of 50 if the score is 5 or more; and those over aged 50 if the score is 4 or more.

Another tool allied to the Beighton score is the Hypermobility Questionnaire (Box 2), which can be used instead of the Beighton score as a quick screen for generalised joint hypermobility [5]. An answer of 'yes' to two or more of the questions gives a very high prediction of the presence of hypermobility, with 85% sensitivity and specificity against the Beighton score.

Box 2: The Hypermobility Questionnaire

1. Can you now (or could you ever) place your hands flat on the floor without bending your knees?
2. Can you now (or could you ever) bend your thumb to touch your forearm?
3. As a child did you amuse your friends by contorting your body into strange shapes OR could you do the splits?
4. As a child or teenager did your shoulder or kneecap dislocate on more than one occasion?
5. Do you consider yourself double-jointed?

It is important however to note that the Beighton score is best used as a screening tool. A positive score indicates it is highly likely an individual is hypermobile. A low score does not rule out generalized, mono, pauci, or regional hypermobility. Other joints should be examined for hypermobility, such as the temporomandibular joint, cervical spine, shoulders, thoracic spine, hips, ankles and feet to gain appropriate insight into the relationship between joint pain and injury and joint hypermobility.

Two other scoring systems have been validated, and, are used most often in specialist medical and therapy assessments. These are the Upper Limb Hypermobility Assessment Tool (ULHAT) [6] and the Lower Limb Assessment Score (LLAS) for children [7] and more recently validated in adults [8]. They are more complex to apply than the screening tools above, and, require more than a general level of skill in musculoskeletal physical examination. The ULHAT for example includes assessment of the shoulder, forearm rotation and the wrist; and the LLAS the hip, ankle, and mid and forefoot.

Joint Subluxation and Dislocation

In addition to the wider range of movement, joint instability may arise in the form of subluxations and/or dislocations. Subluxation describes the phenomenon where the articular surfaces of a joint are partially displaced from their normal alignment with each other as the joint goes through its range of movement. At all times at least some of the joint's surface-to-surface remains in contact. In a dislocated joint the articular surfaces are no longer in contact with each other at all; they have fully misaligned with each other, the joint out of its socket.

Ease of subluxations and dislocations and the related injury are a feature of hypermobility-related disorders, and arise to varying degrees; subluxation is likely to be the more common concern.

Dislocations are readily identified on physical assessment or imaging. It is more difficult to identify subluxations as this requires a more than general knowledge of joint examinations. That being said, at certain sites (such as the base of the thumb, the wrists, the shoulders, the hips, and the kneecaps) it can be clear by manipulating the joint for its stability that the joint is unstable.

Hypermobility-Related Disorders—HSD and hEDS

The most common diagnosis of a hypermobility-related disorder was previously called Joint Hypermobility Syndrome (JHS) [9]. The JHS diagnostic criteria covered a wide group of patients some of whom had signs and symptoms that might equally be described as the Hypermobile variant of Ehlers-Danlos syndrome (EDS) [10]. In 2017 new criteria addressed this by giving clarity to the criteria for Hypermobile EDS (hEDS), and the term JHS was dropped [11]. However, as described above, not all individuals with JHS would have had hEDS, nor would they have had any other Heritable Disorder of Connective Tissue. As such, descriptions were required for where an individual has hypermobility-related musculoskeletal concerns but does not appear to have EDS or other HDCT. In this situation the diagnosis Hypermobility Spectrum Disorder (HSD) is given [1]. A further important consideration is that HSD can apply to concerns where there is mono, pauci, peripheral, or generalised joint hypermobility present. In hEDS the joint hypermobility is generalised in its distribution.

In both HSD and hEDS musculoskeletal symptoms can be mild to moderate to severe; hEDS in this sense is not more severe than HSD. Equally, studies are beginning to show that both can have relatively mild complications or very complex associated symptoms. For example, both HSD and hEDS individuals experience high levels of pain and symptoms of autonomic dysfunction [11].

There are no 'criteria' for HSD. It is defined by the presence of hypermobility-related musculoskeletal concerns in the absence of a HDCT or other condition causing hypermobility [1].

The criteria for diagnosing hEDS are shown in Box 3 below. An individual must fulfil each of the 3 domains. In the second domain they must fulfil 2 of the 3 descriptors (A, B and C) by achieving sufficient scores where relevant. By studying the criteria one can see that hEDS is a condition of the musculoskeletal system, skin, and other structural tissues. There are at this time no known genetic markers for hEDS, unlike the other 13 variants of EDS where the genetics and pathophysiology have been well elucidated. However, the inheritance pattern in hEDS does appear to behave in a dominant way.

Box 3: Domains defining hEDS diagnostic criteria

Domain 1: The presence of generalised joint hypermobility

Domain 2: (A) Skin or fascia signs and/or pelvic floor concerns; OR Marfanoid features;

(B) a family history AND;

(C) the presence of mechanical musculoskeletal symptoms and/or evidence of joint instability/subluxation/dislocations

Domain 3: The absence of any other underlying Heritable Disorder of Connective Tissue including other variants of EDS

Box 4: The 2017 International Criteria for the diagnosis of Hypermobile EDS

Criterion 1, 2 and 3 must be met.

Criterion 1: Generalized Joint Hypermobility (GJH)

The International Consortium on the Ehlers–Danlos Syndromes proposed the following Beighton score cutoffs

Pre-pubertal children and adolescents = 6

pubertal men and women up to the age of 50 = 5

>50 years of age for hEDS = 4.

An additional point is added to the score if the 5-point questionnaire is positive.

Criterion 2: Two or more of the Following Features (A–C) MUST Be Present (e.g.: A and B; A and C; B and C)

Feature A: systemic manifestations of a more generalized connective tissue disorder (a total of five must be present)

- Unusually soft or velvety skin
- Mild skin hyperextensibility
- Unexplained striae such as striae distensae or rubrae at the back, groins, thighs, breasts and/or abdomen in adolescents, men or prepubertal women without a history of significant gain or loss of body fat or weight
- Bilateral piezogenic papules of the heel
- Recurrent or multiple abdominal hernia(s) (e.g., umbilical, inguinal, crural)
- Atrophic scarring involving at least two sites and without the formation of truly papyraceous and/or hemosideric scars as seen in classical EDS
- Pelvic floor, rectal, and/or uterine prolapse in children, men or nulliparous women without a history of morbid obesity or other known pre-disposing medical condition
- Dental crowding and high or narrow palate
- Arachnodactyly, as defined in one or more of the following: (i) positive wrist sign (Steinberg sign) on both sides; (ii) positive thumb sign (Walker sign) on both sides
- Arm span-to-height $\geq$ 1.05
- Mitral valve prolapse (MVP) mild or greater based on strict echocardiographic criteria
- Aortic root dilatation with Z-score $\geq$ 2

Feature B: positive family history, with one or more first degree relatives independently meeting the current diagnostic criteria for hEDS.

Feature C: musculoskeletal complications (must have at least one):

- Musculoskeletal pain in two or more limbs, recurring daily for at least 3 months
- Chronic, widespread pain for > 3 months
- Recurrent joint dislocations or frank joint instability, in the absence of trauma (a or b)

a) Three or more atraumatic dislocations in the same joint or two or more atraumatic dislocations in two different joints occurring at different times
b) Medical confirmation of joint instability at two or more sites not related to trauma

Criterion 3: All the Following Prerequisites MUST Be Met

1. Absence of unusual skin fragility, which should prompt consideration of other types of EDS
2. Exclusion of other heritable and acquired connective tissue disorders, including autoimmune rheumatologic conditions. In patients with an acquired connective tissue disorder (e.g., lupus, rheumatoid arthritis, etc.), additional diagnosis of hEDS requires meeting both Features A and B of Criterion 2. Feature C of Criterion 2 (chronic pain and/or instability) cannot be counted towards a diagnosis of hEDS in this situation.
3. Exclusion of alternative diagnoses that may also include joint hypermobility by means of hypotonia and/or connective tissue laxity. Alternative diagnoses and diagnostic categories include, but are not limited to, neuromuscular on evidence-based management of the symptoms in the context of hEDS.

Pictures

Pictures of the skin and piezogenic papules

Cardiovascular Autonomic concerns in HSD and hEDS

Individuals with HSD and hEDS report fainting or feeling faint, palpitations, chest tightness, or shortness of breath in the absence of asthma or cardiac disease. Often these symptoms are identifiable as autonomic disturbances or orthostatic intolerance (OI), and most often postural tachycardia syndrome (PoTS) in both children and adults [12–14].

Several possible mechanisms continue to be explored as explanations for the association between HSD, hEDS and autonomic dysfunction (Fig. 1). As more is understood of these mechanisms so it should be possible to tailor treatment to an individual's needs, but in general all treatment modalities used to treat OI are in general appropriate to use in people with HSD or hEDS, assuming no specific contraindication in an individual.

Mechanisms that have been explored and continue to be studied include:

- Low blood pressure
- Increased peripheral venous dilation and blood pooling
- Low circulating blood volume
- Elevated circulating catecholamines (such as adrenaline (epinephrine))
- Autoimmunity. Autoantibodies directed against receptors which play a role in the regulation of heart rate and blood pressure
- Medications with side effects that trigger or impair autonomic responses, e.g. tricyclics such as amitriptyline
- Excess levels of histamine, and
- Brainstem or cervical cord impingement from Chiari malformation or cranio-cervical instability.

It is suggested that an excess of stretch or 'give' in larger veins or their ability to expand because of loose supporting connective tissue may be a cause for pooling of blood in the pelvis and the legs. This pooling in the lower half of the body, could lead to lightheadedness, fast heart rate to compensate for lower volumes of blood returning to the heart and sometimes fainting when standing up.

Medications taken for the management of pain may also cause side effects of low blood pressure and fast heart rate. It is always important to read the side effect information leaflet for any medication, but the more common ones used for pain relief and to reduce anxiety that tend to induce low blood pressure or fast heart rate include the neuroleptic drugs (e.g. pregabalin), anti-depressants as analgesics (e.g. amitriptyline), and opioid medications (e.g. codeine and morphine).

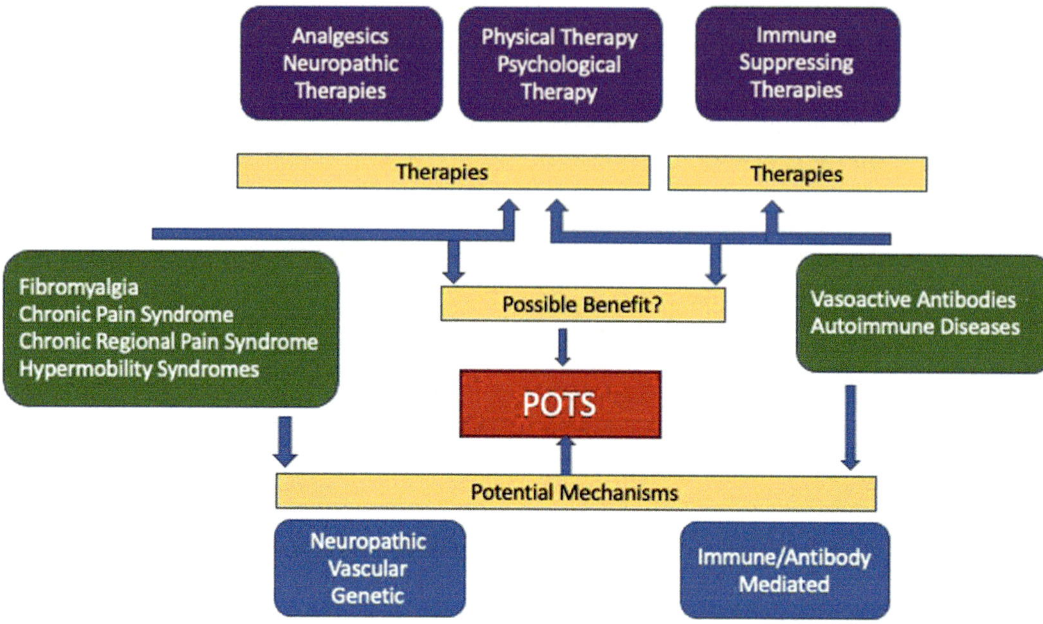

Fig. 1 Summary of the possible mechanisms and potential modes of therapy for Postural Orthostatic Tachycardia Syndrome (PoTS) associated with rheumatological conditions. The therapies listed are associated with benefits with the individual conditions in the green boxes but the link between the mechanisms, therapies and their effects on PoTS remains speculative

Nerve damage has also been suggested as a cause for low blood pressure although the exact mechanisms are not clear at this time. Nerve damage might include changes to the autonomic nerves themselves. Very rarely there may be compression of the brain stem arising from instability of the joints at the skull base and top of the neck (cranio-cervical junction and atlanto-axial instability).

Some people with HSD or EDS may have problems with excessive mast cell activation. Mast cells are immune system cells which help regulate allergic responses. When the mast cells respond to an allergic trigger, they release histamine and many other substances that can influence heart rate and blood pressure.

Management of Joint Hypermobility, Hypermobility Spectrum Disorders and Hypermobile Ehlers Danlos Syndrome: Considerations for Physiotherapy, Occupation therapy and Podiatry

Jane V. Simmonds

Introduction

Current best practice management of Joint Hypermobility, Hypermobility Spectrum Disorders (HSD) and hypermobile Ehlers Danlos Syndrome (hEDS) is essentially a problem solving, patient empowerment approach underpinned by the best available evidence. Ideally a multidisciplinary team will include the General Practitioner, Paediatrician, Rheumatologist, Physiotherapist, Psychologist, Occupational Therapist, Podiatrist, Occupational Health Practitioners, Teachers and Fitness and Exercise Instructors. When co-morbidities are present such as PoTS or orthostatic intolerance, gastrointestinal dysmotility, bladder dysfunction and psychiatric illness, aditional system specialists are also needed in the team.

Education and Family Support

Condition-specific patient education and shared decision-making forms the basis of empowerment based self-management for long term conditions such as HSD and hEDS [15]. In addition to face to face education in clinic, individuals and families can be directed to helpful evidence based information provided by patient support group organisations such as the HMSA www.hmsa.org, EDS Support UK https://www.ehlers-danlos.org and The Ehlers Danlos Society https://www.ehlers-danlos.com/.

Postural Education, Exercise and Functional Rehabilitation

Back pain associated with suboptimal posture and segmental instability is a common clinical finding. Individually tailored posture re-education programmes have shown good improvement in pain and quality of life [16, 17]. An eight week spinal stabilization exercise programme improved back pain, trunk muscle endurance and balance [18]. Patients with musculoskeletal pain have also been shown to have functional changes in the representation of affected muscles on the somatosensory cortex and that these cortical neuroplastic changes, associated with pain, can be reversed by motor-skill training. Boudreau and colleagues [19] suggest several important components to maximize rehabilitative success.

Posture, Motor Control and Principles of Exercise

- Exercises should target a specific component of movement which requires greater skill and precision.
- Motor-skill training should be pain-free. Pain rapidly alters the excitability of the motor cortex and contributes to protective motor control strategies and so hinders learning. Where pain is persistent, exercise should be at a level which does not exacerbate pain.
- Rehabilitation exercises should be goal-orientated or 'cognitive' to enhance cortical neuroplastic changes.
- Quality is preferable to quantity to prevent fatigue and pain interfering with improvements in task performance.

Joint Protection, Splinting and Occupational Therapy

Joint protection is an essential part of management; individuals need to be taught to avoid unhelpful postures [20] and to self-manage subluxations and dislocations. This can avoid repeated attendances at Accident and Emergency centres and unnecessary radiological investigations and the provision of high strength pain medications.

Improving dynamic control of movement and strength to compensate for the ligamentous insufficiency and tackle instability through carefully planned exercise programmes can help to minimize risk of injury, subluxation, dislocation and trauma to joints. If an individual is experiencing significant pain, exercise may start with isometric activation and inner range exercise before progressing to large amplitude resisted work using elastic bands and light weights. Many adults with HSD and hEDS have reported that they find low impact exercise in water, swimming, walking and Pilates helpful [21].

Weight management is another important factor for protecting against musculoskeletal injury and pain. In one large study in the West of England, where adolescents with generalised joint hypermobility were followed up over a 5 year period, being overweight increased the risk of musculoskeletal pain injury 12 fold [22]. Therefore dietary control and judicious participation in physical activity including sport, dance and Physical Education should be encouraged. While sports participation clearly has many benefits for hypermobile individuals, additional care needs to be taken when playing contact sports as there is an increased risk of knee injury [23]. For those with HSD and hEDS, intense physical activity can exacerbate pain, fatigue and PoTS symptoms and therefore activity needs to be carefully paced. Each case should be individually assessed and where necessary adjustments to frequency, intensity and type of physical activity can be made.

Occupational therapists and hand therapists can provide invaluable advice and provision of wrist and hand splints and rehabilitation as well as ergonomic adaptations for the home, school and workplace. Splinting of hypermobile joints should be used judiciously to avoid over-dependence. Specific activity related finger and hand splints (Fig. 2) can be very helpful for specific tasks, for example practicing a musical instrument, opening a jar and prolonged periods of typing or writing. Back supports and knee braces are often helpful after an injury and an acute exacerbation of pain or during early rehabilitation. Tape can also be beneficial to help support a vulnerable joint and also to help facilitate proprioception and postural control [20]. The provision of mobility aids such as crutches and wheelchairs requires careful consideration by the multidisciplinary team.

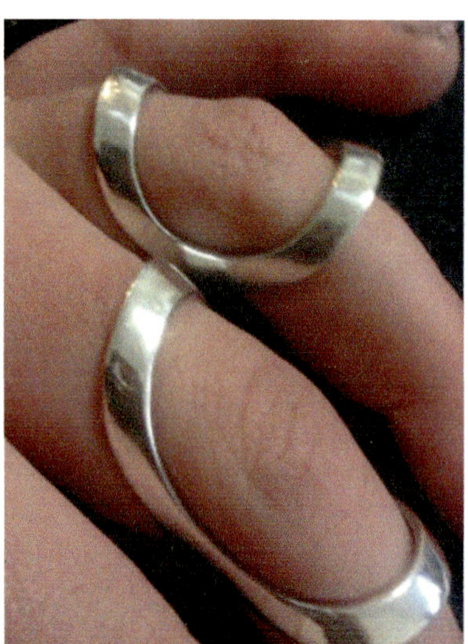

Fig. 2 Ring splints

Gait Re-education and Podiatry

A combination of altered biomechanics, reduced proprioception, poor motor control, weak muscles and reduced stamina frequently affect gait [24–26]. Hypermobile individuals commonly present with over-pronated hind feet, a flattened medial longitudinal arch and sometimes inefficient Tibialis Posterior muscle function. This may lead to an altered gait pattern and subsequent foot, ankle, leg and back pain. Heal and arch raising exercises are often helpful and in many cases correcting the biomechanics of the ankle/foot complex with supportive footwear and/or orthotics significantly optimises function and reduces pain. There is some research evidence for the effectiveness of orthotics in gait for children with Developmental Coordination Disorder and HSD/hEDS [27]. As yet there is no research evidence that orthotics are helpful for adults with HSD or hEDS, however anecdotal reports are positive. Where more complex ankle and foot issues are present, an assessment by an experienced podiatrist is recommended as there needs to be careful consideration of the biomechanical correction and materials used for the orthotics.

Proprioception, Balance and Functional Rehabilitation

Given that proprioception and balance impairments are common in both children and adults with HSD and hEDS, specific balance and proprioceptive exercises need to be incorporated into rehabilitation and fitness programmes.

Carefully prescribed open and closed chain exercise (Figs. 3 and 4) have been shown to be effective for reducing pain, improving strength, proprioception and balance [18, 28–30]. Enhancing sensory input by the use of 'hands on' movement facilitation [21], tape and wearing of tight fitting lycra garments during specific exercise or functional rehabilitation sessions is reported to be helpful by expert clinicians and patients [31]. Exercise which is carefully graduated into the hypermobile range was shown to benefit children in terms of pain reduction and muscle strength. Moreover, from the parents' perspective, exercising into the hypermobile range was helpful in terms of self-esteem [23].

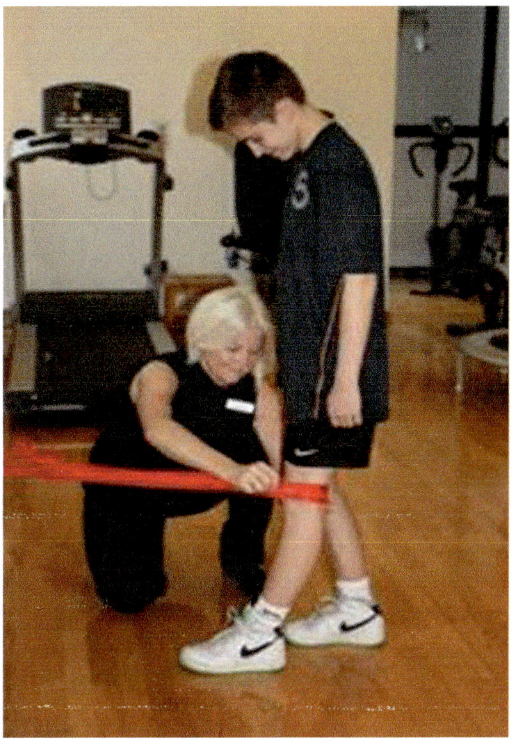

Fig. 3 Closed chain knee strengthening exercise

Single leg standing exercises, progressing to more dynamic balance activities using a balance (wobble) board, to provide a further challenge, as well as exercises in four-point kneeling, can be useful progressions for combined upper and lower limb proprioception and strengthening. Exercises may also include the use of foam rolls and large gym balls. Hydrotherapy has been reported by patients to be helpful [21] and is perceived to be effective by paediatric therapists [32]. Later stage rehabilitation involves more advanced integrated open chain strength and cardiovascular training in line with American College of Sports Medicine (ACSM) guidelines for children [33, 34] and adults [35], in order to improve functional fitness and to facilitate participation in sporting and performing arts activities. A note of caution, exercise progressions should be carefully monitored to ensure the individual can cope with the intensity. A graduated return to higher level sport or dance is recommended and training loads should be observed to ensure adequate recovery.

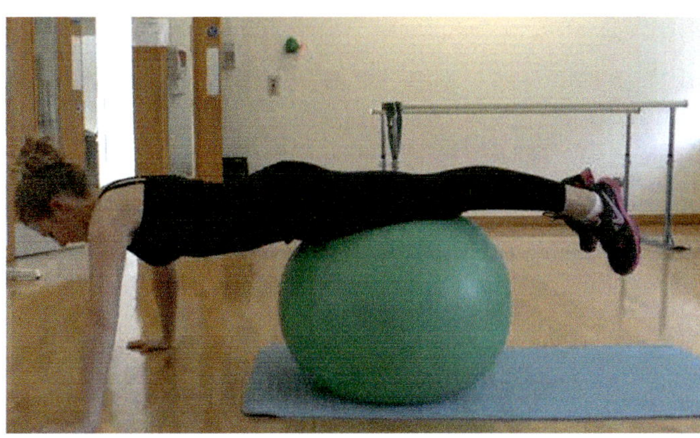

Fig. 4 Closed chain upper quadrant trunk exercise

Pain and Fatigue Management

Individuals with HSD and hEDS may present with a mixture of acute, mechanical and chronic pain with both peripheral and central sensitization often present [36]. Fatigue is a common debilitating symptom [37]. Understanding the mechanism for the fatigue and treating the cause is key. For example, there may be biomechanical causes associated with muscle weakness, joint alignment and poor kinematics. Nutritional and metabolic factors may play a role, such as inadequate hydration, low vitamin D and ferritin levels and poor fitness levels. Low mood and anxiety and other systemic symptoms such as gastrointestinal dysmotility and cardiac dysautonomia may limit exercise tolerance and require adaptation of therapy.

Experts report that a range of treatments can be beneficial for the short term relief of pain, for example ice, heat, gentle manual therapy for stiff joints (usually the thoracic area) and soft tissue massage. Trigger point work and myofascial release can also alleviate pain associated with muscle spasm [38]. Where there is evidence of pathoneurodynamics, neural mobilisation techniques may be helpful. Acupuncture and transcutaneous electrical nerve stimulation (TENS) is useful for some individuals. Higher frequency TENS settings of 120–150 Hz which are thought to activate the descending opioid pathways [39] have been most helpful. All therapies should be applied carefully to avoid exacerbation of pain as peripheral and central sensitization is commonly observed [36]. Learning to pace activity is an important management strategy for tackling persistent pain and fatigue. Additionally, graded functional activity exposure [40] and carefully monitored cardiovascular, strength—endurance programmes and other forms of low impact rhythmical exercise such as Nordic pole walking or tai chi may help to modulate widespread persistent pain and fatigue [41]. Physical reconditioning is also important for managing PoTS symptoms (see chapter "Exercise Guidelines for Postural Tachycardia Syndrome"). For individuals where persistent pain and fatigue impact significantly on functional capacity and maladaptive beliefs are behaviours are recognised, involvement of clinical psychology is recommended (see psychology section, Chapter 40).

Immune and Inflammatory Rheumatic Diseases, Fibromyalgia, CRPS and PoTS

Arvind Kaul

Introduction

This section will critically review the current evidence that PoTS may be associated with mechanisms common to autoimmune conditions, Fibromyalgia and Chronic Regional Pain Syndrome (CRPS), although this is clearly an evolving field which will be significantly added to in the coming years. In common with the above conditions, PoTS is most common in young women between the ages of 15–50. In addition, these conditions share common features including dysautonomia, cognitive impairment, fatigue, sensory changes consistent in some cases with proven small fibre neuropathy and allergic symptoms, possibly consistent with mast cell degranulation.

Autoimmune Rheumatic Conditions and PoTS

There is circumstantial evidence that not only does PoTS have an autoimmune basis in some individuals but may be associated with autoimmune conditions seen in rheumatology practice.

Wang et al. [42] in one pilot study of 17 patients (7 control, 10 PoTS) found a variety of IgG antibodies in PoTS patients which cross-reacted with cardiac proteins including those involved with cell survival (laminin), structural integrity of cardiac muscle (filamin) and cardiac hypertrophy (mimecan, myozenin) amongst others. Furthermore, in another study,

14/14 patients with PoTS exhibited activating antibodies to α1-adrenergic and β1/2 adrenergic receptors [43]. In a follow up study, 12/17 PoTS patients had antibodies to the Angiotensin II Type 1 Receptor (AT1R) with none found in control patients with vasovagal syncope or healthy controls [44].

Gunning et al. [45] found that 50–55 PoTS patients studied had autoantibodies against 4 subtypes of G-protein coupled adrenergic receptors and 5 subtypes of G-protein coupled muscarinic acetylcholine receptors by ELISA. Controls and 5 PoTS patients had no autoantibodies. PoTS patients also exhibited multiple symptoms including fatigue (94.5%), myalgias (83.6%), Raynaud's phenomenon (49.1%) and depression (34.5%). However, there was no attempt to classify these symptoms as being due to any other condition and they may be due to other conditions either related or unrelated to PoTS.

In addition, an 11-year experience with 152 unselected POTS patients demonstrated 86% were female with a mean age of 30.2 years. Of the 42 patients tested, 6 (14.2%) had ganglionic anti-acetylcholine receptor antibodies (G-AchR) in a low positive titre [46]. These antibodies are very specific for autoimmune autonomic ganglionopathy and are not seen in either healthy individuals or patients with Myasthenia Gravis [47].

Li et al. [43] suggested that because a proportion of patients with PoTS have a precipitant such as a presumed viral infection, a form of molecular mimicry may induce PoTS via an autoimmune phenomenon. In a small cohort of 14 PoTS patients and 10 healthy controls, they studied whether PoTS patients may harbour functional antibodies to adrenergic receptors (α1AR, β1AR and β2AR). Their findings suggested that PoTS patients have elevated α1AR autoantibodies which exert a partial peripheral antagonist effect. This leads to a compensatory activation of α1AR and concurrent β1AR mediated tachycardia.

Wang et al. [48] found the presence of autoantibodies to lipid rafts in PoTS patients. Lipid rafts are glycosphingolipid-protein complexes in plasma membranes important in cell signalling and transduction.

The data presented above suggest an autoimmune basis for PoTS. As autoimmune conditions often co-exist it is therefore not surprising that autoantibodies associated with other autoimmune conditions are found in PoTS and may point to a secondary cause. Blitshtyen [49] studied 100 consecutive patients with PoTS of whom 91 were female. Of these, 25% had a positive ANA, 7% had at least one positive antiphospholipid antibody test with 5% fulfilling criteria for full-blown antiphospholipid syndrome (APS). Other specific antibodies such as anti-SSA (most commonly found in Sjögren's Syndrome and SLE) and dsDNA (usually found in SLE) were less frequent but in total, 31% of PoTS patients had positive autoantibodies. It should be noted however, that estimates for the prevalence of ANA can vary and approach between 8 and 40% in some populations. In addition, positive antibodies do not necessarily mean that the patient has a defined active autoimmune disease.

However, in this study, up to 20% of patients had a co-morbid autoimmune disorder, most commonly Hashimoto's Thyroiditis (11%), Antiphospholipid Syndrome (5%), Rheumatoid Arthritis (4%) and SLE (2%). These features were suggested to be at a higher prevalence than then the general population, but larger numbers are needed to clarify this association.

The Antiphospholipid Syndrome (APS) has been associated with pregnancy loss and thrombosis with the presence of either anticardiolipin antibodies or lupus anticoagulant positivity. In one study of 15 APS patients with PoTS or other forms of dysautonomia, retrospective chart reviews revealed the autonomic symptoms improved with anticoagulation or intravenous immunoglobulin in some patients [50].

Given the wide array of autoantibodies detected in PoTS, it is very likely that more than one mechanism is likely to be involved in aetiology. Vasoactive antibodies associated with PoTS may be critical in pathogenesis, but their exact roles are not clear, and it is important to remember that the presence of an antibody does not prove causality.

While there is circumstantial evidence for a link between PoTS and rheumatic immune-mediated disease, much more work is required to clarify any association before any firm conclusions can be drawn.

Chronic Fatigue Syndrome and PoTS

Chronic Fatigue Syndrome (CFS, see chapter "Chronic Fatigue Syndrome") is defined by the International CFS Working Group's 1994 Chronic Fatigue Syndrome Case Definition criteria [51] and may affect 2.5 million people in the USA [52]. It has been suggested that CFS be reclassified as Systemic Exertional Intolerance Disease (SEID) with new diagnostic criteria including (1) unexplained fatigue leading to a disability and lasting more than 6 months, (2) Post exertional Malaise (PEM), (3) unrefreshing sleep, (4) plus one of either cognitive impairment or orthostatic intolerance, the latter the most prominent symptom in patients with SEID/CFS.

In SEID, the commonest forms of OI are PoTS and neurally-mediated hypotension. SEID orthostatic intolerance (OI) is defined by dizziness, lightheadedness, blurred vision, and near syncope worse in the upright posture, improved by lying down. CFS/SEID patients have significantly higher frequency of standing and recumbent dizziness and lightheadedness but these symptoms are not always attributed to PoTS, being found in 6/39 (15%) CFS patients and 1/25 (4%) controls [53].

Despite this, the dysautonomic changes exhibited in PoTS and CFS patients can be similar [54] (see chapter "Chronic Fatigue Syndrome"). Orthostatic intolerance can be detected in patients with CFS on tilt-table testing [55]. Patients with CFS may exhibit higher standing heart rates than age and sex-matched controls with 27% of CFS patients with PoTS compared with 9% of controls in one study [56]. While PoTS patients with CFS had greater orthostatic tachycardia and more labile blood pressure than patients without CFS, the majority of non-CFS POTS patients also fulfilled the criteria for CFS exemplifying the difficulties in interpreting study conclusions [57].

The issue of whether common immune-mediated mechanisms are important in CFS much as they seem to be in PoTS is unclear, making associations between the two conditions difficult to extrapolate currently. In one systematic review of 15 studies, no firm conclusions could be drawn on whether cytokines and by inference, an immune-mediated response, were associated with CFS [58].

Studies show variability in the frequency of orthostatic intolerance and PoTS in CFS and use small numbers of patients. Larger multicentre studies are required to clarify whether PoTS has a significant association with CFS before any conclusions can be drawn on management.

Fibromyalgia and PoTS

In common with many patients with CFS, patients with Fibromyalgia (FM) often complain of similar symptoms including dizziness and lightheadedness.

Fibromyalgia is a condition of chronic diffuse pain associated with fatigue, sleep disturbance and cognitive dysfunction. FM is common, affecting perhaps 1–2% of the UK population [59]. It can be classified according to the American College of Rheumatology (ACR) 2016 revised criteria [60] but recent attempts have aimed to consolidate criteria based around pain, fatigue and sleep disturbance [61].

Very few studies looking at FM and PoTS exist and to add to the confounding effects, some symptoms of FM inevitably overlap with CFS. Dissociative disorders involve problems with memory, identity, emotion, perception, behaviour and sense of self. In one study, 21 FM patients and 22 healthy controls, each participant completed the Dissociative Experiences Scale [62]. Patients with fibromyalgia reported both significantly greater dissociative experiences and more symptoms of orthostatic intolerance than controls. The relationship between fibromyalgia and dissociation remained significant after adjusting for the gender but was rendered non-significant when adjusted for symptoms of orthostatic intolerance. These results suggested that the dissociation symptoms were largely attributable to orthostatic intolerance. However, a clear diagnosis of PoTS was not provided making conclusions difficult to draw.

Tang et al. [63] found that neurally mediated hypotension (NMH), a form of orthostatic intolerance, was common in patients with SLE being found in 47.9% of the 48 patients who had tilt table testing. Although the frequency of PoTS alone was not stated, 14.6% of patient did have both NMH and PoTS while 23.7% of the patients fulfilled criteria for FM. However, the authors were not able to show an association between FM and NMH in SLE although symptoms of FM were reproduced during tilt table testing in some patients. In addition, NMH did not have any significant impact on quality of life measures over and above those due to the FM but data for PoTS was not presented.

In summary, while FM is a common condition of pain, very few studies have proved a causal link between FM and PoTS. Symptoms of orthostatic intolerance may be common in FM but clearly larger controlled studies are needed to determine any link between PoTS and criteria diagnosed FM.

Chronic Regional Pain Syndrome, Dysautonomia and PoTS

Complex regional pain syndrome (CRPS) is characterised by pain and is most commonly found in women. It usually affects one limb (e.g. arm, leg, hand, or foot). CRPS is associated with sensory, autonomic and motor abnormalities with trophic changes including skin colour, temperature, with or without swelling in the affected area.

Two CRPS types currently exist, CRPS-I and CRPS-II. Individuals without a confirmed nerve injury are classified as having CRPS-I (previously known as reflex sympathetic dystrophy syndrome). However, there is evidence of nerve fibre changes in C and Aδ fibres in CRPS-I and so classification criteria are not absolute. CRPS-II (previously known as causalgia) is associated with confirmed nerve injury.

CRPS starts after minor or moderate injury such as wrist fracture. The injured limb is often warm, swollen and very painful. Both allodynia and hyperalgesia may be associated, and pain usually persists and may extend with the limb eventually becoming cold. CRPS symptoms vary in severity and duration, although some cases are mild and eventually go away. In more severe cases, individuals may not recover and may have long-term disability.

The link between PoTS and CRPS is indicated by the finding that CRPS may be associated with autoantibodies against differentiated autonomic neurons. The mechanisms may involve $\beta_2$adrenergic receptor and/or the muscarinic-2 receptor antibodies [64]. In addition, chronic CRPS is associated with activating autoantibodies against alpha-1α adrenoceptors [65]. This raises the possibility that CRPS associated with PoTS may be amenable to immunomodulation and intravenous immunoglobulin has been used in this setting.

There has also been concern about the possibility of HPV vaccination inducing CRPS and PoTS. In 2013, Kinoshita [66] reported 44 Japanese females (aged 11–17 years), 12 of whom developed orthostatic hypotension or PoTS after HPV vaccination. Eighteen were diagnosed with CRPS. The authors noted that HPV vaccination might be a common mechanism in causation of CRPS and PoTS since the average time to onset was 5.47 months ± 5 months post-vaccination.

In 2015, Brinth [67] reported 35 Danish women aged 23.3 ± 7.1 years, 21 of whom fulfilled the criteria for PoTS, who developed dysautonomic symptoms within two months after vaccination for HPV. Chandler [68] cluster analysed the WHO database for HPV vaccine adverse events using data from VigiBase, comprising 10.3 million reports globally. While the majority of clusters of adverse events (71% of the total cases) were expected and reported in the product label, small numbers of cases (total 694) contained four significant clusters reporting adverse events of fatigue, syncope, dizziness and headache. It was suggested that these symptoms overlap with diagnoses including PoTS, CFS and CRPS.

However, the reporting was not explicit enough to suggest that these diagnoses were based on specific criteria. The European Medicines agency (EMA) also reviewed the WHO data and concluded that the reported cases of PoTS, CRPS or CFS were at levels expected in the general population using population estimates [69]. They concluded that there was no evidence of HPV inducing these conditions and recommended continued vigilance.

While there is good evidence that PoTS is linked in some cases to positive autoimmune tests, a specific mechanism to explain all of the symptoms is as yet lacking. Furthermore, it is unclear whether CFS and CRPS, while seemingly associated with PoTS with similar symptoms, are part of the same spectrum, associated or share similar symptoms. There are many strategies to provide symptom control but none yet which could potentially address the possible autoimmune causes.

Management of Patients with Autoimmune Rheumatic Diseases, CFS, FM, CRPS and Suspected PoTS.

Although there is some evidence for a link, the exact relationship between PoTS, FM, CFS, CRPS and autoimmune disorders has not been determined yet in large controlled studies. Therefore, potential PoTS patients with rheumatic disorders must be thoroughly questioned and investigated to determine any possible link.

History

- Specific symptoms such as joint pain and swelling, Raynaud's phenomenon, photosensitivity, recurrent oral ulcers, increased hair fall and sicca symptoms may be important in the diagnosis of autoimmune conditions such as SLE, Sjögren's Syndrome or Rheumatoid Arthritis
- Additionally, triggers that are common to patient groups, including medications such as amitriptyline, dietary factors or other stressors may be relevant.

Examination

- All systems should be scrutinised for abnormalities.
- Skin: malar rash, discoid patches, scarring alopecia, livedo reticularis, Raynaud's
- Cardiovascular: lying/standing blood pressure, auscultation for murmurs
- Gastrointestinal: abdominal tenderness, ascites
- Musculoskeletal: Joint hypermobility, swelling, tenderness
- Respiratory systems. Auscultation for crackles or dullness indicating interstitial lung changes or pleural effusions
- Neurological: Cranial or peripheral neuropathies, weakness/power deficit indicating myopathy

Investigations

If an autoimmune connective tissue disorder such as lupus, Sjogren's Syndrome or APS is suggested, investigations should include:

- FBC, urea and electrolytes, LFT, ESR, CRP
- ANA including pattern and titre
- Extractable nuclear antigens (ENA)
- dsDNA: specific for SLE
- Rheumatoid factor and anti-CCP antibodies
- Antiphospholipid antibody screen (Lupus anticoagulant, IgM and IgG anti-cardiolipin antibodies and IgM and IgG β_2-Glycoprotein-1. If positive, repeat in 12 weeks)
- Immunoglobulins (often high in disease, occasionally low), complement (often low in disease, especially C4)

- As evidence accumulates and tests become more routinely available, this set of tests is likely to expand given the evidence for other autoantibodies in PoTS patients.

Further important investigations which the GP or Rheumatologist should request include.

- Chest xray: interstitial lung disease, pleural or pericardial effusion
- Echocardiogram: Valvular structure (Libman-Sachs vegetations, mitral valve prolapse), pericardial inflammation or effusion.
- Cardiac 24 hr monitor: to exclude obvious cardiac arrhythmias as a cause for presyncopal episodes

Therapeutic options

- There is very little data as yet to justify the routine use of immune modulating drugs to treat patients for symptoms of PoTS associated potentially with any rheumatic disease.
- The rheumatic disease itself may be the target of these drugs (e.g. SLE) but much more research is needed to clarify whether this strategy helps PoTS.
- In some circumstances, the distinction between fibromyalgia, inflammatory arthritis and JHS/EDS can be a difficult one and the use of immune modulating drugs such as hydroxychloroquine, methotrexate, cyclosporin or other drugs needs to be carefully balanced against potential side effects.
- CFS and FM often rely on exclusion of other conditions and utilise exercise therapy and drug therapy with amitriptyline, duloxetine or gabapentin.

Important referrals

- Physiotherapist: As part of the multidisciplinary process, specialist and regional physiotherapy can help joint pains and fatigue. Other forms of physical therapy include hydrotherapy to promote reduction of pain and strength in areas such as the spine and pelvis.
- Cardiologist/Specialist in PoTS: Autonomic function tests and cardiac tilt table testing should rely on initial history, clinical examination including lying and standing blood pressure and pulse rate measurements to clarify the nature of any orthostatic intolerance and referral directed if required to specialist clinics.

References

1. Castori M, Tinkle B, Levy H, Grahame R, Malfait F, Hakim A. A framework for the classification of joint hypermobility and related conditions. Am J Med Genet C Semin Med Genet. 2017. https://doi.org/10.1002/ajmg.c.31539.
2. Singh H, McKay M, Baldwin J, Nicholson L, Chan C, Burns J, Hiller CE. Beighton scores and cut-offs across the lifespan: cross-sectional study of an Australian population. Rheumatology (Oxford). 2017;56(11):1857–64.
3. Beighton PH, Solomon L, Soskolne CL. Articular mobility in an African population. Ann Rheum Dis. 1973;32(5):413–7.
4. Carter C, Wilkinson J. Persistent joint laxity and congenital dislocation of the hip. J Bone Jt Surg. 1964;46-B:40–45.
5. Hakim AJ, Grahame R. A simple questionnaire to detect hypermobility: an adjunct to the assessment of patients with diffuse musculoskeletal pain. Int J Clin Pract. 2003;57(3):163–6.
6. Nicholson LL, Chan C. The upper limb hypermobility assessment tool: a novel validated measure of adult joint mobility. Musculoskelet Sci Pract. 2018;35:38–45.
7. Ferrari J, Parslow C, Lim E, Hayward A. Joint hypermobility: the use of a new assessment tool to measure lower limb hypermobility. Clin Exp Rheumatol. 2005;23(3):413–20
8. Meyer KJ, Chan C, Hopper L, Nicholson LL. Identifying lower limb specific and generalised joint hypermobility in adults: validation of the Lower Limb Assessment Score. BMC Musculoskelet Disord. 2017;18(1):514.
9. Grahame R, Bird HA, Child A, et al. The revised (Brighton 1998) criteria for the diagnosis of benign joint hypermobility syndrome (BJHS). J Rheumatol. 2000;27(7):1777–9.
10. Tinkle B, Castori M, Berglund B, Cohen H, Grahame R, Kazkaz H, Levy H. Hypermobile Ehlers-Danlos syndrome (a.k.a. Ehlers-Danlos syndrome Type III and Ehlers-Danlos syndrome hypermobility type): clinical description and natural

history. Am J Med Genet C Semin Med Genet. 2017. https://doi.org/10.1002/ajmg.c.31538.

11. Malfait F, Francomano C, ByersP T, et al. international classification of the Ehlers-Danlos syndromes. Am J Med Genet C Semin Med Genet. 2017;2017(175):8–26.
12. Copetti M, Morlino S, Colombi M, et al. Severity classes in adults with hypermobile Ehlers-Danlos syndrome/hypermobility spectrum disorders: a pilot study of 105 Italian patients. Rheumatology. 2019;58:1722–30.
13. Hakim A, O'Callaghan C, De Wandele I, Stiles L, Pocinki A, Rowe P. Cardiovascular autonomic dysfunction in Ehlers-Danlos syndrome-hypermobile type. Am J Med Genet C Semin Med Genet. 2017. https://doi.org/10.1002/ajmg.c.31543.
14. Roma M, Marden CL, De Wandele I, Francomano CA, Rowe PC. Postural tachycardia syndrome and other forms of orthostatic intolerance in Ehlers-Danlos syndrome. Auton Neurosci. 2018;215:89–96.
15. Bodenheimer T, et al. Patient self-management of chronic disease in primary care. J Am Med Assoc. 2002;288(19):2469–75.
16. Booshanam DS, et al. Evaluation of posture and pain in persons with benign joint hypermobility syndrome. Rheumatol Int. 2011;31(12):1561–5.
17. Boudreau SA, Hennings K, et al. The effects of training time, sensory loss and pain on human motor learning. J Oral Rehabil. 2010;37(9):704–18.
18. Celeney T, Kaya O. Effects of spinal stabilization exercises in women with benign joint hypermobility syndrome: a randomized controlled trial. Rheumatol Int. 2017;37:1461. https://doi.org/10.1007/s00296-017-3713-6
19. Boudreau SA, Farina D, et al. The role of motor learning and neuroplasticity in designing rehabilitation approaches for musculoskeletal pain disorders. Man Ther. 2010;15(5):410–4.
20. Keer R, Simmonds J. Joint protection and physical rehabilitation of the adult with hypermobility syndrome. Curr Opin Rheumatol. 2011;23(2):131–6.
21. Simmonds J, Herbland A, Hakim A, Ninis N, Lever W, Aziz Q, Cairns M. Attitudes, beliefs and behaviours towards exercise amongst individuals with joint hypermobility syndrome/Ehlers Danlos syndrome—hypermobility type. Disabil Rehabil. 2019;41(4):445–55. https://doi.org/10.1080/09638288.2017.1398278.
22. Tobias J, Deere K, Palmer S, Clinch J. Joint hypermobility is a risk factor for musculoskeletal pain during adolescence: findings of a prospective cohort study. 2013;65:1107–15.
23. Pacey V, et al. Exercise in children with joint hypermobility syndrome and knee pain: a randomised controlled trial comparing exercise into hypermobile versus neutral knee extension. Pediatr Rheumatol Online J. 2013;11(1):30.
24. Murray KJ. Hypermobility disorders in children and adolescents. Best Pract Res Clin Rheumat. 2006;20(2):329–51.
25. Fatoye FA, et al. Gait kinematics and passive knee joint range of motion in children with hypermobility syndrome. Gait Posture. 2011;33(3):447–51.
26. Bates AV, Alexander CM. Kinematics and kinetics of people who are hypermobile. A systematic review. Gait Post. 2015;41(2):361–9.
27. Morrison SC, et al. Assessment of gait characteristics and orthotic management in children with Developmental Coordination Disorder: preliminary findings to inform multidisciplinary care. Res Dev Disabil. 2013;34(10):3197–201.
28. Ferrell WR, et al. Musculoskeletal reflex function in the joint hypermobility syndrome. Arthritis Rheum. 2007;57(7):1329–33.
29. Sahin N, et al. Evaluation of knee proprioception and effects of proprioception exercise in patients with benign joint hypermobility syndrome. Rheumatol Int. 2008;28(10):995–1000.
30. Schubert-Hjalmarsson E, et al. Pain, balance, activity, and participation in children with hypermobility syndrome. Pediatr Phys Ther. 2012.
31. Simmonds JV, Keer RJ. Hypermobility and the hypermobility syndrome. Man Ther. 2007;12(4):298–309.
32. Billings S, Deane J, Bartholomew J, Simmonds JV. Paediatric physiotherapists perception of Joint Hypermobility Syndrome: a national survey. Physiother Pract Res. 2015;36(1):33–41.
33. Faigenbaum AD, et al. Youth resistance training: updated position statement paper from the national strength and conditioning association. J Strength Cond Res. 2009;23(5 Suppl):S60–79.
34. Faigenbaum AD, Myer GD. Pediatric resistance training: benefits, concerns, and program design considerations. Curr Sports Med Rep. 2010;9(3):161–8.
35. Garber CE, Blissmer B, Deschenes MR, Franklin BA, Lamonte MJ, Lee IM, Nieman DC, Swain DP, American College of Sports Medicine. American College of Sports Medicine position stand. Quantity and quality of exercise for developing and maintaining cardiorespiratory, musculoskeletal, and neuromotor fitness in apparently healthy adults: guidance for prescribing exercise. Med Sci Sports Exerc. 2011;43:1334–59.
36. Rombaut L, Malfait F, Cools A, De Paepe A, Calders P. Musculoskeletal complaints, physical activity and health-related quality of life among patients with the Ehlers-Danlos syndrome hypermobility type. Disabil Rehabil. 2010;32:1339–45.
37. de Wandele I, Rombaut L, Malfait F, De Backer T, De Paepe A, Calders P. Clinical heterogeneity in patients with the hypermobility type of Ehlers-Danlos Syndrome. Res Dev Disabil. 2013;34:873–81.

38. Engelbert RH, Juul-Kristensen B, Pacey V, de Wandele I, Smeenk S, Woinarosky N, Sabo S, Scheper MC, Russek L, Simmonds JV. The evidence-based rationale for physical therapy treatment of children, adolescents, and adults diagnosed with joint hypermobility syndrome/ hypermobile Ehlers Danlos syndrome. Am J Med Genet. 2017;175:158–67.
39. Sluka KA, Walsh D. Transcutaneous electrical nerve stimulation: basic science mechanisms and clinical effectiveness. J Pain. 2003;4(3):109–21.
40. Moseley GL. A pain neuromatrix approach to patients with chronic pain. Man Ther. 2003;8(3):130–40.
41. Busch AJ, et al. Exercise therapy for fibromyalgia. Curr Pain Headache Rep. 2011;15(5):358–67.
42. Wang XL, Chai Q, Charlesworth MC, Figueroa JJ, Low P, Shen W, Lee HC. Autoimmunoreactive IgGs from patients with postural orthostatic tachycardia syndrome. Proteomics Clin Appl. 2012;6:615–25.
43. Li H, et al. Autoimmune basis for postural tachycardia syndrome. J Am Heart Assoc. 2014;3:e000755. https://doi.org/10.1161/JAHA.113.000755.
44. Yu X, Li H, Murphy TA, Nuss Z, Liles J, Liles C, Aston C, Raj SR, Fedorowski A, Kem DC. Angiotensin II type 1 receptor autoantibodies in postural tachycardia syndrome. J Am Heart Assoc. 2018;7:e008351. https://doi.org/10.1161/JAHA.117.008351.
45. Gunning WT III, Kvale H, Kramer PM, Karabin BL, Grubb BP. Postural orthostatic tachycardia syndrome is associated with elevated G-protein coupled receptor autoantibodies. J Am Heart Assoc. 2019;8:e013602. https://doi.org/10.1161/JAHA.119.013602.
46. Thieben MJ, Sandroni P, Sletten DM, Benrud-Larson LM, et al. Postural orthostatic tachycardia syndrome: the Mayo clinic experience. Mayo Clin Proc. 2007;82:308.
47. Sandroni P, Low PA. Other autonomic neuropathies associated with ganglionic antibody. Auton Neurosci. 2009;146:13–7.
48. Wang X-L, Ling T-Y, Charlesworth MC, Figueroa JJ, Low P, Shen W, Lee HC. Autoimmunoreactive IgGs against cardiac lipid raft-associated proteins in patients with postural orthostatic tachycardia syndrome. Transl Res. 2013;162:34–44.
49. Blitshteyn S. Autoimmune markers and autoimmune disorders in patients with postural tachycardia syndrome (POTS). Lupus. 2015;24:1364–9.
50. Schofield JR, Blitshteyn S, Shoenfeld Y, Hughes GRV. Postural tachycardia syndrome (POTSPOTS) and other autonomic disorders in antiphospholipid (Hughes) syndrome (APS). Lupus. 2014;23:697–702.
51. Fukuda K, Straus S, Hickie I, et al. The chronic fatigue syndrome: a comprehensive approach to its definition and study. International Chronic Fatigue Syndrome Study Group. Ann Intern Med. 1994;121: 953–9.
52. Institute of Medicine, (National Academy of Medicine), Key Facts Leaflet. 2015.
53. Garner R, Baraniuk JN. Orthostatic intolerance in chronic fatigue syndrome. J Transl Med. 2019;17:185.
54. Stewart JM. Autonomic nervous system dysfunction in adolescents with postural orthostatic tachycardia syndrome and chronic fatigue syndrome is characterized by attenuated vagal baroreflex and potentiated sympathetic vasomotion. Pediatr Res. 2000;48:218–26.
55. Bou-Holaigah I, Rowe PC, Kan J, Calkins H. The relationship between neurally mediated hypotension and the chronic fatigue syndrome. JAMA. 1995;274:961–7.
56. Hoad A, Spickett G, Elliott J, Newton J. Postural orthostatic tachycardia syndrome is an under-recognized condition in chronic fatigue syndrome. Q J Med. 2008;101:961–5.
57. Okamoto LE, Raj SR, Peltier A, Gamboa A, et al. Neurohumoral and haemodynamic profile in postural tachycardia and chronic fatigue syndromes. Clin Sci (Lond). 2012;122:183–92.
58. Corbitt M, Eaton-Fitch N, Staines D, Cabanas H, Marshall-Gradisnik S. A systematic review of cytokines in chronic fatigue syndrome/myalgic encephalomyelitis/systemic exertion intolerance disease (CFS/ME/SEID). BMC Neurol. 2019;19:207.
59. Rahman A, Underwood M, Carnes D. Fibromyalgia. BMJ. 2014;348:28–32.
60. Wolfe F, Clauw DJ, Fitzcharles MA, et al. 2016 Revisions to the 2010/2011 fibromyalgia diagnostic criteria. Semin Arthritis Rheum. 2016;46:319–29.
61. Arnold LM, Bennett RM, Crofford LJ, Dean LE, Clauw DJ, Goldenberg DL, Fitzcharles M-A, Paiva ES, Staud R, Sarzi-Puttini P, Buskila D, Macfarlane GJ. AAPT diagnostic criteria for fibromyalgia. J Pain. 2019;20:611–28.
62. Eccles JA, Aslanyan D, Harrison NA, Davies KA, Critchley HD. Dissociative experiences in patients with fibromyalgia are mediated by symptoms of autonomic dysfunction. J Neurol Neurosurg Psychiatry. 2017;88(8):e21.
63. Tang S, Calkins H, Petri M. Neurally mediated hypotension in systemic lupus erythematosus patients with fibromyalgia. Rheumatol. 2004;43:609–14.
64. Kohr, D, Singh P, Tschernatsch M, Kaps M, Pouokam E, Diener, M, Kummer W, et al. Autoimmunity against the β2 adrenergic receptor and muscarinic-2 receptor in complex regional pain syndrome. Pain. 2011;152:2690–700.
65. Dubuis E, Thompson V, Leite MI, et al. Longstanding complex regional pain syndrome is associated with activating autoantibodies against alpha-1α adrenoceptors. Pain. 2014;155:2408–17.

66. Kinoshita T, Abe R-T, Hineno A, Tsunekawa K, Nakane S, Ikeda S. Peripheral sympathetic nerve dysfunction in adolescent Japanese girls following immunization with the human papillomavirus vaccine. Intern Med. 2014;53:2185–200.
67. Brinth LS, Pors K, Theibel AC, Mehlsen J. Orthostatic intolerance and postural tachycardia syndrome as suspected adverse effects of vaccination against human papilloma virus. Vaccine. 2015;33:2602–5.
68. Chandler R, Juhlin K, Fransson J, Caster O, Edwards IR, Norén GN. Current safety concerns with human papillomavirus vaccine: a cluster analysis of reports in VigiBase. Drug Saf. 2017;40:81–90.
69. Review concludes evidence does not support that HPV vaccines cause CRPS or POTS European Medicines Agency. EMA/714950/2015.

Headache in Postural Tachycardia Syndrome

Linda D'Antona and Manjit Matharu

Introduction

Patients with postural tachycardia syndrome (PoTS) have been reported to suffer headaches in up to 94% of the cases [1]. Among the myriad of symptoms that PoTS patients can be affected by, headache is very prevalent and has been reported as one of the five most common symptoms in PoTS by various authors [1–3]. In a large international survey on 4835 patients with PoTS, Shaw et al. highlighted that the most common comorbidity in PoTS is migraine (40%) [1]. Moreover, PoTS has been found to overlap with other comorbidities typically characterised by head and facial pain such as spontaneous intracranial hypotension and temporomandibular dysfunction [4, 5]. Headache in PoTS has diverse characteristics and it can be either a manifestation of the orthostatic intolerance secondary to PoTS or due to other underlying primary and secondary forms of headache. On occasions, headaches with different aetiologies can manifest in the same patient. The presence of headache in a PoTS patient can therefore pose diagnostic and therapeutic challenges: How can we differentiate between headache secondary to PoTS and other causes of headache? What is the best treatment strategy to manage PoTS patients with headache? Despite the rapidly increasing number of PoTS cases reported in the literature [6], only a few authors have provided a detailed description of the headache characteristics in their case series. In this chapter we summarise the current evidence on headache in PoTS patients and aim to provide information useful for the differential diagnosis and management of patients with headache and PoTS.

Prevalence of Headache in PoTS

The prevalence of headache as a symptom of PoTS has been reported to be between 28 and 100% [7, 8]. This sizeable range could be attributed to the diverse designs of the different studies. A summary of the articles reporting data on the prevalence of the headache in PoTS is provided in Table 1.

Since 2011, three single centre surveys and one international survey on the clinical presentation of PoTS have been published [1, 2, 8, 9]. Shaw et al. recently reported the results of an international online cross-sectional survey conducted involving a total of 4835 participants with a diagnosis of PoTS [1]. According to this study, headache was among the five most common symptoms of PoTS with a prevalence of

L. D'Antona · M. Matharu (✉)
Headache and Facial Pain Group, UCL Queen Square Institute of Neurology and The National Hospital of Neurology and Neurosurgery, Queen Square, London WC1N 3BG, UK
e-mail: m.matharu@uclmail.net

N. Gall et al. (eds.), *Postural Tachycardia Syndrome*, https://doi.org/10.1007/978-3-030-54165-1_13

Table 1 Prevalence of headache in patients with postural orthostatic tachycardia syndrome (POTS) reported in the literature

Author (Year)	Population studied	Type of study	Headache
Shaw et al. (2019) [1]	4835 patients diagnosed with POTS	International survey	3797 patients (94%)
Deb et al. (2015) [2]	39 patients diagnosed with POTS	Single centre survey	34 patients (87%)
Ohja et al. (2011) [9]	53 paediatric and 53 adult patients diagnosed with POTS	Single centre survey (Ohio Dysautonomia Survey ODYSA)	50 patients (54%)
Boris et al. (2018) [3]	708 paediatric patients diagnosed with POTS	Single centre retrospective study	142 patients as presenting symptom (20%) 644 patients as subsequent symptom (91%)
Jiawei et al. (2014) [11]	150 paediatric patients diagnosed with POTS	Single centre retrospective study	52 patients (35%)
Heyer et al. (2013) [8]	70 adolescent patients investigated with tilt table testing for POTS (37 confirmed diagnosis of POTS)	Single centre prospective survey	37 patients (100%)
Thieben et al. (2007) [10]	152 patients diagnosed with POTS	Single centre retrospective study	42 patients (28%)

94% following light-headedness (99%), tachycardia (97%), presyncope (94%) and difficulty concentrating (94%). A combination of all these five symptoms was reported by 83% of the participants [1]. Similarly, Deb et al. conducted a standardised survey in 39 patients with PoTS and found that headache had a high prevalence (87%) and was the third most common symptom following palpitations (92%) and fatigue (90%) [2].

Ojha et al. and Heyer et al. used surveys to investigate the clinical presentation of PoTS in the paediatric population and found a headache prevalence of 45.5% and 100%, respectively [8, 9]. Ojha et al. reported the results of the Ohio Dysautonomia Survey in 53 patients and only considered patients as having headaches if they complained of headache episodes with a duration of 4–72 hours (if untreated); this might be the reason why the headache prevalence they reported is lower when compared to other studies based on surveys. The headache was described as pulsating, one-sided, moderate or severe in intensity and worse with movement in most patients [9].

The two articles reporting the lowest headache prevalence are by Thieben et al. and Li et al., they are single centre retrospective studies on large cohorts of patients with PoTS (152 and 150 patients respectively) [7, 10–12]. These authors report a headache prevalence of 28 and 35%, respectively, which is significantly lower when compared to other studies based on standardised surveys. As a history of headaches had not been systematically sought in these patients, these prevalence figures are likely to be an under-representation of the actual prevalence of headache disorders.

In 2018, Boris et al. conducted a large retrospective study on 708 PoTS patients in the paediatric population. They reported that headache had a prevalence of 91% and was the second most common symptom after dizziness (95%). In addition, headache was the presenting symptoms for PoTS in 20% of the patients [3].

Apart from the work by Boris et al. and Heyer et al., studies based on surveys tended to give a higher prevalence of headache in PoTS when compared to retrospective studies. In a prospective study investigating the prevalence of headache in patients affected by severe autonomic failure, Robertson et al. reported that in their clinical experience only 25% of the patients voluntarily report this symptom [13]. These results imply that many patients with PoTS will report headaches only when asked about it thereby underlining the importance of actively asking about this symptom.

Migraine as a Comorbidity of PoTS

Migraine is an extremely common comorbidity in PoTS and has been reported to affect 28–40% of patients [1, 7]. According to a recent international survey conducted on 4835 patients, migraine is the most common comorbidity in PoTS [1]. In 2011, Khurana and Eisenberg investigated the clinical characteristics of a group of 24 patients with PoTS and reported that 23 out of 24 (96%) fulfilled the International Classification of Headache Disorders (ICHD) diagnostic criteria for migraine or probable migraine [14]. Their reported prevalence of migraine could however have been overestimated due to the nature of the study which only included patients referred to their highly specialised tertiary referral centre.

Another important observation supporting the association among these diseases, is that patients with migraine often suffer symptoms of autonomic impairment [15]. The population-based CAMERA study demonstrates that migraineurs have a higher prevalence of syncope, frequent syncope (five or more attacks) and orthostatic intolerance compared to control subjects [16].

Patients with migraine have been found to have a dysregulation of the sympathetic activity with downregulation in the interictal period (associated with low plasma norepinephrine) leading to an up-regulation of the post-synaptic adrenergic receptors. This up-regulation of post-synaptic adrenergic receptors results in hypersensitivity and an exaggerated sympathetic response to stimuli during the ictal period [15]. While there is still uncertainty regarding what may be the cause of this chain of events, this mechanism could explain why patients with migraine often present with symptoms such as nausea, vomiting, hyperhidrosis, flushing, and palpitations besides several other autonomic symptoms.

One of the reasons why migraine and PoTS often coexist in the same patients, may simply reside in the fact that these diseases tend to affect patients with similar demographic characteristics: young and female [1, 17]. However, the prevalence of migraine in PoTS patients clearly exceeds the prevalence of migraine in the general population, the latter being 6.5% in male and 18.2% in female subjects [17]. This suggests that there are fundamental aetiological drivers underlying the connection between these two diseases rather than a mere coincidental co-occurrence.

Our ability to identify a clear reason for this association is limited by the lack of knowledge of the aetiology and pathophysiology of PoTS as well as our partial understanding of the exact pathophysiology of migraine. Current theories recognise the role of intracranial hypersensitivity and deconditioning as potential linking mechanisms between migraine and POTS [7, 14, 15, 18]. According to Khurana and Eisenberg, migraine could induce central somatic and visceral sensitization in PoTS patients [14]. It should also be considered that migraine and the other often associated PoTS comorbidities (e.g. chronic fatigue syndrome, fibromyalgia, hypermobility syndromes) can significantly affect the patients' level of physical activity and lead to physical deconditioning, which could be an important factor in the development of orthostatic intolerance [15, 18].

Management of Migraine in PoTS

A diagnosis of migraine in patients with PoTS contributes to the overall disability; therefore, its treatment is essential. The management options for migraine are outlined in Table 2. As suggested by Khurana and Eisenberg, beta-blockers should be considered in patients with coexisting migraine and PoTS as both diseases can benefit from them though they have to be used

Table 2 Treatment options in the management of migraine

	Oral/Nasal	Injectable	Neurostimulation
Acute	• Oral and Intranasal Triptans • High dose NSAIDS • Paracetamo • Antiemetics	• Subcutaneous sumatriptan	• Transcranial magnetic stimulation • External trigeminal nerve stimulation (Cefaly) • Vagal nerve stimulation
Preventive	• Beta-blockers: Propranolol, Metoprolol, Timolol, Atenolol, Nadolol • Anticonvulsants: Topiramate, Valproate • Tricyclics: Amitriptyline • SNRI: Venlafaxine • Angiotensin pathway blockers: Lisinopril, Candesartan • Calcium channel blockers: Flunarizine • Nutraceuticals: Riboflavin, Coenzyme Q10, Magnesium, Feverfew	• Onabotulinumtoxin A • CGRP-pathway monoclonal antibodies	• External trigeminal nerve stimulation (Cefaly) • Transcranial magnetic stimulation • Occipital nerve stimulation • High cervical spinal cord stimulation
Transitional	• Corticosteroids	• Greater occipital nerve block • Multiple cranial nerve blocks • Intravenous dihydroergotamine • Intravenous lidocaine	

CGRP Calcitonin gene related peptide; *NSAIDS* Non-steroidal anti-inflammatory drugs; *SNRI* Serotonin and noradrenergic release inhibitors

judiciously as high doses can exacerbate hypotensive episodes [14]. Similarly, candesartan can also lead to hypotension and needs to be used cautiously.

Orthostatic Headache in PoTS: A Diagnostic Challenge

Most authors reporting the prevalence of headache as a symptom of PoTS do not provide an in-depth description of the headache characteristics. For this reason, information regarding the prevalence of orthostatic versus non-orthostatic headache in the PoTS population is limited. While the presence of orthostatic headache can raise the suspicion of PoTS, we do not have enough information to decide on the predictive and diagnostic value of this symptom. The importance of this issue is underlined by the fact that there are other conditions that can present with or mimic an orthostatic headache.

In 2013, Heyer et al. investigated the predictive value of orthostatic headache for the diagnosis of PoTS in a group of adolescent patients who underwent tilt table testing. Of the 70 investigated patients, 37 had a confirmed diagnosis of PoTS while the remaining 33 did not fulfil the diagnostic criteria [8]. Orthostatic headache was present in 89% of the patients with a final diagnosis of PoTS and 21% of the patients who did not have PoTS. According to their results, the report of orthostatic headache could predict a diagnosis of PoTS with a sensitivity and specificity of 89.2% and 78.8% respectively. The authors also found that orthostatic headache was typically preceded or triggered by dizziness in most patients with PoTS [8]. These findings suggest that the presence of orthostatic headache should raise the suspicion of PoTS and trigger further investigations. As stated by the authors, the main limitation of this study is the fact that only adolescent patients referred for tilt table testing were included, therefore we do not know if these predictive values would be applicable to a general population. In fact, a retrospective study by Graf et al. reports very different results, with a prevalence of orthostatic headache in PoTS of only 27% [19]. According to Khurana and Eisenberg instead, 62.5% of the patients with PoTS develop orthostatic headache during head-up tilt test [14]. These discrepancies point out the need for further evidence including in-depth characterisation of the headache in PoTS patients.

The reason why patients with PoTS present with orthostatic headache is unclear. Khurana and Eisenberg noticed that most of the patients with PoTS in their study had an underlying diagnosis of migraine and they suggested that migraine could predispose PoTS patients to orthostatic headache by inducing intracranial hypersensitivity; however there is no clear evidence that patients with PoTS and orthostatic headache have an underlying diagnosis of migraine [14]. Another interesting theory is proposed by Mokri who suggests that patients with PoTS may be affected by a relative CSF hypovolemia and that this is the cause of their orthostatic headache [5].

Orthostatic Headache Due to PoTS or Low CSF Pressure/Volume Syndrome?

The presence of orthostatic headache is not necessarily indicative of PoTS and it is in fact a typical symptom of low cerebrospinal fluid (CSF) pressure/volume syndromes such as spontaneous and iatrogenic intracranial hypotension (SIH). Two authors have highlighted a significant overlap among these conditions and the diagnostic challenge that this creates [5, 19].

In a small case series, Mokri describes four patients with orthostatic headache due to PoTS who received extensive investigations for a suspected CSF leak before reaching a correct diagnosis [5]. A recent study by Graf et al., also highlights an overlap between the clinical presentation and diagnosis of patients with PoTS and SIH [19]. The authors retrospectively looked at the results of the autonomic tests of a group of 57 patients who had a final diagnosis of CSF leak or PoTS. They found that orthostatic headache was more typical of CSF leaks than PoTS; this symptom was in fact present in all cases of CSF leak and only 27% of PoTS cases [19].

Graf et al. also found that every patient diagnosed with a CSF leak fulfilled the diagnostic criteria for PoTS according to head-up tilt test results. It is unclear why patients with a definite CSF leak should fulfil the PoTS diagnostic criteria although one hypothesis is that the presence of a CFS leak could be responsible for a significant reduction in physical activity and therefore lead to PoTS through a deconditioning mechanism. Another hypothesis comes from the observation that the hypermobile variant of Ehlers-Danlos Syndrome (hEDS) is associated with both PoTS and low CSF volume syndromes [1, 20, 21]. hEDS could have a role in the pathogenesis of both PoTS and low CSF volume/pressure syndromes and this would explain why some patients fulfil criteria for both diagnoses.

Another interesting outcome from the study by Graf et al. is the fact that neck stiffness was only present in CSF leaks patients and had a high specificity but low sensitivity; hence, the presence of neck stiffness in a patient with orthostatic headache could be suggestive of a low CSF pressure/volume syndrome rather than PoTS [19]. The headache location could also help differentiating PoTS from CSF leaks. According to Schievink, patients with low CSF pressure/volume syndromes frequently present with occipital headache (33%), while orthostatic headache caused by PoTS seems to more frequently have a frontal distribution [14, 22]. Khurana and Eisenberg's study reports that patients with orthostatic headache caused by PoTS tended to have a frontal, fronto-temporal or holocranial distribution, but not occipital [14].

While a diagnosis of PoTS can be achieved with relatively non-invasive investigations, the identification of a CSF leak (or SIH) often requires a number of invasive exams including brain and spinal MRIs, lumbar punctures and spinal imaging with intrathecal contrast [23].

Moreover, an incorrect diagnosis of SIH could lead to invasive procedures such as multiple epidural blood patches. For these reasons, it is paramount that any physician taking care of a patient with suspected low CSF pressure/volume syndrome should consider a potential diagnosis of PoTS, especially if other typical symptoms or demographic characteristics of PoTS are present and initial imaging investigations for SIH did not demonstrate positive findings.

In summary, the presence of orthostatic headache in a patient with suspected PoTS can create a diagnostic challenge for the physician. According to the available evidence and the authors' experience the following conclusions can be drawn:

- Low CSF pressure/volume syndromes are an important differential diagnosis in patients with suspected PoTS manifesting orthostatic headache.
- In patients with suspected CSF leaks, PoTS should be investigated before any invasive procedure, especially if other characteristics point towards a diagnosis of PoTS.
- PoTS and low CSF pressure/volume syndromes can coexist in the same patient [19].

Management of Orthostatic Headache Secondary to PoTS

The management of orthostatic headache secondary to PoTS is centred on treating the cardiovascular symptoms with lifestyle advice, volume expansion and pharmacological treatments (see chapters "Non-pharmacological Management (Hydration, Diet and Compression), Exercise Guidelines for Postural Tachycardia Syndrome, Medication in PoTS: An Overview, Midodrine, Ivabradine, β-blockers, Fludrocortisone, Octreotide, Clonidine and Other Medications: Desmopressin, Pyridostigmine Erythropoietin and SSRIs"). The outcomes of these treatments have not been systematically studied and thus are scarcely reported in the literature. Mokri and Low reported in their small case series of four patients that patients respond at least partially to these treatments [5]. The authors experience is that while the majority of patients report partial or complete resolution of orthostatic headaches following management of PoTS, a minority continue to have significant orthostatic headaches despite optimual management of the cardiovascular symptoms and the exclusion of a CSF leak.

Management of Orthostatic Headache Due to Spontaneous Intracranial Hypotension

In patients suspected of having SIH, magnetic resonance imaging (MRI) of the brain with gadolinium in considered the initial study for confirming the presence of SIH. MRI does not detect all cases of SIH and does not usually demonstrate the location of the CSF leak. Lumbar puncture with a low CSF opening pressure (<60 mmH_2O) is a confirmatory finding, but intracranial pressure can be normal in patients with SIH. Therefore, most experts defer lumbar puncture in the workup of SIH. Computed tomographic (CT) myelography is generally considered the best test to detect dural defects causing CSF leak, though dynamic CT myelography, magnetic resonance myelography and digital subtraction myelography can be helpful for localising the site of the CSF leak [24, 25].

Acute (<2 weeks), uncomplicated SIH is initially managed conservatively, with bedrest. Epidural blood patch (EBP) is considered first-line therapy in people who fail to respond to conservative management. Lumbar blood patches are often effective even with more cranially located defects. Blood patches targeted at the site of the CSF leak, fibrin sealant, or surgical closure may be needed in refractory cases [24, 25].

Headache in Patients with Hypermobility Syndromes and PoTS

The term hypermobility syndrome indicates conditions characterised by a heritable connective tissue disorder causing joint hypermobility and other manifestations of excessive connective tissue laxity [26]. Hypermobility syndromes have been found to be associated with PoTS in 25–49% of the patients and have been reported as one of the most common comorbidities in patients with PoTS [1, 20]. This association has important clinical implications as patients affected by hypermobility syndromes often present with headaches and this can further complicate the clinical picture of a patient with PoTS [27].

Castori et al. highlight the diverse potential causes of headache in patients with Ehlers-Danlos Syndromes (EDS) [27]. Besides migraine and orthostatic headache secondary to PoTS and CSF leaks, headaches can occur in EDS patients due to tension-type headache, new daily persistent headache, medication-overuse headache, temporomandibular dysfunction and cervicogenic headache. These conditions should therefore be considered as potential causes for headache in patients with PoTS especially if the patients present signs of joint hypermobility or connective tissue disorders.

Temporomandibular Dysfunction

EDS is believed to cause TMJ disorders through TMJ hypermobility and instability, however strong evidence supporting a clear association between the two conditions is still lacking [28]. The prevalence of TMJ disorders in PoTS was investigated by Durham et al. in 2015. The authors assessed the presence of a temporomandibular disorder in a cohort of 36 patients with confirmed diagnosis of PoTS and they found that 47% of the patients had a positive screening result. Though not all their patients complained of headache (only 39% reported headache) and only 2 patients had a diagnosis of EDS, they concluded that temporomandibular disorders are prevalent in PoTS patients [4].

Headache due to TMJ disorders should be suspected when the pain is aggravated by jaw motion or provoked by physical examination (temporalis muscle palpation, passive movement of the jaw), especially if located temporally [29]. These characteristics could help the clinician identify a potential component of TMJ disorder headache in patients with PoTS and treat them accordingly.

Headaches Due to Disorders of the Neck

Cervical spine hypermobility has been reported to cause cervicogenic headache [25]. Cervicogenic headache is caused by a disorder of the cervical spine and its component bony, disc and/or soft tissue elements, usually but not invariably accompanied by neck pain. The ICHD-3 diagnostic criteria require clinical and/or imaging evidence of a disorder or lesion within the cervical spine or soft tissues of the neck, known to cause headache [29]. Furthermore, the headache needs to develop in temporal relation to the cervical disorder, improve or resolve in parallel with improvement of the cervical disorder, demonstrate reduction in range of motion of the neck, worsen with provocation manoeuvres and be abolished following a diagnostic cervical block. Though a diagnosis of cervicogenic headache is frequently made in patients with hypermobility syndromes and neck pain, the authors' experience is that the vast majority do not fulfil the ICHD-3 diagnostic criteria as the neuroimaging is normal.

The cause of headaches and neck pain in these patients may be compression of the lesser and greater occipital nerves by the posterior cervical muscles and their fascial attachments at the occipital ridge with subsequent local perineural inflammation [30]. The resulting pain is typically in the sub-occipital and occipital location, and, via anatomic connections between extracranial and intracranial nerves, may radiate frontally to trigeminal-innervated areas of the head. Migraine-like features of photophobia and nausea may occur with frontal radiation. Occipital allodynia is common, as is spasm of the cervical muscles. Centrally acting membrane-stabilizing agents, which are often ineffective for migraine, are similarly generally ineffective for these patients. Extracranially-directed treatments such as occipital nerve blocks, cervical trigger point injections and botulinum toxin which act primarily in the periphery and may provide substantial relief.

Conclusions

Headache is an extremely common symptom in patients with PoTS and can have diverse pathogenetic mechanisms: it can be a manifestation of PoTS or due to a variety of other primary and secondary causes of headache. Diverse headache forms can occur at different times and can occasionally occur at the same time in patients with PoTS. For these reasons, the differential diagnosis can be quite challenging in PoTS patients. This review has highlighted the need for in-depth assessment of the headache phenotype in PoTS to aid the diagnostic process, thereby to guide the treatment and ultimately improve patient outcomes and quality of life. Finally, further research is needed to investigate the pathophysiology of the various headache disorders in PoTS and hypermobility syndromes as well as develop better treatments as there is a large unmet need.

References

1. Shaw BH, Stiles LE, Bourne K, Green EA, Shibao CA, Okamoto LE, et al. The face of postural tachycardia syndrome—insights from a large cross-sectional online community-based survey. J Intern Med. 2019;286(4):438–48.
2. Deb A, Morgenshtern K, Culbertson CJ, Wang LB, Hohler AD. A survey-based analysis of symptoms in patients with postural orthostatic tachycardia syndrome. Proc (Bayl Univ Med Cent). 2015;28(2):157–9.
3. Boris JR, Bernadzikowski T. Demographics of a large paediatric postural orthostatic tachycardia syndrome program. Cardiol Young. 2018;28(5):668–74.
4. Durham J, McDonald C, Hutchinson L, Newton JL. Painful temporomandibular disorders are common in patients with postural orthostatic tachycardia syndrome and impact significantly upon quality of life. J Oral Facial Pain Headache. 2015;29(2):152–7.
5. Mokri B, Low PA. Orthostatic headaches without CSF leak in postural tachycardia syndrome. Neurology. 2003;61(7):980–2.
6. Brinth L, Pors K, Spahic JM, Sutton R, Fedorowski A, Mehlsen J. Postural Orthostatic Tachycardia Syndrome (POTS) in Denmark: increasingly recognized or new epidemic? Auton Neurosci. 2018;213:92–5.
7. Thieben MJ, Sandroni P, Sletten DM, Benrud-Larson LM, Fealey RD, Vernino S, et al. Postural orthostatic tachycardia syndrome: the Mayo clinic experience. Mayo Clinic Proc. 2007;82(3):308–13.
8. Heyer GL, Fedak EM, LeGros AL. Symptoms predictive of postural tachycardia syndrome (POTS) in the adolescent headache patient. Headache. 2013;53(6):947–53.
9. Ojha A, Chelimsky TC, Chelimsky G. Comorbidities in pediatric patients with postural orthostatic tachycardia syndrome. J Pediatr. 2011;158(1):20–3.
10. Thieben MJ, Sandroni P, Sletten DM, Bernrud-Larson LM, Shen W, Low PA. Postural orthostatic tachycardia syndrome: the Mayo clinic experience. Mayo Clin Proc. 2007;82(3):308–13.
11. Jiawei L, Qingyou Z, Hongjun H, Hongfang J, Junbao D. Clinical features and management of postural tachycardia syndrome in children: a single-center experience. Chin Med J. 2014;127(21):3684–9.
12. Li J, Zhang Q, Hao H, Jin H, Du J. Clinical features and management of postural tachycardia syndrome in children: a single-center experience. Chin Med J (Engl). 2014;127(21):3684–9.
13. Robertson D, Kincaid DW, Haile V, Robertson RM. The head and neck discomfort of autonomic failure: an unrecognized aetiology of headache. Clin Auton Res. 1994;4(3):99–103.
14. Khurana RK, Eisenberg L. Orthostatic and non-orthostatic headache in postural tachycardia syndrome. Cephalalgia. 2011;31(4):409–15.
15. Miglis MG. Migraine and autonomic dysfunction: which is the horse and which is the jockey? Curr Pain Headache Rep. 2018;22(3):19.
16. Thijs RD, Kruit MC, van Buchem MA, Ferrari MD, Launer LJ, van Dijk JG. Syncope in migraine: the population-based CAMERA study. Neurology. 2006;66(7):1034–7.
17. Lipton RB, Stewart WF, Diamond S, Diamond ML, Reed M. Prevalence and burden of migraine in the United States: data from the American Migraine Study II. Headache. 2001;41(7):646–57.
18. Benarroch EE. Postural tachycardia syndrome: a heterogeneous and multifactorial disorder. Mayo Clinic Proc. 2012;87(12):1214–25.
19. Graf N, Fernandes Santos AM, Ulrich CT, Fung C, Raabe A, Beck J, et al. Clinical symptoms and results of autonomic function testing overlap in spontaneous intracranial hypotension and postural tachycardia syndrome. Cephalalgia Rep. 2018;1:1–6.
20. Kavi L, Gammage MD, Grubb BP, Karabin BL. Postural tachycardia syndrome: multiple

symptoms, but easily missed. Br J Gen Pract. 2012;62(599):286–7.

21. Liu FC, Fuh JL, Wang YF, Wang SJ. Connective tissue disorders in patients with spontaneous intracranial hypotension. Cephalalgia. 2011;31(6):691–5.
22. Schievink WI, Maya MM, Louy C, Moser FG, Sloninsky L. Spontaneous intracranial hypotension in childhood and adolescence. J Pediatr. 2013;163(2):504–10.
23. Kranz PG, Gray L, Amrhein TJ. Spontaneous intracranial hypotension: 10 myths and misperceptions. Headache. 2018;58(7):948–59.
24. Kranz PG, Gray L, Malinzak MD, Amrhein TJ. Spontaneous intracranial hypotension: pathogenesis, diagnosis, and treatment. Neuroimaging Clin N Am. 2019;29(4):581–94.
25. Mokri B. Spontaneous intracranial hypotension. Continuum. 2015;21(4 Headache):1086–108.
26. Castori M, Tinkle B, Levy H, Grahame R, Malfait F, Hakim A. A framework for the classification of joint hypermobility and related conditions. Am J Med Genet C Semin Med Genet. 2017;175(1):148–57.
27. Castori M, Morlino S, Ghibellini G, Celletti C, Camerota F, Grammatico P. Connective tissue, Ehlers-Danlos syndrome(s), and head and cervical pain. Am J Med Genet C Semin Med Genet. 2015;169C(1):84–96.
28. Dijkstra PU, Kropmans TJ, Stegenga B. The association between generalized joint hypermobility and temporomandibular joint disorders: a systematic review. J Dent Res. 2002;81(3):158–63.
29. Headache Classification Subcommittee of the International Headache Society. The international classification of headache disorders, 3rd edition. Cephalalgia. 2018;38:1–211.
30. Blake P, Burstein R. Emerging evidence of occipital nerve compression in unremitting head and neck pain. J Headache Pain. 2019;20(1):76.

Postural Tachycardia Syndrome and Sleep

Guy Leschziner

Introduction

Sleep complaints and fatigue are almost universal in patients with postural tachycardia syndrome (PoTS). Fatigue is reported by 97% of patients, 83% of patients complain of unrefreshing sleep and over 60% complain of sleep maintenance and sleep initiation difficulties [1].

Despite these extremely high levels of subjective sleep disturbance, the relationship between PoTS and sleep disturbances remain unclear. Very few patients with sleep disturbance seek out medical attention for this aspect of their condition, and there is often discordance between subjective reports of sleepiness and objective testing. Some authors conclude, usually from relatively small studies, that PoTS patients differ from normal controls only in their subjective reports of fatigue and sleepiness, but not objective measures of sleepiness or sleep architecture, and that sleep-related complaints in PoTS are not directly attributable to the underlying pathophysiology of the condition, but are multifactorial, related to chronic pain, fatigue, bladder disturbance or other symptoms [2, 3].

G. Leschziner (✉)
Department of Neurology and Sleep Disorders Centre, Guy's and St Thomas' NHS Foundation Trust, London, UK
e-mail: Guy.Leschziner@gstt.nhs.uk

Department of Basic and Clinical Neuroscience, Institute of Psychiatry, Psychology and Neuroscience, King's College London, London, UK

Nevertheless, some studies have demonstrated objective differences. PoTS patients have been shown to have a higher proportion of stage II sleep, and differential changes in heart rate variability in different stages of sleep [4]. Our own research has demonstrated an association between subjective sleepiness and enhanced activation of the parasympathetic nervous system [5], although once again we did not find evidence of objective sleepiness or abnormal sleep architecture. A further study has once again confirmed no significant differences in objective measures of sleep in PoTS patients but has suggested that sympathetic activation may contribute to the hyperarousal state and thus worsen the subjective experience of sleep [6].

Despite the dearth of systematic evidence in this field, clinical experience suggests that improvement of sleep quality in PoTS firstly improves quality of life, but may also improve other facets of the condition, such as pain, fatigue, headache and mood disturbance. Therefore, in a condition where successful treatment can be problematic, efforts to identify and treat sleep disturbance may result in significant improvements.

Types of Sleep Disturbance in PoTS

It once again needs to be stressed that the evidence base for sleep disturbance in PoTS remains extremely limited. Therefore, much of

N. Gall et al. (eds.), *Postural Tachycardia Syndrome*, https://doi.org/10.1007/978-3-030-54165-1_14

this chapter relates to clinical experience in the sleep clinic setting. Obviously, patients with PoTS may also experience any of the sleep pathologies that the normal population experiences, but there are certain sleep pathologies that seem to be more frequently encountered in patients with PoTS.

Patients with PoTS exhibit a number of patterns of sleep disturbance. Perhaps the commonest is that of sleep initiation insomnia [7]. This group of patients typically describes lying awake in bed for hours, with major difficulty getting off to sleep. They will complain of a racing, active mind, mental rumination and steadily increasing anxiety about the process of getting off to sleep. On waking, they will feel extremely unrefreshed and fatigued. Despite the extremely short sleep opportunity and profound feelings of sleepiness, they will find it impossible to nap during the day. This group of patients is usually suffering from psychophysiological insomnia, the commonest form of insomnia seen in the general population. Psychophysiological insomnia is characterised by frustration with the process of going to sleep, hyperarousal, rumination and anxiety and pre-occupation regarding the process of going to sleep. The hyperarousal state is often driven by a vicious cycle of anxiety regarding the daytime consequences of poor sleep, resulting in patients trying to actively manage the problem of going to sleep, which worsens failure of mental relaxation and exacerbates the insomnia. The state of hyperarousal is present during the day as well, which explains the difficulty napping during the day as well. It is easy to understand why patients with PoTS, who may already be in a hyperarousal state, are more likely to develop this disorder.

Occasionally some patients may complain of severe sleep initiation or sleep maintenance insomnia, but objective measurements of sleep architecture show normal sleep. This is termed paradoxical insomnia, or sleep state misperception. It is not clear if this is related to lack of awareness of sleep state or due to an underlying sleep pathology that remains to be elucidated.

Less frequently, patients with PoTS may complain of sleep initiation insomnia due to an alternative cause. Clinical features that should raise the possibility of an alternative underlying cause include high measures of subjective sleepiness during the day, reports of napping (rather than simply resting) by family members, or a very late waking time. Restless legs syndrome (RLS) is an extremely common finding in the PoTS population, although it should be stressed that it is extremely common in the general population too [8]. This neurological disorder is characterised by an urge to move the body, typically but not invariably the legs, often associated with unpleasant sensations. The urge to move is under circadian influence and is worse in the evening or night. It is also worsened by immobility and improved either partially or transiently by movement of the affected body parts. Patients will often describe involuntary movements of the lower legs, either in wakefulness in the evening, or arising from sleep, termed periodic limb movements. The sensory symptoms often give rise to sleep initiation issues, and the periodic limb movements of sleep can generate sleep maintenance insomnia or extremely unrefreshing sleep. In contrast to patients with psychophysiological insomnia however, patients with RLS will often report high levels of sleepiness in the day, since the RLS symptoms are absent or far less pronounced in the daytime. In practice, RLS may sometimes be difficult to distinguish from the positional discomfort patients with PoTS often complain of, but the clear circadian fluctuation of symptoms should be a red flag for RLS.

Another cause of apparent sleep initiation insomnia is delayed sleep phase syndrome (DSPS), a circadian rhythm disorder where the onset of sleepiness and wakefulness is much later than the general population. Patients will not feel sleepy until late in the night or even in the small hours of the morning, and will want to wake up extremely late, sometimes well into the afternoon. When allowed to do so, they will sleep for a normal duration, and will be refreshed on waking. Thus, while overtly exhibiting sleep initiation difficulties, they will simply state they do not feel tired or sleepy at "normal" bedtime. DSPS may be genetically driven but may also be related to bright light exposure late in the evening.

A second pattern of sleep disturbance is that of severe sleep maintenance insomnia. Once again, the commonest cause in PoTS is that of a hyperarousal state generating psychophysiological insomnia, although again, periodic limb movements of sleep (PLMS) may be an alternative explanation. Whilst PLMS are almost invariably found in the presence of symptoms of RLS, some 50% of patients with PLMD will not exhibit RLS symptoms. Thus, the presence of sleep maintenance insomnia in the context of subjective excessive daytime sleepiness, even in the absence of symptoms of RLS, should lead the clinician to consider the possibility of PLMS. Other causes of sleep maintenance insomnia include joint pain, urinary frequency or waking with a tachycardia in a high arousal state, but also non-PoTS-associated conditions such as obstructive sleep apnoea (OSA). Anecdotally, OSA in PoTS is rarer than in the general population, perhaps largely due to OSA being associated with male gender, increasing age, and obesity.

The final pattern of sleep disturbance seen is that of excessive sleepiness during the day in the context of a very prolonged unbroken sleep duration. In the absence of PoTS or any other medical or psychiatric condition, this would be termed idiopathic hypersomnia, an extremely rare central hypersomnia. In the context of PoTS however, this may also represent psychiatric hypersomnolence related to depression [9], or sleep state misperception; patients may report unbroken deep sleep during the night or in daytime naps, but objective PSG recordings may show EEG evidence of wakefulness.

Evaluation of Sleep Disturbance in PoTS

For the vast majority of patients, investigations are unnecessary and unsuccessful. Patients with psychophysiological insomnia tolerate polysomnography poorly, and frequently do not sleep at all when admitted for sleep studies. Referral to a sleep service and polysomnography should be reserved for patients in whom there is a realistic expectation of identifying specific sleep pathology. Therefore, patients who describe poor quality sleep or insomnia, in the absence of excessive daytime sleepiness or any other features suggestive of other sleep pathologies, should not be routinely investigated. A number of validated questionnaires can be used to assess sleep quality, to identify particular sleep problems or to assess subjective sleepiness, with the Epworth sleepiness scale and the Pittsburgh Sleep Quality Index being amongst the most widely used. The mean Epworth score in the general population is 5 or 6, and typically patients with organic sleep pathology will have scores above this, while patients with psychophysiological or paradoxical insomnia will usually describe Epworth scores of less than this.

Restless legs syndrome is a clinical diagnosis and does not rely upon polysomnography, although a sleep study may be helpful in determining the presence of periodic limb movements in sleep in a patient in whom the nature of their sensory symptoms is uncertain. Investigations in RLS should be directed towards excluding underlying causes of symptomatic RLS, such as ensuring that renal function is normal and that iron levels are adequate. It is recommended that patients with RLS should be treated with iron supplementation until serum ferritin is over 75 mcg/L, since lower levels are associated with the condition and increase the risk of augmentation—where dopa agonists in the long-term drive a worsening of the RLS—resulting from treatment [8].

Polysomnography is indicated for patients with suspected periodic limb movement disorder in the absence of RLS, sleep apnoea, unusual behaviours at night (parasomnias), or who are excessively sleepy during the day. If a central hypersomnia is being considered, polysomnography should be performed alongside a multiple sleep latency test, to confirm objective excessive sleepiness. Actigraphy should be performed for those patients in whom a circadian rhythm disorder is being considered. Patients will frequently utilise commercially available sleep trackers. While these are generally not recommended for insomnia, due to concerns regarding reliability of sleep staging and detecting awakenings at night, they can be helpful in determining sleep onset and sleep offset. Therefore, they may provide useful data when evaluating for a circadian rhythm disorder.

Treatment of Sleep Disturbance in PoTS

Due to the nature of this multifaceted disorder, pharmacological management of sleep disorders can exacerbate other aspects of PoTS and the treatment of other symptoms can dramatically influence sleep. Therefore, perhaps even more so than in the general population, sleep issues should be dealt with using non-pharmacological therapies as much as possible. For any patient with a sleep disorder, the first step is to ensure optimal sleep hygiene. Patients should be made aware of the behaviours that improve and reduce the quality of sleep. Alcohol, caffeine and tobacco should be avoided, a relaxing bedtime routine should be initiated, and exposure to bright light in the evening should be limited; the latter is of particular importance for patients with delayed sleep phase syndrome. The bedroom should be a place for sleep, not any other activities, with an aim of building positive associations between the bedroom environment and sleep. Evidence points to cognitive behavioural therapy for insomnia (CBTi) being a useful non-pharmacological therapy, with better long-term outcomes than drug-based treatments in isolation. Anecdotally, patients with PoTS respond to CBTi extremely well.

Efforts should be made to remove drugs that may worsen sleep. Particular culprits in PoTS include drugs that are prescribed for mood disturbance, pain relief and co-morbid mast cell activation syndrome. Antidepressants, beta blockers and antihistamines can precipitate or worsen RLS, and if RLS and associated sleep initiation insomnia are very prominent, the use of these drugs should be reconsidered. For patients with significant day-time sleepiness, iatrogenic causes should be borne in mind. Gabapentin, pregabalin, tricyclics and opiates in particular can cause significant sedation, and the relationship between dose and sedating effect is extremely variable between individuals.

Prescribing in PoTS should be undertaken cautiously and slowly. For sleep initiation or sleep maintenance insomnia without any underling organic sleep pathology, melatonin can be prescribed as an adjunct to CBTi. It is extremely well-tolerated, and while not effective for all, can have dramatic effects on sleep for some. There is no significant evidence of dependency, and in view of its safety profile and tolerability, should be considered first-line, if pharmacological therapy is being considered. Melatonin can also be helpful in the shifting of sleep phase, but this should be undertaken by an experienced sleep physician, as the direction of shift is dependent on when the melatonin is given in relation to the patient's endogenous circadian rhythm. Light therapy may also help, particularly when delivered by a high lux light box, but once again, timing is crucial. For RLS, dopa agonists are licensed in the UK, but gastrointestinal side effects and postural hypotension can limit their use in PoTS. Drugs such as gabapentin and pregabalin can very extremely useful in this context, since they are effective for RLS, periodic limb movements of sleep, help musculoskeletal pain associated with sleep, and have beneficial effects on sleep architecture. Where migraine is a prominent feature alongside sleep disturbance, pizotifen may provide some mild sedative effects and is usually well tolerated in PoTS.

The use of stimulant drugs should be very limited in PoTS. Drugs such as modafinil and methylphenidate have a role in patients with demonstrable objective excessive sleepiness, for which no other cause has been identified, but do not generally have any major impact on fatigue and should not be used in this context. Furthermore, the side effect profile of these drugs is particularly problematic in PoTS, as they can cause tachycardia, anxiety, headache, palpitations and gastrointestinal problems. They should only be initiated after a full evaluation by an experienced sleep clinician.

Conclusions

Sleep disturbance is an extremely common feature in PoTS, although the association between PoTS and specific sleep pathologies remains under investigation. Addressing these sleep complaints however can improve multiple aspects of PoTS, including fatigue, pain, headache and mood. A proper evaluation of sleep is important, and management needs to be appropriately tailored to avoid exacerbating other features of the syndrome.

References

1. Xu X, Huang H, Sethi S, Zuzuarregui JR, Weinberg J, Hohler AD. A survey based study on sleep disturbance in postural tachycardia syndrome. J Neurol Sci. 2016;365:199–202.
2. Bagai K, Wakwe CI, Malow B, Black BK, Biaggioni I, Paranjape SY, et al. Estimation of sleep disturbances using wrist actigraphy in patients with postural tachycardia syndrome. Auton Neurosci. 2013;177(2):260–5.
3. Miglis MG, Muppidi S, Feakins C, Fong L, Prieto T, Jaradeh S. Sleep disorders in patients with postural tachycardia syndrome. Clin Auton Res. 2016;26(1):67–73.
4. Mallien J, Isenmann S, Mrazek A, Haensch CA. Sleep disturbances and autonomic dysfunction in patients with postural orthostatic tachycardia syndrome. Front Neurol. 2014;5:118.
5. Pengo MF, Higgins S, Drakatos P, Martin K, Gall N, Rossi GP, et al. Characterisation of sleep disturbances in postural orthostatic tachycardia syndrome: a polysomnography-based study. Sleep Med. 2015;16(12):1457–61.
6. Bagai K, Peltier AC, Malow BA, Diedrich A, Shibao CA, Black BK, et al. Objective sleep assessments in patients with postural tachycardia syndrome using overnight polysomnograms. J Clin Sleep Med. 2016;12(5):727–33.
7. Winkelman JW. CLINICAL PRACTICE. Insomnia Disorder. N Engl J Med. 2015;373(15):1437–44.
8. Leschziner G, Gringras P. Restless legs syndrome. BMJ. 2012;344:e3056.
9. Plante DT. Sleep propensity in psychiatric hypersomnolence: a systematic review and meta-analysis of multiple sleep latency test findings. Sleep Med Rev. 2017;31:48–57.

Investigations of Endocrinopathies

Abbi Lulsegged

Introduction

The symptoms of neurocardiogenic conditions such as postural tachycardia syndrome overlap with a considerable number of endocrine conditions. Some of these such as Addison's disease and phaeochromocytoma are fortunately rare, but nevertheless important diagnoses. Others, such as thyroid dysfunction, are more common and likely to contribute to the symptom burden. The aim of this chapter is to familiarise health care practitioners with these endocrine conditions, including investigations employed to rule them out.

Phaeochromocytoma/Paraganglioma

Definition

Phaeochromocytoma: tumour arising from adrenomedullary chromaffin cells, commonly secrete catecholamines (epinephrine, norepinephrine or dopamine).

Paraganglioma: tumour arising from extra-adrenal chromaffin cells, which may or may not secrete catecholamines.

Very rare: incidence approximately 1 per million per year. The incidence seems to be rising, but possibly as a result of better detection rates [1].

The vast majority arise from the adrenal glands and are benign. Extra-meduallary phaeochromocytomas are more likely to be malignant.

Clinical Features

Approximately 50% are asymptomatic. Clinical features include palpitations, high blood pressure, fever, headaches, breathlessness, tremor, and pallor. These symptoms can be episodic.

Spells can be triggered by certain events such as surgery, anaesthesia, labour, medications (sympathomimetics such as ephedrine, opioids, anti-depressants, neuromuscular blockers).

Beta-blockers can precipitate a crisis if they are given without adequate alpha-blockade.

Clinical pearls:

1. The triad of palpitations, sweating and headaches in a patient with hypertension increases the likelihood of a phaeochromocytoma [2].
2. Patients might have episodic surges in blood pressure.

Screening

Case finding (who to screen) [3]:

- Patients with signs and symptoms, especially with hypertension, which might be episodic.
- Adrenal incidentaloma, with or without hypertension.
- Family history of phaeochromocytoma or paraganglioma.

A. Lulsegged (✉)
HEALTH121 Ltd, London, UK
e-mail: admin@health121.co.uk

N. Gall et al. (eds.), *Postural Tachycardia Syndrome*, https://doi.org/10.1007/978-3-030-54165-1_15

- Past history of phaeochromocytoma or paraganglioma.
- Young patient (<40 years of age) with hypertension.
- Resistant hypertension (BP still elevated despite taking 3 or more antihypertensive agents).

Measurement
Single fractionated Plasma metanephrines is the test of choice [4].

Do not request urinary catecholamines or Vanillylmandelic Acid as they are not as accurate.

24-hour urine fractionated metanephrines are an acceptable alternative.

Procedure for Measurement of Plasma Metanephrines
The patient should fast overnight.

Encourage the patient to avoid the following for 48 hours prior to the test: caffeine, decaffeinated products, spicy food, bananas, cheese, citrus fruits, alcohol, cigarette smoking.

Patient must be supine for a minimum of 30 minutes before blood is taken.

Highly sensitive test—increased risk of false positive.

Refer urgently to Endocrinology if positive.

False Positives
Note medications associated with elevated plasma metanephrines, especially certain antidepressants and midodrine [5].

Other medications include:

Falsely elevated normetanephrine: paracetamol, alpha-methyldopa, tricyclic antidepressants, MAO inhibitors, cocaine, sulphasalazine, levodopa

Falsely elevated metanephrines: buspirone, MAO inhibitors, sympathomimetics, cocaine, levodopa.

Discuss with Biochemistry Consultant or Endocrinologist if any doubt. Do not discontinue medications without consulting with prescribing physician where relevant.

Neuroendocrine Tumours

Definition
Heterogenous group of tumours that arise from enterochromaffin cells of the endocrine and nervous systems. They are classified according to the degree of differentiation as opposed to anatomical location.

Carcinoid tumours are those that arise from the gastrointestinal tract cells. The majority of carcinoid tumours are discovered coincidentally, for example, during surgery, are non-functional and do not produce symptoms. Approximately 10% however secrete hormones and peptides associated with symptoms.

Carcinoid Syndrome
Characterised by classical signs and symptoms associated with excessive production of hormones and peptides by cells of the gastrointestinal tract but especially those of the small intestine. Functional tumours of the jejunoileum, appendix and ascending colon ("mid-gut") are most likely to over secrete Serotonin.

Clinical features

Flushing (typically dry, pink to purple in colour affecting the face and upper torso, lasting a few minutes to a few hours)
Palpitations
Abdominal pain
Diarrhoea
Wheezing
Hepatomegaly
Anaemia
Congestive cardiac failure
Valvular disorders—tricuspid regurgitation.

Carcinoid crises are characterised by labile blood pressure, palpitations, tachycardia, profound flushing and wheezing.

Investigations
Serum Chromogranin A(CgA): glycoprotein expressed by neuroendocrine cells. CgA can be elevated in a wide range of neuroendocrine conditions. However, it is also elevated by renal failure, proton pump inhibitors and by non-functioning tumours so caution is required when interpreting results [6].

Serum chromogranin B: this is rarely elevated in the presence of a neuroendocrine tumour when the CgA might be normal and so the two are requested together especially if there is a strong index of suspicion. It is less likely to be affected by renal impairment.

24-hour urine for 5-Hydroxyindoleacetic acid (5HIAA). Elevated levels have a high sensitivity and specificity. Needs to be collected in an acidic container. 5-HIAA are affected by certain foods and substances which should be avoided for at least 48 hours prior to collection. These include pineapples, plums, kiwi, avocados, bananas, walnuts, tomatoes, nicotine, paracetamol, 5-HTP supplements and cough remedies.

Management
Refer to Endocrinology if CgA or 24-hour urinary 5HIAA are elevated or the patient has signs and symptoms.

Adrenal Insufficiency

Potentially catastrophic condition.

Presentation includes abdominal pain (which might be unexplained), nausea, dizziness, light-headedness, weight loss, increased pigmentation (especially of sun-exposed areas), salt craving.

Clinical features of an acute adrenal crises include collapse, significant weakness, hypotension, reduced level of consciousness, acute abdominal signs including guarding and tenderness.

Contiguous deletion of *CYP21A2* (gene that codes 21-OH hydroxylase implicated in adrenal deficiency associated with congenital adrenal hyperplasia) and *TNXB* (gene that codes for a connective tissue extracellular matrix protein implicated in a joint hypermobility syndrome) has been described and provides a potential important connection [7].

One of the most common causes of adrenal deficiency is exogenous steroids—including inhaled steroids and this is under-appreciated.

Screening
If there is any doubt, test adrenal function.

Signs and symptoms:

Hypotension especially if it is associated with abnormal biochemistry—see below.

Fever, abdominal pain, excess pigmentation, hypoglycaemia (particularly in younger patients).

Potential clues from Biochemistry and haematology results:

Hyponatraemia—can be a late feature
Hyperkalaemia (not present in hypoadrenalism caused by pituitary/hypothalamic disease or secondary to exogenous steroids)
Normocytic anaemia
Metabolic acidosis
Eosinophilia.

Testing
Serum cortisol:

Ideally after an overnight fast.
Exclude exogenous steroid use which can be in the form of a recent intra-articular injection (and therefore, the patient might not think to report this), steroid creams, inhalers and tablets.

Importantly, the blood test needs to be taken before 9 a.m. in view of the circadian rhythm.

Hormone replacement therapy or oral contraceptive pill can increase total cortisol levels and needs to be discontinued for 6 weeks before testing. Ensure adequate contraceptive is substituted if this is advised.

Interpretation:

Pre-9 a.m. cortisol readings below 140 nmol/L—hypoadrenalism likely. Refer urgently to Endocrinology. Also, refer for admission urgently if patient is unwell, vomiting or has diarrhoea. In these circumstances immediately administer hydrocortisone 100 mg IM stat.

In one study, a basal cortisol less than 420 nmol/L had 100% sensitivity and 54% specificity for failing a short synacthen test while a baseline cortisol below 142 nmol/L had a 100% specificity and 35% sensitivity for failing the short synacthen test [8].

Therefore, a short synacthen test is unnecessary if the baseline cortisol taken at 9 a.m. is above 420 nmol/L. A pre-9 a.m. cortisol value between 140 and 420 lies in the "grey zone" and it is important to assess each case individually. A low threshold for referring for a short synacthen test should be considered for those with unusual features such as unexplained abdominal complaints, unintentional weight loss and/or hyperpigmentation. If there is any doubt, discuss with Endocrine colleagues.

If in doubt, discuss with Endocrinology

Protocol for Short synacthen test:
0900: Take blood for cortisol and ACTH.
Give Tetracosactride (ACTH) 250 mcg intravenously (can be given intramuscularly) [9].
0930: Take blood for 30-minute cortisol.
1000: Take blood for 60-minute cortisol.
Interpretation of short synacthen test:

Peak cortisol level below 500 nmol/L at 30 minutes or 60 minutes requires referral to Endocrinology.

Thyroid Dysfunction

A lot of the symptoms attributable to PoTS overlap with symptoms of thyroid dysfunction. This includes cold intolerance, difficulty regulating body temperature, palpitations, fatigue and weakness. Therefore, testing for thyroid dysfunction is almost mandatory.

Hypothyroidism is relatively common.

Routinely, enquire about a family history or past medical history of thyroid dysfunction.

Investigations
Thyroid function tests to include thyroid antibodies if family history or past medical history of thyroid dysfunction present.

Possible Abnormalities
Subclinical hypothyroidism or very early primary thyroid failure.

TSH elevated; normal free thyroid hormone/within reference range.

Not all cases require treatment as elevations in TSH can be transient.

Therefore, arrange repeat tests in the first instance.

Treatment indicated if TSH persistently elevated >10–20 miu/L, especially if associated with positive thyroid antibodies.

Overt Hypothyroidism
Elevated TSH associated with reduced free T4 level.

Treatment almost always indicated.

This can be initiated in primary care with the advice to titrate the dose of Levothyroxine to achieve an TSH no higher than 3 miu/L in young patients and no higher than 4.5 miu/L in elderly patients.

Isolated Hypothyroxinaemia
Differential diagnoses include assay interference, central hypothyroidism e.g. secondary to pituitary tumour (and therefore a potentially important cause) and iodine deficiency.

Discuss with/refer to Endocrinology if confirmed on repeat test.

Referral to, or discussion with Endocrinology is indicated in the following scenarios in which the thyroid function tests are abnormal:

(1) Unusual thyroid function tests e.g. low free T4 but normal TSH or raised TSH and free T4.
(2) Female planning pregnancy.
(3) Patients with pre-existing cardiac disease.

(4) Medication induced thyroid dysfunction e.g. amiodarone or immune modifying drugs.
(5) Patients with a goitre.
(6) Suspected viral thyroiditis (neck tenderness, raised inflammatory markers, abnormal thyroid function tests).
(7) Suspected adrenal dysfunction—do not start thyroxine until this has been confirmed and treated.

Reactive Hypoglycaemia

Definition

Four key components:

1. Hypoglycaemia, ideally, measured by lab glucose. The exact cut-off for hypoglycaemia will vary but typically laboratory glucose below 3 mmol/L
2. Presence of symptoms subdivided into (i) adrenergic symptoms such as palpitations, sweating, tremor, anxiety and (ii) neuroglycopenic/cholinergic including confusion, blurred vision, fatigue, hunger pangs, sensory symptoms.
3. Onset of hypoglycaemia and symptoms following a precipitating meal.
4. Resolution of symptoms with correction of hypoglycaemia.

Importance

1. Anecdotal experience that reactive hypoglycaemia is common in patients with PoTS. Discriminating questions include dips in energy levels mid-morning and/or mid-afternoon (can be profound) and sugar cravings/improvement in symptoms on consuming carbohydrate based snacks [10].
2. Signs and symptoms considerably overlap with those of PoTS including pallor.
3. Likely significant cause of symptom burden.
4. Addressing condition is potentially rewarding.

Testing

Recommended gold standard test: Mixed Meal 5-hour prolonged glucose tolerance test.

Alternative: 5-hour Prolonged Oral Glucose Tolerance Test [11].

Needs to be performed with trained, ideally experienced nurse in attendance.

Do not perform the test in patients with a history of, or suspicion of, periodic paralysis. Refer to Endocrinology if any doubt.

Cautions

Patients with history of heart disease, epilepsy or suspected epilepsy.

Encourage patients to remain hydrated before and during the test, otherwise there is a high likelihood of worsening PoTS-related symptoms during the test.

Treatment

Avoidance, especially, of high glycaemic index foods.

Ideally, a low carbohydrate, high fat diet is excellent for rapidly controlling symptoms of reactive hypoglycaemia. Persistence of symptoms after 4 weeks of implementing a very low carbohydrate diet is unlikely to be due to reactive hypoglycaemia.

Caution with Low Carbohydrate Diet

Transient side effects during the first 2 weeks including osmotic diuresis, constipation, weakness, irritability and headaches.

Patients with histamine intolerance.

Pre-existing fat malabsorption.

Refer

Patients with symptoms suggestive of spontaneous hypoglycaemia (to exclude rare causes such as insulin producing tumour).

Persistent symptoms despite implementing treatment.

Difficulty with implementing diet.

References

1. Berends AMA, Buitenwerf E, de Krijger RR, Veeger NJGM, van der Horst-Schrivers ANA, Links TP, Kerstens MN. Incidence of pheochromocytoma and sympathetic paraganglioma in the Netherlands: a nationwide study and systematic review. Eur J Intern Med. 2018;51:68–73.

2. Pourian M, Mostafazadeh DB, Soltani A. Does this patient have pheochromocytoma? A systematic review of clinical signs and symptoms. J Diabetes Metab Disord. 2016;31(15):11.
3. Jacques W, Lenders M, Duh Q-Y, Eisenhofer G, Gimenez-Roqueplo A-P, Grebe SKG, Murad MH, Naruse M, Pacak K, Young WF. Pheochromocytoma and paraganglioma: an endocrine society clinical practice guideline. J Clin Endocrinol Metabol. 2014;99(6):1915–42.
4. Neumann HPH, Young WF Jr, Eng C. Pheochromocytoma and Paraganglioma. N Engl J Med. 2019;381(6):552–65.
5. Farah G, Grossman A, Lulsegged A, Gall N. Grossly elevated plasma metanephrine levels due to midodrine, an [alpha]1 receptor agonist, in a patient presenting with postural orthostatic tachycardia syndrome. Endocrine Abstracts (2015) 37 EP1237. https://doi.org/10.1530/endoabs.37.ep1237. Accessed 31 Aug 2019.
6. Lawrence B, Gustafsson BI, Kidd M, Pavel M, Svejda B, Modlin IM. The clinical relevance of chromogranin a as a biomarker for gastroenteropancreatic neuroendocrine tumors. Endocrinol Metab Clin N Am. 2011;40:111–34.
7. Miller WL, Merke DP. Tenascin-X, congenital adrenal hyperplasia, and the CAH-X syndrome. Horm Res Paediatr. 2018;89(5):352–61.
8. Kadiyala R, Kamath C, Baglioni P, Geen J, Okosieme OE. Can a random serum cortisol reduce the need for short synacthen tests in acute medical admissions? Ann Clin Biochem. 2010;47(Pt 4):378–80.
9. Dorin RI, Qualls CR, Crapo LM. Diagnosis of adrenal insufficiency. Ann Intern Med. 2003;139:194–204.
10. Goedhart C, Gall N, Lulsegged A. A retrospective observational-cohort study of the relationship between reactive hypoglycaemia to postural orthostatic tachycardia syndrome (PoTS). Endocrine Abstracts (2016) 41 EP235.
11. Cryer, PE, Axelrod L, Grossman AB, Heller SR, Montori VM, Seaquist ER, Service FJ. Evaluation and management of adult hypoglycemic disorders: an endocrine society clinical practice guideline. J Clin Endocrinol Metab. 2009;94:709–28.

Postural Tachycardia Syndrome and the Gut

Alicia Green and Asma Fikree

Introduction

Patients with PoTS can experience multiple gastrointestinal (GI) symptoms. Some of these symptoms occur in the upright position and improve with lying down, others are not related with the orthostatic challenge. General lifestyle modifications recommended in patients with PoTS could improve GI and non-GI symptoms. Moderate to severe postprandial GI symptoms in patients with PoTS may lead to reduced food intake that could cause nutritional deficiencies. In this case, nutritional assessment is recommended. Gastrointestinal investigations and management are indicated when GI symptoms are severe and impact significantly on quality of life.

Key Points

- PoTS is associated with a range of gastrointestinal (GI) symptoms affecting any part of the gut, most commonly abdominal pain, nausea, bloating and altered bowel habit.
- GI dysmotility is common in patients with PoTS—this does not appear to be the sole cause of GI symptoms.
- Organic conditions which may mimic symptoms of PoTS e.g. phaeochromocytoma, carcinoid, adrenal insufficiency and thyroid disease need to be considered and excluded before diagnosing functional GI disorders in PoTS.
- The presence of flushing, diarrhea, nausea and multiple intolerances may be a sign of underlying mast cell dysfunction and treatment with antihistamines and mast cell stabilisers should be considered.
- GI physiology testing can help in refractory cases to define the GI phenotype and guide management strategies.
- There are no established guidelines for the management of GI symptoms in PoTS and patients are therefore treated symptomatically.

Symptoms

Gastrointestinal Symptoms in PoTS

Gastrointestinal disturbances are common in patients with a prevalence of 70–90% [1–6]. More than two-thirds of the patients experience nausea (which can be refractory), abdominal pain, (which can be persistent) bloating and constipation. Around 50% of patients present with heartburn and diarrhoea. The most common symptoms are shown in Table 1.

A. Green · A. Fikree (✉)
Department of Gastroenterology, Royal London Hospital, Barts Health NHS Trust, London, UK
e-mail: asma.fikree@nhs.net

N. Gall et al. (eds.), *Postural Tachycardia Syndrome*, https://doi.org/10.1007/978-3-030-54165-1_16

Table 1 Gastrointestinal symptoms in patients with postural tachycardia syndrome

GI symptoms in PoTS	Range (%)	Dysmotility/functional causes	Reference
Nausea	75–90	Gastroparesis Functional dyspepsia Chronic idiopathic nausea	[1–6]
Abdominal pain	70–90	IBS Visceral hypersensitivity Food intolerance	[1–6]
Constipation	50–71	Slow transit constipation Dyssynergic defaecation	[1–6]
Bloating	55–90	IBS SIBO Food intolerance	[1–6]
Heartburn	27–64	Reflux hypersensitivity Oesophageal hypomotility Gastro-oesophageal reflux disease	[1–6]
Diarrhoea	33–69	IBS SIBO MCAS Food intolerance	[1–6]

IBS irritable bowel syndrome; *SIBO* small intestinal bacterial overgrowth; *MCAS* mast cell activation syndrome

Gastrointestinal symptoms in patients with PoTS have two different presentations:

1. Symptoms that are triggered by standing up and that improve in the recumbent position—most commonly nausea, vomiting and abdominal pain [7, 8]. These may be secondary to PoTS and can be ameliorated by treating PoTS [9].
2. Symptoms that are present independently of the body position. For example, abdominal pain associated with bloating, diarrhoea or constipation and which is not related to orthostasis may be a manifestation of irritable bowel syndrome (IBS) or underlying dysmotility. These would not be relieved by treating the PoTS and instead management would be directed at managing symptoms (e.g. pain) or pathology e.g. dysmotility. Consequently, it is crucial to differentiate whether the GI symptoms in patients with PoTS are related or not with the orthostatic challenge as the management would differ in each case [9].

Course of GI Symptoms and Associated Complications

Although most patients experience that their symptoms either improve or remain stable over time, 40% of patients describe that symptoms worsen over the years [5]. The presence of gastrointestinal and other non-orthostatic symptoms and comorbidities worsens what is already a poor quality of life in patients with PoTS [10].

The presence of postprandial symptoms of nausea, vomiting, abdominal pain and altered bowel habit can be severe enough to impact on feeding and nutrition, which could lead to weight loss and nutritional deficiencies [11]. This can further worsen GI symptoms and orthostatic intolerance and set up a vicious cycle.

Pathophysiology

The pathophysiology of GI symptoms in PoTS remains unclear. Some symptoms seem to be secondary to the orthostatic challenge while the majority of them seem to be caused either by GI dysmotility, functional gastrointestinal disorders or by comorbidities associated with PoTS. Most medications used for PoTS can also cause GI symptoms.

Physiological or psychological stress appears to be an important trigger of symptoms with patients reporting the initial onset of symptoms within 3 months after an acute stressor such as pregnancy, surgery or infection and less commonly, vaccination, an accident, emotional stress and trauma [5, 12]. Acute exercise, heat, dehydration, alcohol, menstruation and prolonged recumbency can exacerbate symptoms in PoTS patients [12].

Pathologies Underlying GI Symptoms in PoTS

GI Dysmotility

In patients whose GI symptoms are directly related to orthostasis, the exact mechanism for GI symptoms has not been elucidated; however dysmotility seems to be involved. In a study of children with orthostatic intolerance, tilt table testing reproduced symptoms of orthostasis, nausea, vomiting and abdominal pain and these were associated with abnormal antroduodenal manometry e.g. dysmotility of the stomach and duodenum [4, 7, 13]. Symptoms improved with hydration and fludrocortisone (i.e. treatment of PoTS).

Dysmotility of the oesophagus, stomach, small bowel and colon have been documented in patients with PoTS [2–4, 8, 14–18]. It is unknown whether symptoms are directly related to dysmotility as treating this does not always alleviate symptoms.

Gastroduodenal abnormalities (neuropathic pattern) have been documented in patients with dyspepsia i.e. abdominal pain, nausea, vomiting, bloating.

Oeosphageal hypomotility is present in the majority of patients with oesophageal symptoms e.g. heartburn and dysphagia [2].

Delayed colonic transit is present in those with constipation.

Gastric emptying abnormalities are present in 30% with postprandial symptoms.

Two-third of these patients show rapid gastric emptying—this can induce a dumping-syndrome-like reaction which causes symptoms of epigastric pain, bloating, nausea, vomiting and diarrhea, as well as lightheadedness, fatigue and headaches soon after meal intake [19, 20]. Late symptoms of confusion, headaches, weakness and syncope can arise if reactive hypoglycaemia is present [21].

A third of patients present with delayed gastric emptying [3, 14, 15]—this is associated with postprandial symptoms of early satiety, fullness, nausea, vomiting, bloating, epigastric pain or epigastric burning. The severity of gastroparesis does not necessarily correlate well with the severity of symptoms [16].

Gastric myoelectrical (pacemaker) activity has also been shown to be abnormal in PoTS patients compared to healthy controls. They show more variability in the gastric slow wave frequency and this is increased postprandially in those with postprandial symptoms [17]. Gastric arrhythmias such as bradygastria and tachygastria have been shown to be increased in patients with PoTS [18].

Functional Diagnoses Are Common in Patients with PoTS

Functional gastrointestinal disorders (FGIDs) are conditions which cause symptoms in the absence of abnormalities on biochemical, radiological or endoscopic testing. The pathophysiology of these disorders includes visceral hypersensitivity, low grade immune activation, altered mucosal integrity (i.e. leaky gut), altered microbiota and abnormalities in the communication between the brain and the gut (brain-gut axis) [22]. The most common functional disorders seen in patients with PoTS are IBS, functional dyspepsia and abdominal distension/bloating.

Irritable Bowel Syndrome (IBS): Around a third of patients with PoTS experience symptoms of IBS [5]—recurrent abdominal pain at least one day per week in the last three months, which is related to defaecation and associated with a change in the frequency or form of stool. IBS is further characterized by the predominant bowel habit; IBS-D (diarrhoea), IBS-C (constipation), IBS-mixed (alternating diarrhoea and constipation) or unclassified IBS. In the absence of red flag symptoms, the management would focus on the most prominent symptom e.g. antispasmodics for pain, imodium for diarrhoea, laxatives for constipation.

Functional Dyspepsia: This causes similar symptoms to those of gastroparesis (see above) but there is little or no delay in gastric emptying. Symptoms are caused either by impaired accommodation of the stomach (reduced relaxation of the proximal stomach in response to a meal) or by hypersensitivity to gastric distension. Treatment is directed at any of those underlying physiological mechanisms e g prokinetics in the presence of delayed gastric emptying, mirtazapine for abnormal accommodation and visceral hypersensitivity.

Bloating and Abdominal Distension: this is due to a variety of causes including constipation, food intolerances e.g. FODMAPS (fermentable oligosaccharides, disaccharides, monosacharides and polyols), gluten and dairy, small intestine bacterial overgrowth (SIBO) and carbohydrate malabsorption [23].

Small intestinal bacterial overgrowth (SIBO) refers to the relative overabundance of bacteria in the small intestine which causes fermentation of ingested products leading to gas production i.e. bloating and pain. It can also lead to maldigestion and malabsorption of fat, proteins or carbohydrates with secondary diarrhoea and potentially deficiency of vitamin B12, iron, protein, albumin and fat-soluble vitamins depending on the degree of malabsorption [11].

Comorbidities in PoTS and How They Impact on GI Symptoms

A recent cross-sectional online community-based survey including almost 4000 participants with PoTS diagnosed by a physician, found that 83% of responders reported comorbid conditions, most commonly migraine headaches (40%), IBS (30%) Ehlers-Danlos syndrome (25%) fibromyalgia (20%), and mast cell activation disease (MCAD) (9%)—see Table 2 [5]. In addition, there are recent reports of an association with median arcuate ligament syndrome [24]. All these comorbidities can be associated with their own set of GI symptoms and can alter the presentation of the patient with PoTS.

Hypermobile Ehlers-Danlos syndrome (hEDS) hEDS is associated with a range of GI symptoms most commonly dyspepsia, abdominal pain, alternating bowel habit with a tendency to constipation, and reflux. hEDS is associated with functional GI disorders, notably functional dyspepsia and irritable bowel syndrome. Visceral hypersensitivity is common in hEDS and contributes to the development of pain syndromes. The presence of PoTS in hEDS is associated with increased incidence of GI dysmotility and worse quality of life.

Mast cell activation disorder (MCAD) can occur in patients with PoTS, typically causing symptoms of flushing, dizziness, lightheadedness, headache, urinary irritability and gastrointestinal symptoms such as nausea, diarrhoea and abdominal cramping. GI symptoms caused by MCAD respond well to treatment for MCAD e.g. antihistamines, and mast cell stabilisers [25].

Table 2 GI symptoms associated with non GI comorbidities in PoTS [5]

Comorbidity	Prevalence (%)	GI involvement
Migraine	40	Nausea, vomiting (cyclical vomiting), abdominal pain (abdominal migraine)
Hypermobile Ehlers-Danlos syndrome	25	Gastro-oesophageal reflux disease, functional dyspepsia, IBS, constipation
Fibromyalgia	20	IBS
Mast Cell Activation Syndrome	9	Nausea, diarrhoea, abdominal pain
Hashimoto Thyroiditis	6	Constipation
Coeliac disease	3	Any GI symptom, malabsorption, anaemia, nutritional deficiencies
Inflammatory connective tissue disorders eg SLE, Sjogrens	2–3	GI dysmotility

IBS Irritable bowel syndrome

Median arcuate ligament syndrome (MALS) also called coeliac artery compression syndrome has been reported in up to 50% of patients with PoTS in one study [24]. This causes chronic and recurrent postprandial abdominal pain associated with **weight loss**, nausea, vomiting or diarrhoea and is related to compression of the celiac artery and/or celiac plexus by the median arcuate ligament [24, 26]. Diagnosis is made radiologically, typically with CT/MR angiography or duplex ultrasound. Similar radiological findings can also be seen with significant weight loss and so it is important to be cautious when considering this diagnosis and discuss it in an MDT forum. In a case series, surgical division of the median arcuate ligament improved GI symptoms, orthostatic symptoms and quality of life [11].

Medications and GI Symptoms in PoTS

Most medications, which are used to treat PoTS or its allied conditions, are associated with GI symptoms

See Table 3.

Assessment

A thorough medical history, systems review, detailed drug history, and physical examination are essential to rule out important differentials:

- Endocrine problems such as thyroid problems, adrenal insufficiency, diabetes
- Inflammatory connective tissue disorders
- Coeliac disease
- Inflammatory bowel disease eg Crohn's disease and ulcerative colitis
- Malignancy
- Infections
- Neuroendocrine tumours e.g. carcinoid
- Drug effects e.g. opiates can produce bowel dysfunction and worsen abdominal pain.

Diagnostic Testing and GI Evaluation in PoTS Patients Depends on:

- Severity of GI symptoms and effect on quality of life
- Presence of alarm symptoms. If they have alarm symptoms these have to be investigated to exclude an underlying malignancy:
  - Rectal bleeding
  - Weight loss
  - Iron deficiency anemia
  - Nocturnal symptoms
- Family history
- Previous investigations
- Response to treatments.

Initial Testing to Rule Out Organic Causes:

- Blood testing for FBC, U&E, LFTs, ESR, CRP, thyroid function, coeliac serology and autoimmune screen as an initial blood screen.
- When patients have a very restrictive diet, excessive vomiting and/or diarrhea and or weight loss we recommend monitoring of micronutrients e.g. iron, B12, folate, clotting, Vitamin D.

Table 3 Gastrointestinal symptoms cause by medications

Medication	GI side effects
Opiates	Nausea, vomiting, constipation
Fludrocortisone	Nausea, GI discomfort, peptic ulcer
Midodrine	Nausea, GI discomfort, diarrhoea
Ivabradine	Abdominal pain, constipation, diarrhoea
Clonidine	Constipation, nausea, vomiting
Pyridostigmine	Abdominal pain, diarrhoea, nausea, vomiting
Octreotide	Cholelithiasis and cholecystitis, constipation, diarrhoea, abdominal pain, vomiting

- Stool test for faecal calprotectin in those with diarrhea to rule out underlying colonic inflammation.
- Endoscopies: gastroscopy to rule out inflammatory or structural causes of upper GI symptoms e.g. nausea, vomiting, reflux. Colonoscopy to investigate altered bowel habit in the presence of red flags or raised faecal calprotectin.
- Radiology: cross sectional imaging to investigate anaemia, weight loss, severe abdominal pain.

Simple and Safe Treatments that Might Help

Dietary and Lifestyle Modifications

Ingestion of food is a major trigger for GI symptoms in patients with PoTS. Despite the lack of strong available evidence to support specific dietary modifications our experience suggests that dietary alteration can improve symptoms.

Obtain a proper dietary history; ask the patient to keep a food intake diary—this will help to identify specific triggers and avoid unnecessary dietary restrictions.

In patients with rapid gastric emptying and postprandial hypoglycemia we recommend the following:

- Eat small and frequent meals
- Eat slowly and chew food thoroughly
- Opt for low-glycemic-index food
- Increase fat and protein intake to balance energy requirements
- Separate intake of liquids from solids, avoiding liquids for half an hour before and after meals
- Lie down for 30 minutes after meals—this can reduce postprandial symptoms e.g. palpitations, flushing or dizziness
- Increasing intake of salt and water appears to improve symptoms of nausea.

In patients with gastroparesis, we recommend:

- Adequate chewing to reduce the size of the food
- Avoid intake of insoluble fiber
- 'Graze'—eat regular small meals
- Reduce fat intake.

An unhealthy lifestyle contributes to GI symptoms so it is important to assess for this and to educate patients accordingly:

- Increase salt and water intake
- Dietary advice
- Optimize sleep
- Physical exercise for conditioning
- Stress management—stress exacerbates (functional) GI symptoms.

When to Refer to the Gastro Clinic?

Patients should generally be referred to a gastroenterology clinic when the patient:

- Presents with alarm symptoms, or difficulty maintaining nutrition with or without nutritional deficiencies
- Has an organic diagnosis that needs to be treated in a specialist setting
- Experiences symptoms severely impacting on QOL
- Needs specialized physiology testing e.g. Motility testing of oesophagus, small bowel or colon, Gastro-oesophageal reflux testing, Gastric emptying test or Hydrogen breath test for investigation of small intestinal bacterial overgrowth.

What Treatment Is Instituted in the Specialist Clinic?

In general the treatment of GI symptoms follows principles for treating functional gastrointestinal disorders, unless there is evidence of a specific dysmotility disorder. Some of the commonly used treatments in functional gut disorders are given in Table 4.

An empathic doctor-patient relationship, as always, is crucial in treating these patients. Adequate time during the consultation needs to be devoted to reassuring the patient about the legitimacy of their symptoms, to explain possible causes and reassure them of the absence of a life-threatening illness. Equally, it is important to explain that the management will require several steps and strategies:

- Lifestyle modification (see above).
- Dietary modification with adequate fluid and salt intake (see above).
- Review medicines and try to reduce polypharmacy and consider GI side effects of medications, particularly opiates that should be avoided.
- Symptom directed pharmacological therapy (Table 1). It is the authors anecdotal experience that in some patients with PoTS their GI symptoms improve following treatment of their main non-GI PoTS symptoms although this has not formally been demonstrated by

Table 4 Pharmacological therapy

Symptom	Type of medication	Examples of medications	Monitoring required	Important side effects
Nausea/Vomiting	Anti-emetics Anti-nausea	Ondansetron Metoclopramide Cyclizine Promethazine Prochlorperazine (can be give sublingual)	Ondansetron need to measure QT interval	Metoclopramide risk of tardive dyskinesia
Gastroparesis	Motility stimulants	Metoclopramide Domperidone Erythromycin Prucalopride	Domperidone and Erythromycin, need to measure QT interval	Erythromycin (short term only due to risk of tachyphylaxis)
Pain	Antispasmodics	Buscopan Mebeverine Peppermint oil Dicycloverine		
	Antidepressants	Amitriptyline/nortriptyline Duloxetine Mirtazapine	Avoid amitriptyline in patients with severe constipation	Weight gain with duloxetine, amitriptyline and mirtazapine
	Pain Modulators	Gabapentin Pregabalin	Measure QT interval	Weight gain
Diarrhoea	Antimotility drugs	Loperamide		
Constipation	Laxatives	Prucalopride Linaclotide Stimulant laxatives e.g. bisacodyl Osmotic laxatives e.g. movicol, up to 8/day Stool softeners e.g. lactulose (this causes bloating) Suppositories e.g. glycerine Rectal irrigation Enemas e.g. phosphate enemas		

systematic research studies and therefore such treatment should only be considered when appropriately clinically indicated.
- Psychological therapy when the patient has difficulty with coping or if stress is thought to trigger symptoms.
- Referral to dietitian for nutritional assessment in those with multiple food intolerances and those with reduced food intake impacting on nutrition and weight e.g. low FODMAP diet in patients with IBS.
- Nutritional supplementation e.g. enteral/ parenteral feeding, has to be considered in patients with weight loss, dehydration and deficiency of micronutrients though the decision to start this needs to be made in an MDT setting.

Ideally, this multidisciplinary input would be provided by a multidisciplinary team including a gastroenterologist/physician with a specialist interest in PoTS, a dietitian, psychiatrist/psychologist and specialist nurse.

Management in Special Situations

- Nausea in patients with PoTS could have several causes:
  - If the symptom worsens in the upright position, we recommend general treatment for PoTS, i.e. increased hydration, salt intake, etc. as the first line treatment.
  - If the nausea appears early in the morning or even during the night, it may be due to delayed gastric emptying and a trial of prokinetics e.g. can be attempted.
  - Episodic nausea and vomiting accompanied with severe headache with light and sound sensitivity should be managed as a migraine.
  - If the patient experiences nausea associated with dyspeptic symptoms in the presence of a normal gastroscopy, treat as per functional dyspepsia. Exclude *H pylori* infection with a stool or breath test and treat it if positive. Treatment with PPIs or H2 blocker for 8 weeks is recommended as initial therapy. If there is no improvement, the patient should be referred to a specialist [9].
  - If rapid gastric emptying is present on gastric emptying tests and the symptoms are suggestive of dumping syndrome the patient can be referred to the endocrine team for a prolonged glucose tolerance test to assess for this. Octreotide can be considered to slow gastric emptying in confirmed symptomatic cases but this should only be initiated in a specialist setting [19].
- In patients with symptoms of mast cell activation a trial of an H1-receptor antagonist, H2-receptor antagonist and cromoglycate or ketotifen (ketotifen is particularly good if they are anxious) is recommended [9, 25].
- Median arcuate ligament syndrome—the decision about surgical intervention should be considered with caution, and not without an MDT discussion [11].
- Psychological therapy i.e. mindfulness meditation, cognitive behavioural therapy or hypnotherapy [27] is indicated for those with high levels of anxiety, depression, stress and those with a history of significant life events.

References

1. Wang LB, Culbertson CJ, Deb A, Morgenshtern K, Huang H, Hohler AD. Gastrointestinal dysfunction in postural tachycardia syndrome. J Neurol Sci. 2015;359(1–2):193–6.
2. Huang RJ, Chun CL, Friday K, Triadafilopoulos G. Manometric abnormalities in the postural orthostatic tachycardia syndrome: a case series. Dig Dis Sci. 2013;58(11):3207–11.
3. Park KJ, Singer W, Sletten DM, Low PA, Bharucha AE. Gastric emptying in postural tachycardia syndrome: a preliminary report. Clin Auton Res. 2013;23(4):163–7.
4. Moak JP, Fabian RR, Clarke LC, Hanumanthaiah S, Desbiens J, Darbari A. Antroduodenal manometry is abnormal in children presenting with orthostatic intolerance and gastrointestinal symptoms. J Pediatr Gastroenterol Nutr. 2016;63(3):329–35.
5. Shaw BH, Stiles LE, Bourne K, Green EA, Shibao CA, Okamoto LE, et al. The face of postural tachycardia syndrome—insights from a large cross-sectional online community-based survey. J Intern Med. 2019.

6. Deb A, Morgenshtern K, Culbertson CJ, Wang LB, Hohler AD. A survey-based analysis of symptoms in patients with postural orthostatic tachycardia syndrome. Proc (Bayl Univ Med Cent). 2015;28(2):157–9.
7. Safder S, Chelimsky TC, O'Riordan MA, Chelimsky G. Autonomic testing in functional gastrointestinal disorders: implications of reproducible gastrointestinal complaints during tilt table testing. Gastroenterol Res Pract. 2009;2009:868496.
8. Fortunato JE, Wagoner AL, Harbinson RL, D'Agostino RB, Shaltout HA, Diz DI. Effect of fludrocortisone acetate on chronic unexplained nausea and abdominal pain in children with orthostatic intolerance. J Pediatr Gastroenterol Nutr. 2014;59(1):39–43.
9. Chelimsky G, Chelimsky T. The gastrointestinal symptoms present in patients with postural tachycardia syndrome: a review of the literature and overview of treatment. Auton Neurosci. 2018;215:70–7.
10. Benrud-Larson LM, Dewar MS, Sandroni P, Rummans TA, Haythornthwaite JA, Low PA. Quality of life in patients with postural tachycardia syndrome. Mayo Clin Proc. 2002;77(6):531–7.
11. DiBaise JK. The POTS (postural tachycardia syndrome) epidemic: hydration and nutrition issues. In: Tisha N, Lunsford LAH, editor. Practical gastroenterology. Nutrition Issues in Gastroenterology, Series #187; 2019. p. 14–26.
12. Raj SR, Stiles LE. Special issue for the silver anniversary of postural tachycardia syndrome. Auton Neurosci. 2018;215:1–2.
13. Fortunato JE, Shaltout HA, Larkin MM, Rowe PC, Diz DI, Koch KL. Fludrocortisone improves nausea in children with orthostatic intolerance (OI). Clin Auton Res. 2011;21(6):419–23.
14. Lawal A, Barboi A, Krasnow A, Hellman R, Jaradeh S, Massey BT. Rapid gastric emptying is more common than gastroparesis in patients with autonomic dysfunction. Am J Gastroenterol. 2007;102(3):618–23.
15. Loavenbruck A, Iturrino J, Singer W, Sletten DM, Low PA, Zinsmeister AR, et al. Disturbances of gastrointestinal transit and autonomic functions in postural orthostatic tachycardia syndrome. Neurogastroenterol Motil. 2015;27(1):92–8.
16. Antiel RM, Risma JM, Grothe RM, Brands CK, Fischer PR. Orthostatic intolerance and gastrointestinal motility in adolescents with nausea and abdominal pain. J Pediatr Gastroenterol Nutr. 2008;46(3):285–8.
17. Seligman WH, Low DA, Asahina M, Mathias CJ. Abnormal gastric myoelectrical activity in postural tachycardia syndrome. Clin Auton Res. 2013;23(2):73–80.
18. Safder S, Chelimsky TC, O'Riordan MA, Chelimsky G. Gastric electrical activity becomes abnormal in the upright position in patients with postural tachycardia syndrome. J Pediatr Gastroenterol Nutr. 2010;51(3):314–8.
19. Berg P, McCallum R. Dumping syndrome: a review of the current concepts of pathophysiology, diagnosis, and treatment. Dig Dis Sci. 2016;61(1):11–8.
20. Zhao XT, Wang L, Lin HC. Slowing of intestinal transit by fat depends on naloxone-blockable efferent, opioid pathway. Am J Physiol Gastrointest Liver Physiol. 2000;278(6):G866–70.
21. Lin HC, Neevel C, Chen PS, Suh G, Chen JH. Slowing of intestinal transit by fat or peptide YY depends on beta-adrenergic pathway. Am J Physiol Gastrointest Liver Physiol. 2003;285(6):G1310–6.
22. Drossman DA. Functional gastrointestinal disorders: history, pathophysiology, clinical features and Rome IV. Gastroenterology. 2016.
23. Azpiroz F, Malagelada JR. Abdominal bloating. Gastroenterology. 2005;129(3):1060–78.
24. Abdallah H. Median arcuate ligament syndrome presenting as POTS. Auton Neurosci. 2015;123.
25. DiBaise JK, Harris LA, Goodman B. Postural tachycardia syndrome (POTS) and the GI tract: a primer for the gastroenterologist. Am J Gastroenterol. 2018;113(10):1458–67.
26. Ashangari C. Median arcuate ligament syndrome in postural orthostatic tachycardia syndrome (POTS). Auton Neurosci. 2015;124–5.
27. Van Oudenhove L, Crowell MD, Drossman DA, Halpert AD, Keefer L, Lackner JM, et al. Biopsychosocial aspects of functional gastrointestinal disorders. Gastroenterology. 2016.

Urological Considerations in PoTS

Visha Tailor and Vik Khullar

Introduction

The heterogenous, multifactorial condition of postural tachycardia syndrome (PoTS) is frequently associated with other conditions, as discussed in earlier chapters. The association of PoTS with hypermobile Ehlers Danlos syndrome (EDS) and mast cell activation syndrome (MCAS) are discussed in depth separately in this book (see Chaps. 12 and 21).

Voiding Dysfunction

Voiding dysfunction is defined as abnormally slow and/or incomplete micturition diagnosed by symptoms and urodynamic investigations [1]. Patients with PoTS are more likely to present with voiding dysfunction with an impaired sensation of bladder fullness and inefficient voiding. They may strain to void with associated chronic retention of urine. In a small study of 21 female PoTS patients, 32% of patients were found to have post-void residual measurements >100 ml [2]. As a result, patients may already have been established on a regime of clean intermittent self-catheterisation, even prior to a formal diagnosis of PoTS; this is the most commonly used treatment method. Changes to the connective tissue in patients with hypermobile EDS may affect bladder wall contractility.

Voiding dysfunction can be associated with urethral kinking and bladder outlet obstruction; in women this may be a result of vaginal pelvic organ prolapse. Voiding dysfunction has been reported in up to 27% of women with stage III or IV vaginal prolapse [3]. Therefore, correction of the vaginal prolapse through the use of vaginal pessaries or surgery may improve voiding dysfunction. However, following the surgical correction of vaginal prolapse, 1.1% may develop de novo voiding dysfunction [3].

There is a role for sacral neuromodulation with stimulation of the sacral nerve roots, through an implanted electrode, in correcting voiding dysfunction particularly if detrusor underactivity is found. Successful treatment of non-obstructive voiding dysfunction with elimination of the need to self-catheterise has been reported in 33–90% of treated patients. Considerations may be needed for patients who may require regular MRI assessment; however MRI-compatible sacral neuromodulation devices are being developed and are now more widely available [4].

V. Tailor
Urogynaecology Department, St Mary's Hospital, Imperial College London, London, UK

V. Khullar (✉)
Subspecialist in Urogynaecology, Urogynaecology Department, St Mary's Hospital, Imperial College London, London, UK
e-mail: vik.khullar@imperial.ac.uk

N. Gall et al. (eds.), *Postural Tachycardia Syndrome*, https://doi.org/10.1007/978-3-030-54165-1_17

Overactive Bladder Syndrome

Patients with PoTS often have a low total blood, plasma and red cell volume. The renin-angiotensin-aldosterone system (RAAS) is a regulator of blood volume and systemic vascular resistance. Abnormalities in the RAAS system in PoTS patients have been documented, with increased levels of angiotensin 2 without an increase in the active angiotensin metabolite. This may encourage urine output and a reduction in circulating volume [5].

Despite its importance in arterial pressure maintenance, results regarding the responses of the RAAS during upright posture in PoTS patients are few and controversial [6]. In patients with hyperadrenergic PoTS it is not unusual for patients to describe urinary urgency on standing for short periods of time [5].

Lower urinary tract symptoms appear to be more common in patients with PoTS, EDS and MCAS. For patients with PoTS, symptoms can begin in childhood with 24% in one study reporting childhood voiding symptoms [2].

Symptoms of overactive bladder syndrome (OAB) include urinary urgency, urgency related urinary incontinence, urinary frequency and nocturia. OAB is a dynamic condition with the prevalence increasing with age and is likely to manifest from a vast array of primary pathologies. The International Continence Society defines OAB when these symptoms present in the absence of pathological or metabolic conditions that might be able to explain them [1].

The prevalence of OAB in the general population has been estimated from 2–53%, with a median prevalence estimate of 16.5% (range 2–35% in men, and 3–41% in women). In more recent studies that include an assessment of severity, less than 10% of people have moderately bothersome OAB [7]. From a survey using a validated symptom questionnaire (OAB-q), 13/19 (68.4%) female PoTS patients met the criteria for a diagnosis of probable overactive bladder by reporting a symptom score ≥ 16 [8]. Similarly, in a large online survey of 4835 patients with PoTS, 68% reported increased urinary frequency [9].

Normal bladder function relies upon sophisticated signalling pathways with somatic (S2–S4 Pudendal nerve) and autonomic (parasympathetic S2–4 and sympathetic L1–L3) innervation [10]. Studies have suggested a potential relationship between autonomic dysfunction and the development of OAB. In one study, those less responsive to medical management with anticholinergic treatment were more likely to have sympathetic autonomic dysfunction [11]. However, the defining factors linking distinct autonomic disorders and resultant lower urinary tract manifestations remain at the early stages of study.

Investigating Lower Urinary Tract Symptoms

The assessment of lower urinary tract function begins with a thorough history and examination of the patient. Abdominal palpation may reveal abdominal distension or suprapubic tenderness. Vaginal examination for women is important to identify vaginal prolapse, pelvic floor muscle spasm or point tenderness and anterior vaginal wall tenderness. Compression of the anterior vaginal wall may reproduce the patient's pain symptoms and is suggestive of bladder inflammation or infection which may be contributing.

A history of multiple, repeated infections should prompt consideration of immunoglobulin quantification and possibly, immunology referral for the evaluation of immunodeficiency [12].

Completion of a bladder diary can help to identify the patient's fluid intake and voiding patterns.

Lower urinary tract symptoms can be further investigated by urodynamic studies. Urodynamic studies (UDS) consist of various components and can include some or all of the following: uroflowmetry, post-void residual measurements, cytometry, pressure flow studies, urethral function tests and in some centres, electromyography and video urodynamic studies. The tests are relatively invasive and therefore often reserved for patients who have not responded to initial medical therapy. As for any patient, urodynamic studies should be considered in PoTS patients with significant lower urinary tract symptoms.

Uroflowmetry or pressure-flow studies can identify a strain pattern to void which is not uncommon in patients with PoTS. Cystometry will identify bladder capacity and filling sensation. Loss of bladder compliance is not thought to be associated with PoTS [2].

Patients with OAB may have associated detrusor overactivity (DO) which is defined as involuntary detrusor contractions during the cystometry; they can be seen through the filling phase or through provocation such as with movement or when listening to water moving. However, approximately half of those presenting with OAB symptoms will not display DO, particularly patients without associated incontinence [13].

Treatment of Overactive Bladder Syndrome and Detrusor Overactivity

Conservative Management

Lifestyle interventions and advice include avoiding caffeinated drinks and alcohol, management of constipation and smoking cessation to improve overactive bladder symptoms. Fluid restriction to 1–1.5 litres a day is commonly advised to help manage frequency symptoms; however, this will probably not be tolerated by many patients with PoTS. Patients presenting with signs and symptoms of histamine intolerance or MCAS should also be advised to follow a modified diet with a trial of antihistamine medication considered. This is discussed later in this chapter.

Further conservative management for overactive bladder symptoms is non-invasive through pelvic floor muscle training exercises and bladder retraining. Practising the exercises aims to strengthen the pelvic floor muscles, provide urethral support to prevent urine leakage, and suppress urinary urgency. The benefits are considered to be greater for patients presenting with stress urinary incontinence compared with urgency related urinary incontinence. Cure or improvement can be seen in 67% of women with urinary incontinence following 3–6 months treatment [14]. For women who have difficulty in carrying out pelvic floor muscle training, biofeedback may be utilised. Outcomes of conservative management have not been specifically reported for women with PoTS; however given the non-invasive nature and safety of this intervention it is often recommended as a first line therapy.

Bladder retraining aims to increase the interval between voiding, bladder capacity and reduce urge incontinence episodes. The retraining is structured around timed voiding, increasing the voiding interval by 15–30 minutes every week until the desired interval is achieved. Good motivation is required but relapse can occur over time.

Medical Management of OAB

Bladder contraction is mediated through para-sympathetic (cholinergic) neurons. Therefore, antimuscarinic agents are often the first line treatment for patients with storage dysfunction and overactive bladder symptoms. However, many medications produce anti-cholinergic side effects including drowsiness, reduced saliva and tear production, urinary retention, constipation and tachycardia [15]; Solifenacin more than oxybutynin and tolterodine may exacerbate constipation. Most anti-muscarinic agents readily cross the blood-brain barrier with the potential for deterioration in cognitive performance, sedation, insomnia and confusion in a susceptible population. Fesoterodine fumerate, trospium chloride and darifenacin are known to have little or no cognitive side effects and can be considered for use in an older population [16]. Prescribers should remain aware of polypharmacy and the anticholinergic burden in older patients.

Active relaxation of muscles in the bladder wall is mediated through beta-3 (noradrenergic) receptors. Mirabegron, a beta-3 agonist, may therefore be helpful on its own or in combination with anti-cholinergics in the management of urinary urgency and frequency. It is often considered second line therapy after a trial of anti-muscarinic treatment or if there are contraindications to anti-muscarinic treatment or if anti-muscarinics are not tolerated.

Treatment of Refractory OAB

Patients not responsive to medical management or who have unsatisfactory improvement or who do not tolerate medical therapies are described as having refractory OAB. For this group of patients, intra-detrusor injection of onabotulinum toxin A at cystoscopy or neuromodulation therapies are alternative treatment options. Local blockade of acetylcholine release effected by onabotulinum toxin can benefit patients for 6–12 months. Risks of the procedure include urinary tract infection in 1 out of 12 cases and the temporary need to carry out intermittent urinary catheterisation in 3–10% of patients. Repeat intra-vesical injections are often required if the toxin effects decrease over time with return of symptoms.

Neuromodulation therapy is well-established to modulate bladder function to improve voiding dysfunction and detrusor overactivity. Animal studies have demonstrated that OAB symptoms may be the result of an alteration in the inhibitory and excitatory signals of the voiding reflex changing the pelvic neuromuscular environment. Over-riding neural messages through the use of sacral nerve stimulators may be very effective in some patients [17]. A stimulator is implanted in the buttock with an electrode (a tined lead) placed alongside the sacral nerves through the S3 sacral foramen. Lead placement is fluoroscopically guided to achieve a specific motor/sensory response with stimulation. Insertion is often a two-step procedure with an initial test phase and external stimulator followed by implantation of the internal pulse generator or stimulator if treatment success with >50% improvement in symptoms is observed during the test period. Following implantation, 67–87% will have successful treatment outcomes with longer term studies reporting 90% benefiting at 77 months [18].

Tibial nerve stimulation is a form of peripheral neuromodulation treatment. The posterior tibial nerve is a distal branch of the sciatic nerve that originates from the L5–S3 spinal roots and descends towards the lower extremities. Peripheral stimulation at the lower leg/ankle to the posterior tibial nerve is thought to deliver retrograde neuromodulation to the sacral nerve plexus. Alteration to nerve signalling is thought to occur with cross-signalling between sympathetic and parasympathetic post-ganglionic nerve terminals and synapses involved in the voiding reflex [17]. This therapy is typically delivered through weekly thirty-minute sessions of percutaneous or transcutaneous posterior tibial nerve stimulation. The treatment is considered less invasive compared with sacral neuromodulation. However long-term maintenance treatments are often required [15]. Newer implantable tibial nerve stimulators are currently in clinical trials and could have the advantage of self-administered treatment [19].

Nocturia

Nocturia can be described as the interruption of sleep one or more times because of the need to micturate [1]. The severity of the symptoms can be quantified using a bladder diary. Nocturia can be associated with OAB but has mixed and multiple aetiologies. Patients with PoTS often have nocturia.

Adopting the supine position at night and thereby reducing the hydrostatic pressure in the legs, results in reabsorption of fluid from peripheral tissues into the bloodstream. The ensuing expansion of intravascular volume increases urine production through both antidiuretic hormone inhibition and increased glomerular filtration rate. These can contribute to worsening of nocturia in patients with PoTS. The use of pressure stockings during the day, raising the head of the bed by approximately 10 cm and leg elevation in the hours prior to retiring to bed can therefore help moderate the volume of urine production overnight [15].

In the absence of chronic bladder inflammation or infection, small doses of desmopressin, a synthetic analogue of vasopressin can be administered to reduce the volume of urine produced overnight by up to 50% to aid in relieving bothersome nocturia symptoms.

Recurrent Urinary Tract Infection and Bladder Pain Syndrome

Recurrent urinary tract infection (UTI) in adults is defined as ≥2 UTI episodes in 6 months or ≥3 symptomatic and medically diagnosed episodes in 1 year. The current gold standard and most commonly used investigation to detect a UTI is through urine culture. Recurrent infections occur in approximately 35–53% of women that were treated for a UTI in the last year [20]. Recurrent UTI is a common cause of female pelvic floor dysfunction and has been reported to affect up to 66% of patients with PoTS attending for lower urinary tract symptom evaluation [2]. The increased risk in PoTS patients may be associated with the need to carry out clean intermittent self-catheterisation (CISC) which affects 25% of people who regularly perform this [21] or due to underlying MCAS or histamine intolerance. Recurrent UTI is associated with chronic bladder inflammation with studies reporting increased urinary nerve growth factor, increased mast cell expression and urothelial apoptosis compared to normal controls [22].

MCAS and histamine intolerance can be associated with recurrent infections including urinary tract infections and bladder pain syndrome/interstitial cystitis (BPS/IC). Recurrent UTI, BPS/IC and overactive bladder syndrome can present with overlapping symptoms including bladder pain, urinary frequency, urinary urgency, dysuria and nocturia. Bladder pain is defined as the complaint of suprapubic or retro-pubic pain, pressure, or discomfort, related to the bladder and usually increases with bladder filling. It may persist or be relieved after voiding. When symptoms are associated with lower urinary tract symptoms such as urgency, frequency and nocturia, the diagnosis of bladder pain syndrome (BPS) is given [23]. International societies vary in their opinion of the duration of symptoms from 6 weeks (American Urological Association [24]) to 6 months (European Society for the Study of Bladder Pain Syndrome 2008 [25]), but all agree the diagnosis is given in the absence of identifiable pathology or causes.

Interstitial cystitis (IC) is considered a subtype under the overall umbrella diagnosis of BPS. The symptom presentation remains the same, however typical bladder ulcerations are seen at cystoscopy. The original description of the ulcers given by Hunner in 1915 is used to diagnose the appearance of patches of red mucosa exhibiting small vessels radiating to a central pale scar [26].

Increased mast cells and their activation may be secondary to chronic infection, alternatively mast cells in the bladder may be reacting to other stimuli such as food allergens, resulting in chronic inflammation. Patients may present with recurrent or constant bladder pain as well as more generalised symptoms of MCAS or histamine intolerance. Flares of dermatographia and flushing associated with episodes of worsening bladder pain and lower urinary tract symptoms can occur with triggers such as the intake of histamine containing or liberating foods.

With prolonged symptoms, BPS/IC can contribute to chronic pelvic pain and has a negative impact on quality of life and sexual function (7). Patients can experience both superficial and deep dyspareunia which can persist after intercourse. This may be related to bladder inflammation or concomitant diagnoses such as endometriosis. For some, intercourse may also trigger a flare of cystitis symptoms (urinary frequency, urgency, nocturia and dysuria) or UTI.

Inflammation in Bladder Pain Syndrome and Interstitial Cystitis

The pathophysiology of BPS/IC is not fully understood and considered to be multifactorial affecting primarily young and middle-aged women. Twin studies have suggested that IC/BPS can be genetically inherited. However, a more favoured aetiology is the dysfunction of the normally impermeable bladder urothelial lining, resulting in increased permeability allowing irritants such as urinary solutes to diffuse across the lining and generate hypersensitivity symptoms. Neurogenic inflammation, infection, chronic autoimmune inflammation and urine abnormalities may contribute to the initial dysfunction. The process in part can be mediated by the activation and proliferation of mast cells [7, 25].

Increased mast cell counts (>28/mm^2) within the bladder mucosa and particularly the detrusor muscle are associated with IC/BPS and can be identified on bladder biopsy [27]. Furthermore, mast cells and inflammation may play a role in the pathophysiology of OAB symptoms. Upregulation of chemo-attractant protein-1 (MCP-1), which causes degranulation of mast cells, has been observed in patients with OAB [28]. Activation of these mast cells leads to histamine release leading to the induction of inflammation and hypersensitivity of the bladder. Infection can be a precipitating event and women with a clinical history of recurrent UTI as children are significantly more likely to have a diagnosis of BPS/IC as adults [29].

A dysfunctional urothelium, in combination with the continuous exposure to toxic urine contents and released inflammatory mediators, such as histamine, cytokines, and proteases, can lead to the sensitisation of peripheral afferent endings. Long term, these have the potential to change neuronal function and neuroplasticity. Animal models of cystitis demonstrate an increase in the urothelial neurotransmitter release of ATP, prostaglandin E2 and cholinergic regulated urothelial nitric oxide release with increased receptor expression. These are also considered to be downstream consequences of inflammation, infection or urothelial breakdown [29].

Histamine binds to four different G-protein couple receptors, H1, H2, H3, H4. Detrusor cells express all four receptor subtypes. However, the functional role of each receptor is not fully understood [28]. All four receptor types have increased expression in patients with BPS/IC compared with healthy controls particularly in the bladder mucosa, and less pronounced surrounding interstitial blood vessels and the detrusor muscles [30]. Studies of porcine urothelium suggest that only the H1 receptor is active in the urothelium, lamina propria and detrusor and is responsible for spontaneous phasic contractions. These contractions increased in frequency when stimulated by histamine and were inhibited in the presence of the H1 agonists pyrilamine, fexofenadine and cephroheptadine. Activation of the H2 receptor conversely inhibits the H1-mediated contractions in the urothelium with lamina propria but not the detrusor [28]. These studies support the use of histamine receptor antagonists in the treatment of BPS/IC.

Investigation with Cystoscopy

Cystoscopy is a useful study for BPS/IC. Other indications include OAB symptoms not responding to medical treatment, voiding dysfunction to assess for obstruction, recurrent urinary tract infections and persistent haematuria.

There is no consensus for diagnostic cystoscopy findings for BPS/IC. However, cystoscopy is recommended to exclude alternative causes of the symptom presentation such as bladder carcinoma, endometriosis, infection and bladder stones [24, 25].

Bladder biopsy may reveal associated histological changes such as a degree of denuded epithelium, ulceration, chronic inflammation and raised mast cell count. The European Society for the Study of Interstitial Cystitis (ESSIC) proposes mast cell counts in the detrusor muscle with a density >28 mast cells/mm^2 as diagnostic criterion for BPS/IC [25]. A standardised method of rigid cystoscopy for the investigation and biopsy sampling has been described by ESSIC [25, 27].

Detection of mast cells in tissue was traditionally studied using Giemsa stain or toluidine blue staining of mast cell granules. Immunohistochemistry methods to identify CD117, a mast cell transmembrane tyrosine kinase receptor, is becoming more commonly used [31]. Alternatively antibodies to human mast cell tryptase to stain mast cell granules has been described with a threshold of 27 mast cells / mm^2 defining significant mastocytosis [27]. This method allows differentiation between activated mast cells with granules outside the cytoplasm and non-activated mast cells, with the granules located within the cytoplasm. Degranulation of mast cells may point towards a hyper-responsive state and patients may benefit from therapy with mast cell stabilizers. However, the most sensitive and accurate immunohistochemical stain available today is CD-117 [32].

Management of Bladder Pain Syndrome and Genitourinary MCAS Symptoms

There is no cure available for PoTS, hEDS and MCAS, therefore management is based on the avoidance of triggers and medication to help to control symptoms and improve quality of life. With the likely multi-factorial aetiology, this results in a wide range of available management options. Treatment is multimodal but should also include a trial of mast cell targeting therapies to address any mast cell or histamine-mediated symptoms. Despite treatment clinically used in this subset of patients, there is limited data on treatment outcomes.

The following are medications used to help control symptoms of MCAS that may influence PoTS and hEDS symptoms as well as associated bladder pain symptoms. The clinical experience of many PoTS specialists suggests that the empiric addition of safe mast cell medications may confer benefit in PoTS patients given that negative testing may not preclude mast cell involvement in symptoms [15]. It is unlikely that mast cell activation is a prominent component in all patients with PoTS and thus empiric treatment with mast cell medications should not be continued indefinitely if no benefit is observed. Given the reasonably low cost and relative safety, consideration should be made for a therapeutic trial with H1 antagonists, H2 antagonists, cromolyn, and montelukast. Even when MCAS is unequivocally present in a patient with PoTS, it is unclear to what degree the PoTS symptoms will respond to mast cell therapy.

It is understood that considerable variation exists in the assessment and treatment of comorbid mast cell activation in PoTS. A suggested approach to treatment would be the addition of the medications in sequential fashion. Each treatment should be assessed for effectiveness and if ineffective consider discontinuation.

Lifestyle and Dietary Changes

General relaxation, stress and pain management, patient education, self-care and behavioural modification can be useful adjunctive treatment to help manage and cope with this chronic condition. Manual physical therapy/trigger point techniques are often a first line non-invasive treatment method for pain symptoms such as vulvodynia or pelvic floor muscle spasm.

Most patients with PoTS and MCAS go through a phase of trying exclusion diets and pro-biotics with variable success. Histamine and other biogenic amines are present to various degrees in many common foods and their presence increases with food maturation. Manipulation of diet by controlling histamine intake can therefore alleviate and stabilise symptoms over time.

Patients with evidence of MCAS can benefit from exclusion of mast cell liberating foods such as egg-white, citrus, chocolate and crustaceans (Table 1) [15, 33]. In general, fresh, unprocessed or basic foods should be better tolerated. Food storage will affect the histamine content of food and therefore it should be refrigerated, ideally uninterrupted before consumption. Fermented or microbe-ripened products (e.g. alcoholic products, vinegar, yeasts), perishable fresh produce with inadequate/uncertain freshness or with an interrupted cooling chain (e.g. seafood) should be avoided. Canned, finished or semi-finished products or foods for reheating with long storage time should also be avoided.

Patients suspected of histamine intolerance due to low serum diamine oxidase will benefit from low dietary intake of amines including histamine (Table 1). A small study of 20 patients

Table 1 Food table for diet modification

Histamine liberating foods	Foods that inhibit DAO
Nuts—walnuts, cashews Cocoa and chocolate Pineapple Citrus fruits Kiwi Strawberries Tomatoes, ketchup, tomato juice Pulses/legumes	Alcohol Cocoa Black tea Green tea Mate tea (chimarrão)
Foods high in histamine	*Foods considered low in histamine*
Pickled foods Matured cheese Hard cheeses Smoked or cured meats Preserved fish products Beans Chickpeas Soy beans and soy products Alcohol—particularly red wine, beer Nuts—peanuts, cashew, walnuts Black and green tea Cocoa and chocolate	Soft cheese Fresh meats Freshly caught seafood Egg yolk Pasta Rice noodles Yeast-free rye bread Oats, oat milk Corn/rice/crisp bread Rice, puffed rice, rice milk Fresh fruit: melon, blueberry, cranberries, lychee, mango, rhubarb, cherries, apricot, apple Fresh vegetables: lettuce, cabbage, beetroot, pumpkin, onion, radishes, lamb's lettuce, carrot, broccoli, potato, cucumber, leek, zucchini/courgette, sweet corn, asparagus, garlic

Note DAO—Diamine Oxidase

with low diamine oxidase activity (<40 HDU/ml) showed an improvement or disappearance of symptoms at 6 months. A relapse in symptoms was noted if a high histamine meal was ingested [34].

A histamine limited diet can impose complex restrictions and can negatively impact the quality of life of patients [35]. Therefore, in the absence of benefit, patients can be encouraged to revert to a healthy, balanced diet if the trial fails to improve symptoms. In the future it may be possible for personalised recommendations for dietary modifications to be developed through the study of an individual's glycaemic and microbiome profile and the response to specific foods [15].

Histamine Receptor Antagonists

Oral medication with both histamine-receptor 1 (H1) and histamine-receptor 2 (H2) antagonists can reduce the histamine burden released by mast cells and provide symptomatic relief. Historically this has been the most frequently used treatment approach. Second generation H1 antagonists such as loratidine, cetirizine, fexofenadine and desloratadine, thought to be less sedating, are now commonly prescribed. There are over 40 preparations available worldwide.

Ranitidine is an H2 antagonist. It is more commonly used to reduce stomach acidity, but it can also be used to target H2 receptors in the bladder to reduce inflammation. Cimetidine is an alternative H2 antagonist although inhibition of diamine oxidase can occur and therefore should be avoided if histamine intolerance is suspected or serum diamine oxidase is found to be low.

Combined treatment with H1 and H2 antagonists are typically prescribed to take on a daily basis for a trial of at least 4 weeks–6 months. Symptom improvement with this treatment supports the diagnosis of MCAS and should be continued to maintain symptom control. However, there is only one randomised controlled trial to support which dose, combination or duration of treatment regime is most efficacious in bladder pain [36].

Sodium Cromoglicate

Sodium cromoglicate or cromolyn disodium inhibits mast cell activation through an elusive and unknown mechanism therefore preventing the release of histamine and tryptase and synthesis of inflammatory prostaglandins and leukotrienes. It has been shown to diminish the early and late phase allergic response by mast cells to antigen challenge. Cromolyn has recently been shown to activate the G protein coupled receptor GPR35. This receptor is present on mast cells, basophils and eosinophils. It is upregulated after mast cell exposure to IgE antibodies but is also described as a Gαi/o—coupled inhibitor of synaptic transmission. Animal studies have suggested an anti-nociceptive effect after agonist binding [37].

Sodium cromoglicate is available as eye drops (for allergic conjunctivitis), intra-nasal spray (for allergic rhinitis), inhaler (for asthma maintenance treatment) and tablet form (for food allergy with diet restriction). Oral administration may be used to treat the gastrointestinal symptoms of MCAS.

Side effects of sodium cromoglycate include an intolerance of the medication, transient bronchospasm with inhaler use, arthralgia, nausea, rash and rarely eosinophilic pneumonia with inhaled use [38].

Ketotifen

Ketotifen is a first generation anti-histamine, with H1 receptor antagonist properties as well as a mast cell stabilising action. It is available as eye drops for allergic conjunctivitis, in tablets or as an oral solution. Common side effects of ketotifen include drowsiness in up to 40% of users [36], gastro-intestinal discomfort and dry mouth. The authors prescribe an increasing dose of ketotifen every 2 weeks commencing with 0.5 mg once at night or twice daily. This is increased to reach up to 2 mg twice daily if benefits are experienced and side effects tolerated.

Montelukast

Montelukast sodium is classically used in the treatment of asthma or allergic rhinitis. It is a selective leukotriene receptor antagonist of the cysteinyl leukotriene 1 receptor (CysLT1R) with no agonist activity. Cysteinyl leukotrienes (LTC 4, LTD 4, LTE 4) are products of arachidonic acid metabolism that are released from mast cells and eosinophils. Inhibition of cysteinyl leukotrienes binding to CysLT1R has reduced neuroinflammation and promoted blood brain barrier function in animal studies. This can make montelukast a useful adjunct for MCAS neurogenesis treatment [37].

Common side effects of montelukast include diarrhoea, headache, gastrointestinal discomfort, nausea, vomiting, upper respiratory tract infection, dry mouth, oedema and rarely neuropsychiatric reactions, including speech impairment and obsessive-compulsive symptoms. Reassuringly studies have shown no significant drug interactions with theophylline, warfarin, fexofenadine and oral contraceptives containing norethindrone 1 mg and ethinyl estradiol 35 mcg [39].

Diamine Oxidase

Patients considered to have histamine intolerance especially with a serum diamine oxidase level of <10 U/mL would benefit from the use of a diamine oxidase supplements in addition to a diet low in histamine.

A non-randomised study using Daosin® (AET Pharma, Italy), diamine oxidase supplementation up to three times a day for 4 weeks in 28 patients presenting with histamine intolerance with serum diamine oxidase <10 U/mL, demonstrated a significant improvement to gastrointestinal, cardiovascular, respiratory and skin symptoms [40]. Similarly, in a small study of 14 patients suspected to have histamine intolerance presenting as food intolerance, 10 were found to have serum diamine oxidase <10 U/mL (mean 7.04 ± 6.90 U/mL). Treatment with Daosin twice daily 15 minutes before food for a minimum of 14 days demonstrated a reduction of at least 1 histamine intolerance associated symptom when combined with a low histamine diet [35].

Histamine intolerance may not always be clear in its presentation and overlap with MCAS and PoTS symptoms; however if suspected a trial of diamine oxidase supplementation my provide benefit. A pilot study using Daosin for thirty days, on twenty patients with chronic urticaria as the main symptom, found no overall significant improvement in 7-day urticarial activity score in patients. However, in the 5 patients with a low serum diamine oxidase (<10 U/mL), treatment with 1 capsule 15 minutes before lunch and dinner produced a significant improvement [41]. Similarly, a larger study using diamine oxidase treatment for 1 month in patients with migraines, found a significant reduction in migraine severity with a decrease in triptan medication use [42].

Of note Daosin contains 0.3 mg of porcine diamine oxidase. Vegetable based diamine oxidase is also available over the counter or from health food shops but to our knowledge have not been formally studied in randomised controlled trials.

Vitamin and Flavonol Supplementation

Histamine degradation can be supported by the administration of oral vitamin C (ascorbic acid) which has mild antihistamine action. Good sources of dietary vitamin C include citrus fruits and strawberries which are high in histamine and have histamine-liberating effects with exclusion from the diet recommended. Therefore, supplementation for this group of patients could be a useful adjunct.

Vitamin C is available in a joint preparation with quercetin, a ubiquitous plant flavonol found in fruit and vegetables. Quercetin is considered to have anti-inflammatory, antioxidative and anti-carcinogenic activity. Its anti-inflammatory action allows it to be a mast cell stabiliser preventing degranulation and inhibits histamine release. In a dose dependent manner, it has also been reported to inhibit tryptase and the transcription of histidine decarboxylase which generates histamine from histadine [43]. The authors in their clinical practice suggest supplementation of quercetin 500 mg twice daily to patients considered to have MCAS.

Diamine oxidase is a vitamin B6 (pyridoxine)-dependent enzyme. Supplementation with vitamin B6 is thought to lead to an increase in diamine oxidase activity and may be a useful adjunct in patients with histamine intolerance [44].

Treatment of Recurrent Urinary Tract Infections

Recurrent urinary tract infection symptoms are a significant bother to patients and can increase in incidence for women over 65 years of age. Women found to have evidence of bacterial infection or chronic bladder inflammation may benefit from treatment to eradicate and supress an infective cause. Acute treatment of a urinary tract infection is with antibiotic medication. Antimicrobial medication as well as non-antibiotic treatment can be considered for prevention. There is considerable overlap in symptom presentation in patients with recurrent UTI and BPS/IC, with both infective and inflammatory pathologies being present. Often treatment of recurrent UTI is complemented with medication to target MCAS or histamine intolerance.

In the era of antibiotic stewardship and the consideration of long-term side effects of antibiotic medication, alternative treatments to prevent recurrent UTI have been studied. The overuse of anti-microbial medication in both human and veterinary medicine has driven the global emergence of urinary pathogens that are resistant to commonly used antibiotics. With our armoury of effective antibiotics being reduced, we must be conscientious prescribers of antibiotic medication.

Antibiotic Treatment

Large reviews have shown that long-term antibiotic prophylaxis, taken for 6–12 months, can significantly reduce clinical recurrences of a UTI comparing with placebo in both pre and post-menopausal women [45, 46]. However, there are no formal recommendations or consensus to guide commencement of treatment or dose regime. There is a concern that prolonged antibiotic treatment can increase urinary and faecal microbial antibiotic resistance with other common side effects including vaginal and oral candidiasis and gastrointestinal symptoms [45]. Furthermore, the beneficial effects are not reported to be long-lasting with a diminished effect once prophylaxis stops. Therefore, a discussion between clinician and patient should be carried out to discuss the risks and benefits of long-term prophylaxis treatment [46].

D-Mannose

D-Mannose is monosaccharide extracted from larch rod. It is rapidly absorbed and excreted by the urinary tract. D-mannose inhibits bacterial adhesion to the bladder urothelium therefore preventing the critical step to initiate a UTI caused by *Escherichia coli (E.Coli)*. D-mannose inhibits the interaction between *E.Coli* FimH adhesion molecules, found at the tip of the *E.Coli* fibrillum, with mannosylated host proteins at the surface of the urothelium by saturating the FimH adhesins. Bacteria bound to D-mannose will remain free in the urine and consequently are expelled from the urinary tract with voiding [20].

D-mannose is available in granule form or tablet (Mannocist® 1.5 g Laboratori Farmaceutici Krymi, Rome, Italy) form. A small study of 43 patients with current UTI demonstrated a reduction in UTI recurrence at 6 months when comparing a treatment and prophylaxis regime of Mannocist with a once only treatment. The treatment included Mannocist twice daily for 3 days, daily for 10 days, followed by prophylaxis with once daily Mannocist one a week every month. 4.5% (n = 1/22) compared with 33% (n = 7/21) of study participants who continued the prophylaxis developed a recurrent UTI at 6 months [47].

A larger study of 308 participants, comparing 2 g D-mannose powder in 200 ml water with daily 50 mg nitrofurantoin and no prophylaxis, showed a significant reduction in recurrent UTI in both the antibiotic and D-mannose groups. At 6 months, 14.6% in the D-mannose group and 20.4% in the nitrofurantoin group, compared with 60% in the untreated group developed recurrent urinary tract infections [48].

The optimal treatment regime is yet to be determined. However, D-mannose is reported to be well tolerated with a good safety profile. For patients who develop recurrent UTI particularly caused by *E.Coli* a trial of D-mannose could be beneficial.

Methenamine Hippurate

Methenamine hippurate has been used as a urinary anti-septic since 1899. It is a cyclic hydrocarbon that is hydrolysed in acidic urine into ammonia and formaldehyde and is considered bacteriostatic. In vitro studies suggest an optimal pH of <5.85 is required to produce the optimal bacteriostatic concentration of formaldehyde from methenamine, and therefore methenamine can be administered with ascorbic acid. Study results are heterogeneous, though some benefit has been noted in patients with recurrent UTI with no renal tract abnormalities [20]. A more recent small retrospective study of 38 renal transplant patients found that 1 g OD of methenamine reduced the risk of recurrent UTI, hospital admissions and length of antibiotic therapy [49].

Methenamine has a low adverse-effect profile and no risk of antimicrobial resistance. This could be a promising non-antibiotic treatment option but should be avoided in patients with severe renal failure (GFR < 10 mL/min) due to the risk of toxic serum levels and hepatic impairment. Optimal regimes have not been established and dosing can range from 1 to 4 g daily. The authors preferred regime is 1 g taken twice a day.

Topical Vaginal Oestrogen

Menopausal women are at increased risk of developing recurrent urinary tract infections. A fall in oestrogen promotes structural changes that can contribute to reduced urinary flow, increased post-void residual volume as well as an increased vaginal pH with the loss of commensal lactobacilli. Replacement of oestrogen with topical oestrogen creams, oestrogen ring or vaginal pessaries aims to modulate the natural defences of the lower urinary tract against UTI [50]. Oestrogen receptors are normally present in the upper vagina, urethra and trigone. Replenishment of vaginal oestrogen in post-menopausal women promotes glycogen storage within the vaginal epithelium which in turn allows lactobacilli to thrive. Lactobaccilli aid in maintaining a low vaginal pH by converting glycogen into lactic acid. An acidic vaginal pH is hostile to uropathogens which can otherwise cause recurrent UTI in post-menopausal women [51, 52].

Vaginal irritation, burning or itching has been reported which can lead to treatment cessation.

Bladder Pain Syndrome Targeted Therapies

Antidepressants such as amitriptyline or duloxetine can help reduce bladder pain symptoms. Gabapentin and pregabalin may also be a useful adjunct to treat chronic pain symptoms.

Pentosan polysulfate (Elmiron®) is licenced for use in the treatment of bladder pain syndrome. However long-term high dose use can rarely cause pigmentary maculopathy and therefore regular ophthalmic examinations during the treatment are recommended. Other common side effects include alopecia, back pain, asthenia, dizziness, gastrointestinal discomfort, diarrhoea, pelvic pain and peripheral oedema.

If oral treatment with antihistamine medication or mast cell stabilising medication is not fully effective additional treatments may be sought to reduced symptom severity. Intravesical treatments with instillations using hyaluronic acid, chondroitin sulfate, dimethyl sulfoxide, corticosteroid (e.g. hydrocortisone, triamcinolone), lidocaine and heparin have been found to be effective in treating symptoms [7], although the best combination, dosage, and frequency is yet to be determined.

Bladder dome or trigone injection with Botulinum toxin A, a neurotoxin, or triamcinolone, particularly in the presence of ulceration, have both been studied. Both have shown treatment benefit with a reduction in bladder pain, but neither are curative and require repeat treatment. Risks of urinary tract infection, dysuria and urine retention have been reported with the use of Botulinum toxin [53].

If ulcerations are identified at cystoscopy, transurethral fulguration, ablation or resection is recommended producing symptom improvement in 50–81% of treated patients [54]. Medically recalcitrant cases may be suitable for sacral neuromodulation and may be of additional benefit in treating pain symptoms as well as lower urinary tract symptoms. Success rates, particularly with optimised protocols to include motor response with low ($\leq$3 V) voltage stimulation can produce clinical benefit with a reduction in visual analogue pain scores and validated symptom questionnaires in up to 95% of patients [55].

Resistant cases may benefit from adjuvant treatment with cyclosporine which inhibits production and release of lymphokines and therefore suppressing cell-mediated immune responses. The last line of treatment is surgery which can include urinary diversion without cystectomy, augmentation ileocystoplasty and cystectomy [56].

Pelvic Floor Muscle Spasm or High Tone Pelvic Floor Dysfunction

Palpable pelvic floor spasm or high tone pelvic floor dysfunction can be a cause of persistent pelvic pain despite optimal management of the underlying causes, for example endometriosis and bladder pain syndrome. Pelvic floor muscle spasm is also a cause of chronic pelvic pain associated with dyspareunia, vaginismus, lower back pain and constipation. It is estimated that 87% of patients with bladder pain syndrome/interstitial cystitis also have concomitant pelvic floor muscle spasm [57].

Chronic pelvic pain is pain that persists in the lower abdomen or pelvis for a minimum of six months that does not occur exclusively with menstruation, pregnancy or intercourse. Chronic pelvic pain can arise from any pelvic structure and is estimated to account for 20–40% of gynaecological consultations [23]. It is likely that both peripheral and central sensitisation sustains chronic pain symptoms. Central sensitisation is associated with the release of pro-inflammatory mediators such as substance P and calcitonin gene-related protein (CGRP). These contribute to the lowered pain thresholds, allodynia, and hyperalgesia that has been demonstrated for fibromyalgia, endometriosis, vulvodynia, and dysmenorrhea. As such, myofascial trigger points and spasm can become present in pelvic floor muscles [58].

Vaginal examination should be carried out in patients presenting with chronic pelvic pain. Pelvic floor muscle spasm or trigger point tenderness can be palpated for. Compression of the anterior vaginal wall may reproduce the patient's pain symptoms and is suggestive of bladder inflammation or infection. Cervical excitation or pain upon movement of the cervix is suggestive of an inflammatory process of the pelvic organs and can be identified through bimanual examination of the cervix and uterus. The finding is classically associated with pelvic inflammatory disease but can be present in endometriosis or acutely with ovarian torsion and appendicitis for example.

Management of pelvic floor muscle spasm is multi-modal. Muscle spasm can be treated through pelvic floor muscle relaxation exercises to relieve pain. Physiotherapists can carry out trigger point stimulation and massage; alternatively, dry needling, or injection of local anaesthetic can be administered. Dry needling is carried out by placing a fine needle into the area of maximal pain or trigger point, using rapid in-and-out manoeuvres. The technique can be as effective as injection with local aesthetic [57].

For patients not responding to the above treatments, injections with onabotulinum toxin A to the pelvic floor muscles are gaining popularity to relieve pelvic floor spasm and associated pain. The Onabotulinum toxin A inhibits acetylcholine release from presynaptic neurons at the nicotinic neuromuscular junction. It is also thought to prevent the release of pain-associated pro-inflammatory neurochemicals, including glutamate, CGRP, and substance P. The treatment benefits have been reported to last 5–11 months. Adverse events are reported to be mild and transient including minor bleeding, constipation, temporary faecal incontinence, urine retention, vaginal heaviness or worsening vaginal prolapse, or worsening or new urinary incontinence [58].

Key Points

- The frequent presentation of the triad of PoTS, hypermobile EDS and MCAS suggests common pathophysiological mechanisms.
- There is a higher prevalence of recurrent urinary tract infections.
- Bladder dysfunction in PoTS patients can lead to voiding dysfunction with an increased post-void residual or urinary retention.
- Bladder dysfunction in PoTS patients can lead to urinary frequency, urgency, nocturia, stress urinary and urgency incontinence.
- Bladder dysfunction in PoTS patients can be associated with bladder pain syndrome/interstitial cystitis.
- Patients with the triad of PoTS, hEDS, MCAS can present with chronic pelvic pain syndromes including pelvic floor dysfunction with spasm and increased pelvic floor tone.

References

1. Haylen BT, Ridder D, Freeman RM, Swift SE, Berghmans B, Lee J, et al. An international urogynecological association (IUGA)/international

continence society (ICS) joint report on the terminology for female pelvic floor dysfunction. Neurourol Urodyn. 2010;29(1):4–20.

2. Walker NF, Feuer J, Taylor, C. Urodynamic evaluation of bladder dysfunction in patients with Postural Orthostatic Tachycardia Syndrome (POTS). BAUS ePoster online library. Taylor C. 2017;177417:P7–11.
3. Lo TS, Shailaja N, Hsieh WC, Uy-Patrimonio MC, Yusoff FM, Ibrahim R. Predictors of voiding dysfunction following extensive vaginal pelvic reconstructive surgery. Int Urogynecol J. 2017;28(4):575–82.
4. Hartigan SM, Reynolds WS, Dmochowski RR. Detrusor underactivity in women: a current understanding. Neurourol Urodyn. 2019;38(8):2070–6.
5. Mustafa HI, Garland EM, Biaggioni I, et al. Abnormalities of angiotensin regulation in postural tachycardia syndrome. Heart Rhythm. 2011;8(3):422–8.
6. Fu Q, VanGundy TB, Shibata S, Auchus RJ, Williams GH, Levine BD. Menstrual cycle affects renal-adrenal and hemodynamic responses during prolonged standing in the postural orthostatic tachycardia syndrome. Hypertension. 2010;56(1):82–90.
7. Abrams P, Cardozo L, Wagg A, Wein A (Eds). Incontinence 6th Edition. ICI-ICS. International Continence Society, Bristol UK. 2017 p 66–77. ISBN: 978-0956960733.
8. Kaufman MR. Chang-Kit L, et al. Overactive bladder and autonomic dysfunction: lower urinary tract symptoms in females with postural tachycardia syndrome. Neurourol Urodyn. 2017;36:610–3.
9. Shaw BH, Stiles LE, Bourne K, et al. The face of postural tachycardia syndrome—insights from a large cross-sectional online community-based survey. J Intern Med. 2019;286(4):438–48.
10. Ochodnicky P, Uvelius B, Andersson KE, Michel MC. Autonomic nervous control of the urinary bladder. Acta Physiol (Oxf). 2013;207(1):16–33.
11. Ates E, Ipekci T, Akin Y, Kizilay F, Kukul E, Guntekin E. Impact of sympathetic dysfunction in the etiology of overactive bladder in women: a preliminary study. Neurourol Urodyn. 2016;35(1):26–8.
12. Goodman BP. Evaluation of postural tachycardia syndrome (POTS). Auton Neurosci. 2018;215:12–9.
13. Digesu GA, Khullar V, Cardozo L, Salvatore S. Overactive bladder symptoms: do we need urodynamics? [published correction appears in Neurourol Urodyn. 2003;22(4):356]. Neurourol Urodyn. 2003;22(2):105–108. https://doi.org/10.1002/nau.10099.
14. Dumoulin C, Cacciari LP, Hay-Smith EJC. Pelvic floor muscle training versus no treatment, or inactive control treatments, for urinary incontinence in women. Cochrane Database Syst Rev. 2018;(10). Article No. CD005654.
15. Wells R, Tonkin A. Clinical approach to autonomic dysfunction [published correction appears in Intern Med J. 2017;47(1):126]. Intern Med J. 2016;46(10):1134–1139.
16. Athanasopoulos A, Giannitsas K. An overview of the clinical use of antimuscarinics in the treatment of overactive bladder. Adv Urol. 2011;2011:820816.
17. Bhide AA, Tailor V, Fernando R, Khullar V, Digesu GA. Posterior tibial nerve stimulation for overactive bladder-techniques and efficacy. Int Urogynecol J. 2019.
18. Tahseen S. Role of sacral neuromodulation in modern urogynaecology practice: a review of recent literature. Int Urogynecol J. 2018;29:1081–91.
19. Te Dorsthorst M, Digesu GA, Tailor V, et al. 3-year follow-up, of a new implantable tibial nerve stimulator for the treatment of overactive bladder syndrome (OAB) [published online ahead of print. 2020]. J Urol. 2020. https://doi.org/10.1097/ju.0000000000001024.
20. Sihra N, Goodman A, Zakri R, Sahai A, Malde S. Nonantibiotic prevention and management of recurrent urinary tract infection. Nat Rev Urol. 2018;15:750–776.
21. Kavi L, Nuttall M, Low DA, et al. A profile of patients with postural tachycardia syndrome and their experience of healthcare in the UK. Br J Cardiol. 2016;23:1–6.
22. Chuang FC, Kuo HC. Increased Urothelial cell apoptosis and chronic inflammation are associated with recurrent urinary tract infection in women. PLoS ONE. 2013;8:5.
23. Doggweiler R, Whitmore KE, Meijlink JM, Drake MJ, Frawley H, Nordling J, Hanno P, Fraser MO, Homma Y, Garrido G, Gomes MJ, Elneil S, van de Merwe JP, Lin ATL, Tomoe H. A standard for terminology in chronic pelvic pain syndromes: a report from the chronic pelvic pain working group of the international continence society. Neurourol Urodyn. 2017;36(4):984–1008.
24. Hanno PM, Erickson D, Moldwin R, Faraday MM, American Urological Association. Diagnosis and treatment of interstitial cystitis/bladder pain syndrome: AUA guideline amendment. J Urol. 2015;193(5):1545–53.
25. van de Merwe JP, Nordling J, Bouchelouche P, et al. Diagnostic criteria, classification, and nomenclature for painful bladder syndrome/interstitial cystitis: an ESSIC proposal. Eur Urol. 2008;53(1):60–7.
26. Hunner GL. A rare type of bladder ulcer in women; report of cases. Boston Med Surg J. 1915;172:660–4.
27. Larsen MS, Mortensen S, Nordling J, Horn T. Quantifying mast cells in bladder pain syndrome by immunohistochemical analysis. BJU Int. 2008;102(2):204–7.
28. Stromberga Z, Chess-Williams R, Moro C. Histamine modulation of urinary bladder urothelium, lamina propria and detrusor contractile activity via H1 and H2 receptors. Sci Rep. 2019;9(1):3899. Published 2019 Mar 7.

29. Grundy L, Caldwell A, Brierley S. Mechanisms underlying overactive bladder and interstitial cystitis/bladder pain syndrome. Front Neurosci. 2018;12(12):931.
30. Shan H, Zhang E, Zhang P, Zhang XD, Zhang N, Du P, Yang Y. Differential expression of histamine receptors in the bladder wall tissues of patients with bladder pain syndrome/interstitial cystitis—significance in the responsiveness to antihistamine treatment and disease symptoms. BMC Urol. 2019;19:115.
31. Bonamichi-Santos R, Yoshimi-Kanamori K, Giavina-Bianchi P, Aun MV. Association of postural tachycardia syndrome and ehlers-danlos syndrome with mast cell activation disorders. Immunol Allergy Clin North Am. 2018;38(3):497–504.
32. Afrin LB, Molderings GJ. A concise, practical guide to diagnostic assessment for mast cell activation disease. World J Hematol. 2014;3:1–17.
33. Izquierdo-Casas J, Comas-Baste O, Latorre-Moratalla ML, Lorente-Gascon M, Duelo A, Soler-Singla L, Vidal-Carou. Low serum diamine oxidase (DAO) activity levels in patients with migraine. J Physiol Biochem. 2018;74:93–99.
34. Mušič E, Korošec P, Šilar M, Adamič K, Košnik M, Rijavec M. Serum diamine oxidase activity as a diagnostic test for histamine intolerance. Wien Klin Wochenschr. 2013;125:239–43.
35. Manzotti G, Breda D, Di Gioacchino M, Burastero SE. Serum diamine oxidase activity in patients with histamine intolerance. Int J Immunopathol Pharmacol. 2016;29(1):105–11.
36. Nurmatov UB, Rhatigan E, Simons FE, Sheikh A. H1-antihistamines for primary mast cell activation syndromes: a systematic review. Allergy. 2015;70(9):1052–61.
37. Doherty TA, White AA. Postural orthostatic tachycardia syndrome and the potential role of mast cell activation. Auton Neurosci Basic Clin. 2018;215:83–8.
38. https://bnf.nice.org.uk/drug/sodium-cromoglicate.html#indicationsAndDoses.
39. https://bnf.nice.org.uk/drug/montelukast.html.
40. Schnedl W, Schenk M, Lackner S, Enko D, Mangge H, Forster F. Diamine oxidase supplementation improves symptoms in patients with histamine intolerance. Food Sci Biotechnol. 2019;28(6):1779–84.
41. Yacoub MR, Ramirez GA, Berti A, Mercurio G, Breda D, Sapriti N, et al. Diamine oxidase supplementation in chronic spontaneous urticaria: a randomized, double-blind placebo-controlled study. Int Arch Allergy Immunol. 2018.
42. Izquierdo-Casas J, Comas-Baste O, Latorre-Moratalla ML, Lorente-Gascon M, Duelo A, Soler-Singla L, Vidal-Carou. Diamine oxidase (DAO) supplement reduces headache in episodic migraine patients with DAO deficiency: a randomized double-blind trial. Clin Nutr. 2019;38:152–8.
43. Shaik Y, Caraffa A, Ronconi G, Lessiani G, Conti P. Impact of polyphenols on mast cells with special emphasis on the effect of quercetin and luteolin. Cent Eur J Immunol. 2018;43(4):476–81.
44. Maintz L, Novak N. Histamine and histamine intolerance. Am J Clin Nutr. 2007;85:1185–96.
45. Ahmed H, Davies F, Francis N, Farewell D, Butler C, Paranjothy S. Long-term antibiotics for prevention of recurrent urinary tract infection in older adults: systematic review and meta-analysis of randomised trials. BMJ Open. 2017;7:e015233.
46. Albert X, Huertas I, Pereiro I, Sanfélix J, Gosalbes V, Perrotta C. Antibiotics for preventing recurrent urinary tract infection in non-pregnant women. Cochrane Database Syst. Rev. 2004;(3). Article No. CD001209.
47. Dominici L, Monti M, Bracchi C, Giorgini M, Colagiovanni V, Muzii L, et al. D-mannose: a promising support for acute urinary tract infections in women: a pilot study. Eur Rev Med Pharmacol Sci. 2016;20(13):2920–5.
48. Kranjčec B, Papeš D, Altarac S. D-mannose powder for prophylaxis of recurrent urinary tract infections in women: a randomized clinical trial. World J Urol. 2014;32:79–84.
49. Hollyer I, Varias F, Ho B, Ison MG. Safety and efficacy of methenamine hippurate for the prevention of recurrent urinary tract infections in adult renal transplant recipients: a single center, retrospective study. Transpl Infect Dis. 2019;21(3):e13063.
50. Mody L, Juthani-Mehta M. Urinary tract infections in older women: a clinical review. JAMA. 2014;311(8):844–54.
51. Stamm WE, Raz R. Factors contributing to susceptibility of postmenopausal women to recurrent urinary tract infections. Clin Infect Dis. 1999;28:723–72.
52. Stapleton AE. The vaginal microbiota and urinary tract infection. Microbiol Spectr. 2016;4(6). https://doi.org/10.1128/microbiolspec.uti-0025-2016.
53. Shim SR, Cho YJ, Shin IS, Kim JH. Efficacy and safety of botulinum toxin injection for interstitial cystitis/bladder pain syndrome: a systematic review and meta-analysis. Int Urol Nephrol. 2016;48(8):1215–27.
54. Crescenze IM, et al. Advanced management of patients with ulcerative interstitial cystitis/bladder pain syndrome. Urology. 2019. pii: S0090-4295(19)30723-X.
55. Marinkovic SP. Improving clinical outcomes with lower motor voltage ($\leq$3 V) during stage 1 sacral neuromodulation for interstitial cystitis or bladder pain syndrome. Neurourol Urodyn. 2019;38(8):2233–41.
56. Redmond EJ, Flood HD. The role of reconstructive surgery in patients with end-stage interstitial cystitis/bladder pain syndrome: is cystectomy necessary? Int Urogynecol J. 2017;28(10):1551–6.

57. Jia X, Rana N, Crouss T, Whitmore KE. Gynecological associated disorders and management. Int J Urol. 2019;26(Suppl 1):46–51.
58. Karp BI, Tandon H, Vigil D, Stratton P. Methodological approaches to botulinum toxin for the treatment of chronic pelvic pain, vaginismus, and vulvar pain disorders. Int Urogynecol J. 2019;30:1071–81.

Gynaecological Considerations in PoTS

Visha Tailor and Vik Khullar

Introduction

The heterogenous, multifactorial condition of postural tachycardia syndrome (PoTS) is frequently associated with other conditions including Ehlers-Danlos syndrome (EDS) and mast cell activation syndrome (MCAS) which are discussed in depth separately in this book. To understand the burden of these associations this chapter will provide a brief overview of these associated conditions to facilitate the understanding of the gynaecological presentation in women with PoTS.

Two large questionnaire-based studies have been carried out to evaluate the presentation, management pathway and common co-morbidities in patients with PoTS. A USA initiated online questionnaire study between 2015 and 2017 of 4835 patients diagnosed with PoTS, found that 25% also had a diagnosis of Ehlers Danlos Syndrome (EDS) and 9% had been diagnosed with mast cell activation syndrome (MCAS) [1]. A similar British study of 779 PoTS patients in the UK identified 49% of patients had associated EDS (using the Villefranche criteria) or generalised joint hypermobility [2].

Studies into the prevalence of PoTS in those diagnosed with hypermobile EDS (hEDS) have identified that 74–94% of patients have orthostatic intolerance and 41–49% have PoTS [3–5]. In comparison, 34% of healthy volunteers also displayed orthostatic intolerance.

hEDS and PoTS have associated co-morbidities, some of which are overlapping, including sleep disturbance, chronic fatigue syndrome/myalgic encephalomyelitis (CFS/ME), anxiety, depression, functional gastrointestinal disorders, chronic pain syndromes such as fibromyalgia, and MCAS [6].

The formal diagnosis of MCAS can be given to patients with symptoms typical for MCAS, laboratory evidence of mast cell activation, and clinical improvement with mast cell directed therapy. Symptoms are often vague and varied and overlap with PoTS and hEDS symptoms. Those particularly suggestive of MCAS in PoTS patients include facial or upper trunk flushing, hives, diarrhoea, itchy skin, and urinary irritability. The clinical manifestation often occurs in flares or bursts produced by episodic release of mast cell mediators in response to specific stimuli. Triggers for symptom flare should be explored and may include normal activities of daily life like exercise, food or alcohol ingestion, medication, or even menstruation in women [7, 8].

Chronic infection may precipitate symptoms and contribute to the pathophysiology in patients

V. Tailor · V. Khullar (✉)
Urogynaecology Department, St Mary's Hospital, Imperial College London, London, UK
e-mail: vik.khullar@imperial.ac.uk

N. Gall et al. (eds.), *Postural Tachycardia Syndrome*, https://doi.org/10.1007/978-3-030-54165-1_18

with hyperadrenergic PoTS and MCAS. These processes can underlie the presentations of bladder pain or pelvic pain to the gynaecology clinic.

Gynaecological Considerations

PoTS has a 5:1 female predominance with the onset or diagnosis most commonly given during the reproductive years between ages 15 and 50 [9]. Given the frequent association of PoTS with joint hypermobility, EDS and MCAS, it is sensible to understand the associated gynaecological and lower urinary tract symptoms that more frequently presents in this group of patients (Table 1).

Menstrual Physiology

Human females experience a highly regulated monthly menstrual cycle that normally allows for the ovulation of one oocyte in each cycle. There is a complex interaction between the hypothalamus, pituitary, ovary and uterus to facilitate this cycle. The length of the cycle is counted from the first day of a period to the first day of the next, typically varying from 21 days to 35 days in an adult. The cycle has three phases involving the ovary (ovarian cycle) and the uterus (uterine cycle). The ovarian cycle is divided into the follicular phase, ovulation and luteal phase. The uterine cycle is divided into menstruation, proliferative phase and secretory phase.

Table 1 Common gynaecological presentations and diagnoses in patients with PoTS, hEDS and MCAS

Menstrual dysfunction	Menorrhagia Intermenstrual bleeding Anovulation Dysmenorrhoea Endometriosis
Fertility considerations	Anovulation Infertility/sub-fertility
Pain syndromes	Dysmenorrhoea Vulvodynia Bladder pain syndrome Fybromyalgia
Infection	Vulval and vaginal infections Urinary tract infections
Urogynaecological	Vaginal prolapse
Bladder	Overactive bladder symptoms Voiding dysfunction Bladder pain syndrome

During the follicular phase the increasing oestrogen levels encourage proliferation of the endometrium following menses and development of ovarian follicles. Approximately mid-cycle ovulation occurs with a fall in oestrogen levels, a surge of luteinizing hormone (LH) and follicle stimulating hormone (FSH), followed by the release of an oocyte from the dominant follicle. LH and FSH can also be described as the gonadotrophin hormones, they are released by the anterior pituitary gland under the influence of gonadotrophin releasing hormone pulses from the hypothalamus. FSH encourages follicle development. LH initiates the final maturation of the oocyte within the follicle. It also induces an inflammatory-type reaction to the apex of the follicle adjacent to the ovarian cortex to enable rupture of the follicle wall for ovulation.

During the luteal phase the dominant follicle remnants form the corpus luteum which releases progesterone causing levels to rise. There is an associated rise in oestrogen until the mid-luteal phase, although not as pronounced as the rise that occurs towards the end of the follicular phase. The endometrium enters the secretory phase in anticipation of implantation of an embryo. In the absence of pregnancy, the corpus luteum involutes, progesterone levels fall, and menstruation follows with the follicular phase beginning again.

Menstruation can be described as an inflammatory event. A complex series of intra-uterine signalling occurs involving metalloproteinase enzymes, prostaglandin release and a release of chemotactic factors to draw leucocytes to the uterus. This invasion of leucocytes leads to release of inflammatory mediators such as prostaglandins E (PGE) and F (PGF). The PGE series stimulates pain, localised oedema, vasodilation and synthesis of interleukin 8 which is an inflammatory and chemotactic mediator. PGF, particularly $PGF_{2\alpha}$ produce myometrial contractions and vasoconstriction. Vasoconstriction leads to localised tissue hypoxia exacerbating inflammatory mediator release [10].

Effects of the Menstrual Cycle in Women with PoTS

Women with PoTS may note an increase in their 'light headedness' during the late luteal phase in the lead up to their menses and peaking in symptom severity during menses. During this time in the menstrual cycle, the effect of oestrogen is impaired by the anti-oestrogen effect of progesterone [11]. A rise towards a peak in oestrogen levels in the follicular phase around ovulation is associated with the improvement noted in 'light-headedness' until ovulation. However, at ovulation there is a sudden drop in oestrogen for 24 hours and ovulation itself is associated with an inflammatory episode to allow the release of the oocyte.

This pattern of light headedness is also reported in healthy women without a diagnosis of PoTS, though to a less severe degree. There is a reported increase in pre-syncopal episodes in both women with and without PoTS in the early follicular phase of the menstrual cycle compared to the mid luteal phase. This suggests a role of both oestrogen and progesterone in promoting orthostatic tolerance in women [12] or as a result of the inflammatory process during menstruation.

The mechanisms and pathophysiology of PoTS is heterogenous. A reduction in blood and plasma volume is thought to contribute to a reduction in stroke volume resulting in reflex tachycardia during orthostasis [13] in a cohort of patients with PoTS. Dysregulation of the renin-angiotensin-aldosterone system may be a cause of or contribute to PoTS symptomology. Similarly, an elevated sympathetic tone can also be seen in PoTS patients which may represent the primary underlying pathophysiology or be secondary to another mechanism such as hypovolaemia or neuropathy [14].

Effects of Oestrogen and Progesterone on the Renin-Angiotensin-Aldosterone System

The renin-angiotensin-aldosterone system (RAAS) has an important role in haemodynamic homeostasis. In patients with PoTS there can be a 'normal' levels of plasma renin activity with low levels of aldosterone. On standing, plasma renin activity can increase, and this has been shown to occur after 2 hours of standing; however a significant rise in aldosterone has not been observed. Patients with PoTS have and maintain a low aldosterone: renin ratio, even in the presence of hypovolaemia [12, 13].

Changes in oestrogen and progesterone levels during the menstrual cycle can impact the RAAS which may contribute to the cyclical nature of the light-headedness or pre-syncope symptoms experienced by PoTS patients and healthy women [12].

Oestrogen decreases the synthesis of renin and angiotensin converting enzyme but increases angiotensinogen synthesis. There are 2 angiotensin II receptors, AT1R and AT2R which are thought to have opposing effects [15]. Oestrogen decreases the expression of AT1R in target tissues which is responsible for the ability of angiotensin II to regulate blood pressure, maintain water-electrolyte balance and promote vasoconstriction. Oestrogen increases the expression of AT2R, activation of which prevents the development of pathological processes such as inflammation, activation of the sympathetic nervous system, apoptotic cell death, autophagy, cardiac fibrosis and arterial stiffness [16].

Endogenous progesterone increases during the luteal phase and acts as a mineralocorticoid receptor antagonist. Aldosterone acts in the kidney to promote sodium and water retention, with concomitant potassium and magnesium loss. Therefore, in the luteal phase antagonist interaction by progesterone prevents sodium retention with a compensatory increase in renin secretion, plasma renin activity, angiotensin II and plasma aldosterone [17].

In healthy women, therefore, the plasma renin activity and aldosterone increase, and plasma norepinephrine decreases during the luteal phase, when oestrogen levels are low and progesterone rising. The renal-adrenal response to orthostatic stress becomes significantly augmented in the luteal phase compared with the follicular phase of the menstrual cycle. Blood pressure, heart rate, and the responses to orthostasis however remains unchanged. Plasma catecholamine concentrations are also not thought to be affected by the menstrual cycle [12].

In comparison, women with PoTS have greater supine plasma renin activity in the mid-luteal phase compared with the early follicular phase, in keeping with the change in oestrogen levels [12]. In the early follicular phase, cardiac output and stroke volume is lower, while total peripheral resistance is greater compared to the mid-luteal phase after 30 min of standing. In a small study of ten patients, women with PoTS were found to have lower average progesterone levels in the mid-luteal phase compared with controls. However, with no direct effect on the length of menses, the full relevance of this is unknown [12]. Lastly, the plasma catecholamine concentrations are not thought to be affected by the menstrual cycle in women with PoTS.

The hormonal changes in the mid-luteal phase are associated with greater increases in renal-adrenal hormones and thought to overall lead to an associated increase in volume retention, and therefore improved late standing tolerance in PoTS patients.

Effect of the Menstrual Cycle on Sympathetic Stimulation

Patients with PoTS can have raised resting sympathetic nerve activity, as measured by microneurography. Microneurography assesses postganglionic efferent nerve discharges leading to the skeletal muscle. Investigations into the role of the sympathetic activity during the menstrual cycle in women with PoTS has yielded mixed results. It has been reported that the menstrual cycle can affect muscle sympathetic nerve activity (MSNA) which is attenuated in the upright position during the early follicular phase of the cycle [18] compared to the mid-luteal phase in healthy women not diagnosed with PoTS. This effect of the menstrual cycle has not been convincingly reproduced [19]. The reason why sex steroid concentrations would be related to MSNA in healthy individuals but not in PoTS patients is also unclear.

The vestibulosympathetic stimulation involved in regulating blood pressure is not thought to be affected by the menstrual cycle [18]. Attenuation of this reflex is more commonly associated with a reduction in arterial pressure that is seen with increasing age [20].

Hormonal Manipulation of the Menstrual Cycle

The menstrual cycle can be manipulated using synthetic hormones, for example the combined oral contraceptive pill, patch or vaginal ring, and progesterone only preparations. Combined oral hormonal replacement most commonly administers ethinylestradiol and a progestogen to inhibit ovulation as the primary effect. In addition, endometrial atrophy, alteration of cervical mucus, altered tubal motility and impaired uterine receptivity to implantation can occur. Desirable side effects as a result include a reduction in dysmenorrhea, menstrual flow, and pre-menstrual symptoms.

An alternative to combined hormonal treatment is the administration of progestogen either orally, via an injectable intra-muscular depot, subdermal implant or using an intra-uterine device system (IUS) (Mirena®, Kyleena® or Jaydess®, Bayer Schering, UK). Progesterone administration can inhibit ovulation to varying degrees, older 1st or 2nd generation progestogen pills in particular inhibit ovulation inconsistently. The IUS causes marked endometrial atrophy with little effect on ovarian activity. For some there is a desirable side effect of amenorrhoea in ~20% using desogestrel, 70% using injectable progestogen, 20% with a subdermal implant, and most patients with an IUS.

Irregular and unscheduled light bleeding is a common side effect of all progestogen use [10]. Women with EDS may find their joint dislocations worsen with progestogens. In this situation a very low dose progestogen intra-uterine coil such as Jaydess® can be used, but a compromise has to be struck as this coil is effective for only 3 years rather than 5 years with the Mirena® coil (which has three times the dose of levonorgestrel).

Given that women with PoTS are more susceptible to orthostatic intolerance when both oestrogen and progesterone levels are low, supplemental hormonal therapy with the combined oral contraceptive treatment, or even behaviour modification during the early follicular phase may improve symptoms. Combined use of oestrogens and synthetic progestogens may therefore enhance the oestrogenic effects on body sodium and blood pressure [17] through potent stimulation of the RAAS, particularly through first-pass hepatic metabolism. Synthetic progestogens with the exception of drospirenone are not mineralcorticoid receptor antagonists.

In contrast to the combined oral contraceptive pill (OCP), combined hormonal contraception administration using the transdermal patch (for example EVRA® Janssen-Cilag, UK) avoids hepatic first-pass metabolism. Theoretically, the contraceptive patch should not stimulate hepatic production of angiotensinogen [21]. Use of the contraceptive patch in normotensive pre-menopausal women is associated with less RAAS activation as well as blunting of the RAAS response to a simulated orthostatic stress. Pre-menopausal women using the contraceptive patch were found to have significantly lower baseline levels of angiotensinogen, angiotensin II and plasma renin activity compared with combined oral contraceptive use [22].

The use of combined oral hormonal treatment is thought to have limited impact on sympathetic neural control in young women and not considered to change basal MSNA levels in menopausal women. Long term transdermal administration of oestrogen however, can suppress basal MSNA without augmentation of arterial baroreflexes [18]. Overall, further research is needed to understand the impact of hormonal manipulation in women with PoTS and which method of administration is best tolerated.

Mast Cells and the Menstrual Cycle

At the end of the luteal phase of the menstrual cycle, luteolysis begins in the absence of implantation of a blastocyst. There is structural and functional degradation of the corpus luteum with a fall in serum oestradiol and progesterone levels. This leads to triggering of a process causing superficial endometrial tissue breakdown. During the normal menstrual cycle there is a marked immune response predominantly involving lymphocytes, macrophages, neutrophils, and natural killer cells. Mast cells are also normally present in the basal endometrium and myometrium with an increased presence during menstruation [23]. Elevated levels of extracellular tryptase in the late secretory phase is suggestive of increased mast cell activation during this time. Tryptase and other mediators including histamines, cytokines and growth factors released by the mast cells, induce tissue oedema and activate proteolytic enzymes and matrix metalloproteinases. Activation of the matrix metalloproteinase cascade results in subsequent degradation of extracellular matrix [24]. Upregulated mast cells and matrix metalloproteinase activation persists during menstruation.

Dysregulation of immune cells during the menstrual cycle is likely to create an inflammatory environment that can interfere with successful embryonic implantation, as well as contribute to other gynaecological pathologies such as heavy menstrual bleeding or even endometriosis.

The role of mast cells specifically during the menstrual cycle is not otherwise fully understood. However increased heparin-like activity has been reported in women with heavy menstrual bleeding. Degranulation of mast cells premenstrually and during menstruation leads to the release of the anti-coagulant heparin. Other mast cell products, including cyclooxygenase

(COX-2) enzymes and prostaglandins, are also increased in the endometrium of this group of women. Whilst prostaglandin production plays an integral role in the inflammatory process of normal menstruation, significantly elevated levels in women with heavy menstrual bleeding may alter the function of surrounding endometrial leukocytes. It has been reported that elevated levels of COX-2 and the resultant upregulated prostaglandins may even adversely affect the numbers and function of other leukocytes and dendritic cell populations [24].

Clinically, in women with MCAS, mast cell activation and symptom flare can occur pre-menstrually and with menstruation in approximately 25% [25]. At the extreme end of the clinical presentation spectrum, there are case reports of women who have experienced anaphylactoid reactions to the menstrual cycle. The reports describe how women develop urticaria, abdominal cramps and bloating after consumption of spice and shellfish, symptoms suggestive of MCAS [26]. It is important to remember that there are both histamine type 1 and 2 receptors present in the uterus and these can be targeted with anti-histamine medication.

Gynaecological Presentations in Women with PoTS

A questionnaire-based study sent to women with PoTS, revealed this group of women are more likely to be diagnosed with gynaecological conditions compared to 'healthy volunteers'. They may present more frequently with dysfunctional uterine bleeding, uterine fibroids, endometriosis, anovulation and ovarian cysts. They were not more likely to experience pre-menstrual symptoms when compared with healthy age matched controls [11, 27].

It is possible that the occurrence of gynaecological diagnoses may be related to the underlying physiological changes of PoTS. However,

Table 2 Food table for diet modification

Histamine liberating foods	Foods that inhibit DAO
Nuts—walnuts, cashews Cocoa and chocolate Pineapple Citrus fruits Kiwi Strawberries Tomatoes, ketchup, tomato juice Pulses/legumes	Alcohol Cocoa Black tea Green tea Mate tea (chimarrão)
Foods high in histamine	**Foods considered low in histamine**
Pickled foods Matured cheese Hard cheeses Smoked or cured meats Preserved fish products Beans Chickpeas Soy beans and soy products Alcohol—particularly red wine, beer Nuts—peanuts, cashew, walnuts Black and green tea Cocoa and chocolate	Soft cheese Fresh meats Freshly caught seafood Egg yolk Pasta Rice noodles Yeast-free rye bread Oats, oat milk Corn/rice/crisp bread Rice, puffed rice, rice milk Fresh fruit: melon, blueberry, cranberries, lychee, mango, rhubarb, cherries, apricot, apple Fresh vegetables: lettuce, cabbage, beetroot, pumpkin, onion, radishes, lamb's lettuce, carrot, broccoli, potato, cucumber, leek, courgette/zucchini, sweet corn, asparagus, garlic

Note DAO—Diamine Oxidase

PoTS is commonly associated with hEDS which is likely to contribute to the wide presentation of gynaecological and genitourinary symptoms, often with more than one symptom reported. It should also be acknowledged that patients with PoTS receive greater medical attention and investigation which may lead to an increase in diagnoses or acknowledgement of symptoms [11].

Gynaecological Presentations in EDS and MCAS

The gynaecological presentations in female patients with EDS have been best described in patients with hEDS and are similar to those described in women with PoTS. The prevalence of gynaecological problems in women with hEDS has been identified through questionnaire or survey-based studies. Approximately a third of women report normal menses [28]. Menstrual disturbances include menorrhagia (32.9–76%), recurrent anovulation (41.3%), irregular menses (28–46.3%), inter-menstrual bleeding (18.6%), endometriosis (15.8%) and dysmenorrhoea (72–92.5%) [28–31].

Menorrhagia or heavy menstrual bleeding is overall experienced by up to 15% of menstruating women; however, the exact pathophysiological mechanisms are largely unknown. In women with the triad of PoTS, hEDS and MCAS, there may be increased mast cell activation and release of heparin which will contribute to this increased prevalence of menorrhagia as well as dyspareunia and vaginitis. A novel treatment modality with diphenhydramine, a first generation H1 antagonist with anticholinergic properties, has been reported. Diphenhydramine administered as a vaginal douche has been successfully used to reduce dysfunctional uterine bleeding in patients diagnosed with MCAS who were not fully responsive to oral administration of H1 and H2 antagonists [32]. Whilst these authors do not recommend this form of treatment at this time, it provides insight into the development of novel future treatment methods.

From a survey of 1225 women with EDS 44.1% self-reported infertility [30]. Anovulation, pelvic pain, sexual dysfunction, vaginal dryness (25%) or the nature of a chronic condition could all be contributing negatively to fertility for these women [28].

Pain is a common symptom in women with PoTS and is associated with other systemic conditions such as fibromyalgia. Related to gynaecology 31.7–77% report dyspareunia and approximately 30% describe vulvodynia [28–31]. This may be related to underlying pathology such as endometriosis, recurrent vaginal infection (53%) or vaginal dryness (25%) [28]. The pain can be described as burning, stinging or irritation that is intermittent, persistent, immediate or delayed. Pain can be felt in the vagina or introitus and can be provoked by touch, pressure or friction in a generalised or localised distribution. Vulvodynia, were pain is triggered by touch of the skin around the vaginal entrance, can also be associated with additional pain syndromes and co-morbidities including high tone pelvic floor dysfunction, fibromyalgia, bladder pain syndrome/interstitial cystitis and irritable bowel syndrome (covered separately) [33].

The presentation of vulvodynia is similar to the nature of symptoms that are associated with MCAS. It is a complex pain syndrome that is poorly understood. However increased mast cells and sensory hyperinnervation of the vulva have been identified. A study of vulval biopsy in patients with vulvodynia identified >60 mast cells/mm^2 (range, 40–120 mast cells) in a sub-epithelial distribution or clustering around the vestibular glands [34]. The majority of these identified mast cells were present in a degranulated or activated state. This chronic inflammation can lead to the development of nociceptive and neuropathic pain over time [35].

Traditionally treatment for vulvodynia has involved systemic tricyclic antidepressants (amitriptyline), gabapentin, topical 2% amitriptyline and 2% baclofen cream or lidocaine. Surgical management has also been described with varying success following vulvar excision and vestibulectomy and is often reserved for women that have failed conservative and medical management. Given the association of POTS with MCAS, a trial of mast cell stabiliser treatments such as histamine type 2 blockers, ketotifen 1 mg at night or rupatadine 10 mg once a day should be considered.

Women with hEDS may also present with labial oedema and erythema which can be triggered by intercourse. It can be associated with pelvic floor muscle spasm, dyspareunia and vulval irritation. The nature of these symptoms is thought to be related to the underlying collagen abnormalities but may also be indicative of mast cell activation. During sexual arousal, blood flow to the genitals increases, leading to genital vasocongestion. PoTS theoretically may influence this process with exaggerated pooling of blood in the lower extremities, combined with tissue laxity which may explain this presentation [36]. It is also useful to explore additional symptoms associated with MCAS to aid symptom management as the oedema and erythema may represent localised intravaginal pressure urticaria related to MCAS [32].

Treatments

Lifestyle and Dietary Changes

General relaxation, stress and pain management, patient education, self-care and behavioural modification can be useful adjunctive treatment to help manage and cope with this chronic condition. Manual physical therapy/trigger point techniques are often a first line non-invasive treatment method for pain symptoms such as vulvodynia or pelvic floor muscle spasm.

Many patients with PoTS and MCAS go through a trial of exclusion diets and pro-biotics with variable success. Histamine and other biogenic amines are present to various degrees in many common foods, and their presence increases with maturation. Manipulation of diet by controlling histamine intake can therefore alleviate and stabilise symptoms over time.

Patients with evidence of MCAS can benefit from exclusion of mast cell liberating foods such as egg-white, citrus, chocolate and crustaceans (Table 2) [37, 38]. In general, fresh, unprocessed or basic foods should be tolerated. Food storage will affect the histamine content of food and therefore it should be refrigerated ideally uninterruptedly before consumption. Fermented or microbially ripened products (e.g. alcoholic products, vinegar, yeast, bacteria), perishable fresh produce with inadequate/uncertain freshness or with an interrupted cooling chain (eg seafood) should be avoided. Canned, finished or semi-finished products or foods for re-heating with long storage time should also be avoided.

Patients suspected of histamine intolerance due to low serum diamine oxidase will benefit from low dietary intake of amines including histamine (Table 2). A small study of 20 patients with low diamine oxidase activity (<40 HDU/ml) showed an improvement or disappearance of symptoms after 6 months of a low histamine diet. A relapse in symptoms was noted if a high histamine meal was ingested [39].

A histamine limited diet can impose complex restrictions and can negatively impact the quality of life of patients [40]. Therefore, in the absence of benefit, patients can be encouraged to revert to a healthy balanced diet if the trial fails to improve symptoms. In the future it may be possible for personalised recommendations for dietary modifications to be developed through the study of an individual's glycaemic and microbiome profile and response to specific foods [37].

Histamine Receptor Antagonists

Oral medication with both histamine-receptor 1 (H1) and histamine-receptor 2 (H2) antagonists can reduced the histamine burden released by mast cells and provide symptomatic relief. Historically this has been the most frequently used treatment approach. Second generation H1 antagonists such as loratidine, cetirizine, fexofenadine and desloratadine, thought to be less sedating, are now commonly prescribed; there are over 40 preparations available worldwide.

Ranitidine is a H2 antagonist. It is more commonly used to reduce stomach acidity, but can also be used to target H2 receptors in the bladder to reduce inflammation contributing to BPS/IC symptoms. Cimetidine is an alternative H2 antagonist. However, inhibition of diamine oxidase can occur and therefore is to be avoided if histamine intolerance is suspected or serum diamine oxidase is found to be low.

Combined treatment with H1 and H2 antagonists is typically prescribed to take on a daily basis for a trial of at least 4 weeks–6 months. Symptom improvement with this treatment supports the diagnosis of MCAS and should be continued to maintain symptoms control. However, there is only one randomised controlled trial to support which dose, combination or duration of treatment regime is most efficacious [41].

Sodium Cromoglicate

Sodium cromoglicate or cromolyn disodium inhibits mast cell activation through an elusive and unknown mechanism therefore preventing the release of histamine and tryptase and preventing the synthesis of inflammatory prostaglandins and leukotrienes. It has been shown to diminish the early and late phase allergic response by mast cells to antigen challenge. Cromolyn has recently been shown to activate the G protein coupled receptor GPR35. This receptor is present on mast cells, basophils and eosinophils. It is upregulated after mast cell exposure to IgE antibodies but is also described as a Gαi/o—coupled inhibitor of synaptic transmission. Animal studies have suggested an anti-nociceptive effect after agonist binding [42].

Sodium cromoglicate is available as eye drops (for allergic conjunctivitis), intra-nasal spray (for allergic rhinitis), inhaler (for asthma) and tablet form (for food allergy with diet restriction). Oral administration may be used to treat the gastrointestinal symptoms of MCAS. Case reports also describe the successful use of inhaled sodium cromoglicate and a selective COX-2 inhibitor (e.g. celecoxib) to reduce pro-inflammatory prostaglandins that modulate mast cell activation to treat anaphylaxis like symptoms during menses in a woman with PoTS and MCAS [26].

Novel use of sodium cromoglycate treatment includes vaginal douching with sodium cromoglycate intended for oral use mixed with warm saline to reduce vulvovaginitis following intercourse in a patient with MCAS [32]. Again, the authors do not currently recommend this practice at present time but acknowledge there may be innovative was to treat seemingly resistant symptoms.

Side effects of sodium cromoglycate include an intolerance of the medication, transient bronchospasm with inhaler use, arthralgia, nausea, rash and rarely eosinophilic pneumonia with inhaled use [43].

Ketotifen

Ketotifen is a first-generation antihistamine with H1 receptor antagonist properties as well as a mast cell stabilising action. It is available as eye drops for allergic conjunctivitis, and as tablets or oral solution. Common side effects of ketotifen include drowsiness in up to 40% of users [41], gastro-intestinal discomfort and dry mouth. The authors prescribe an increasing dose of ketotifen every 2 weeks commencing with 0.5 mg once or twice daily to reach up to 2 mg twice daily if benefits are experienced and side effects tolerated.

Patients with endometriosis in addition to bladder pain syndrome / interstitial cystitis (BPS/IC) with features of MCAS may have additional benefits from the use of ketotifen if tolerated. Animal studies using mice models of endometriosis demonstrated a reduction in hyperalgesia, reduction of mast cells in model endometriotic cysts, down regulation of angiogenesis and reduced serum histamine and TNF-α concentrations in the ketotifen treated mice [44].

Vaginal Prolapse

Pelvic organ prolapse is defined as descent of one or more of the anterior vaginal walls (central, paravaginal or combination cystocele), posterior vaginal wall (rectocele), the uterus and cervix or the apex of the vagina after hysterectomy (vaginal vault). This can be asymptomatic or present as awareness of a bulge or lump in the vagina, vaginal heaviness or discomfort particularly worse on standing, improvement with lying and associated lower back ache. It is particularly common for parous women with an overall estimated prevalence of 37–50% of women on examination, with a lower symptomatic prevalence in 3–8% of women [45]. Common risk factors include increasing age, parity, menopause, obesity and genetic factors.

Clinically significant pelvic organ prolapse is thought to be more prevalent in women with EDS and joint hypermobility. From self-completed surveys, 15.3% of women with hEDS report pelvic organ prolapse [28]. Women with joint hypermobility also have a significantly higher prevalence of genital pelvic organ prolapse in comparison to women with normal mobility with a pooled odds ratio of 2.37 (95% confidence interval 1.54–3.64) [46]. In particular anterior vaginal compartment prolapse may be more common and associated with voiding difficulties [47].

Alterations to collagen metabolism is relevant to the aetiology of pelvic organ prolapse. Collagen types I, III and V are the main providers of strength to soft tissues. Collagen type I is non-elastic and provides resistance to tensile forces and is a major structural component of the vaginal epithelium and endopelvic fascia. Collagen type III has elastic properties and collagen type V, whilst widely distributed is only a minor fibrillar collagen. Increased Type III and type V collagen are more prevalent in flexible tissues [48].

Type III collagen is typically overexpressed in pelvic tissues from women with prolapse and in the hypermobile population. There is an associated decrease in type 1 collagen with an increased type III to type I collagen ratio. This is associated with an overall decrease in tensile strength of connective tissue due to decreased fibre size which can lead to the development of pelvic organ prolapse [48].

The clinical features of EDS are caused by underlying defects in the collagen type I, III and V gene as well as defects in proteins important for the post-translational modifications and processing of these collagens [28] which is thought to contribute to the increased risk of developing genital prolapse in this group of patients.

Treatments for pelvic organ prolapse include conservative measures with weight reduction and pelvic floor muscle exercises, vaginal pessaries and lastly surgery. There is an overall 12.6% lifetime risk for prolapse surgery [21]. Pelvic organ prolapse of the uterus and cervix is an indication for a vaginal hysterectomy. Rates of hysterectomy vary globally and are decreasing, but it is a common operation that more than a third of American women undergo by the age of 60 [49]. It is unclear if this is increased in women with joint hypermobility. To compare, from a self-reported survey, 19% of women with hEDS report undergoing a hysterectomy [29]. There is also thought to be an increased risk of prolapse recurrence following surgical treatment and need for repeat surgery in women with a Beighton score of four or more [49].

Key Points

- The frequent presentation of the triad of PoTS, hypermobile EDS and MCAS suggests common pathophysiological mechanisms.
- Women with PoTS have more frequent menstrual irregularities.
- PoTS symptom flares can be associated with MCAS triggers such as menstruation, ingestion of histamine liberating food or foods high in histamine for example.
- PoTS symptoms can be ameliorated by suppressing the menstrual cycle with progestogens, continuous combined oral contraceptive pills or intra-uterine progestogen releasing coils.

- Women with PoTS have higher prevalence of pelvic pain, dyspareunia and vulvodynia.
- Due to the association with hEDS, women with PoTS are more likely to have vaginal prolapse which is more difficult to treat due to the collagen metabolism abnormalities.

References

1. Shaw BH, Stiles LE, Bourne K, Green EA, Shibao CA, Okamoto LE, et al. The face of postural tachycardia syndrome—insights from a large cross-sectional online community-based survey. J Intern Med. 2019;286(4):438–448.
2. Kavi L, Nuttall M, Low DA, et al. A profile of patients with postural tachycardia syndrome and their experience of healthcare in the UK. Br J Cardiol. 2016;23:1–6.
3. Celletti C, Camerota F, Castori M, et al. Orthostatic intolerance and postural orthostatic tachycardia syndrome in joint hypermobility syndrome/ehlers-danlos syndrome, hypermobility type: neurovegetative dysregulation or autonomic failure? Biomed Res Int. 2017;2017:9161865.
4. De Wandele I, Rombaut L, De Backer T, et al. Orthostatic intolerance and fatigue in the hypermobility type of Ehlers-Danlos syndrome. Rheumatology (Oxford). 2016;55(8):1412–20.
5. De Wandele I, Rombaut L, Leybaert L, et al. Dysautonomia and its underlying mechanisms in the hypermobility type of Ehlers-Danlos syndrome. Semin Arthritis Rheum. 2014;44(1):93–100.
6. Hakim A, De Wandele I, O'Callaghan C, Pocinki A, Rowe P. Chronic fatigue in Ehlers-Danlos syndrome-hypermobile type. Am J Med Genet C Semin Med Genet. 2017;175(1):175–80.
7. Castells M, Austen KF. Mastocytosis: mediator-related signs and symptoms. Int Arch Allergy Immunol. 2002;127:147–52.
8. Thieben MJ, Sandroni P, Sletten DM, Benrud-Larson LM, Fealey RD, Vernino S, Lennon VA, Shen WK, Low PA. Postural orthostatic tachycardia syndrome: the Mayo clinic experience. Mayo Clin Proc. 2007;82:308–13.
9. Low PA, Opfer-Gehrking TL, Textor SC, Benarroch EE, Shen WK, Schondorf R, Suarez GA, Rummans TA. Postural tachycardia syndrome (POTS). Neurology. 1995;45(4 Suppl 5):S19–25.
10. Edmonds K, editor. Dewhursts textbook of obstetrics and gynaecology. 8th ed. UK: Wiley-Blackwell; 2012. p. 487–508.
11. Peggs KJ, Nguyen H, Enayat D, Keller NR, Al-Hendy A, Raj SR. Gynecologic disorders and menstrual cycle lightheadedness in postural tachycardia syndrome. Int J Gynaecol Obstet. 2012;118(3):242–6.
12. Fu Q, VanGundy TB, Shibata S, Auchus RJ, Williams GH, Levine BD. Menstrual cycle affects renal-adrenal and hemodynamic responses during prolonged standing in the postural orthostatic tachycardia syndrome. Hypertension. 2010;56(1):82–90.
13. Mar PL, Raj SR. Neuronal and hormonal perturbations in postural tachycardia syndrome [published correction appears in Front Physiol. 2019;10:978]. Front Physiol. 2014;5:220. Published 2014 Jun 16.
14. Garland EM, Celedonio JE, Raj SR. Postural tachycardia syndrome: beyond orthostatic intolerance. Curr Neurol Neurosci Rep. 2015;15(9):60.
15. Hilliard LM, Sampson AK, Brown RD, Denton KM. The "his and hers" of the renin-angiotensin system. Curr Hypertens Rep. 2013;15(1):71–9.
16. Kaschina E, Namsolleck P, Unger T. AT2 receptors in cardiovascular and renal diseases. Pharmacol Res. 2017;125(Pt A):39–47.
17. Oelkers WK. Effects of estrogens and progestogens on the renin-aldosterone system and blood pressure. Steroids. 1996;61(4):166–71.
18. Fu Q. Microneurographic research in women. Front Physiol. 2012;3:278.
19. Stickford AS, VanGundy TB, Levine BD, Fu Q. Menstrual cycle phase does not affect sympathetic neural activity in women with postural orthostatic tachycardia syndrome. J Physiol. 2015;593(9):2131–43.
20. Ray CA, Carter JR. Vestibular activation of sympathetic nerve activity. Acta Physiol Scand. 2003;177(3):313–9.
21. Temkin SM, Minasian L, Noone AM. The end of the hysterectomy epidemic and endometrial cancer incidence: what are the unintended consequences of declining hysterectomy rates? Front Oncol. 2016;6:89.
22. Odutayo A, Cherney D, Miller J, et al. Transdermal contraception and the renin-angiotensin-aldosterone system in premenopausal women. Am J Physiol Renal Physiol. 2015;308(6):F535–40.
23. Drudy L, Sheppard B, Bonnar J. Mast cells in the normal uterus and in dysfunctional uterine bleeding. Eur J Obstet Gynecol Reproduct Biol. 1991;39:193–201.
24. Salamonsen LA, Woolley DE. Menstruation: induction by matrix metalloproteinases and inflammatory cells. J Reprod Immunol. 1999;44(1–2):1–27.
25. Shibao C, Arzubiaga C, Roberts LJ, Raj S, Black B, Harris P, Biaggioni I. Hyperadrenergic postural tachycardia syndrome in mast cell activation disorders. Hypertension. 2005;45:385–90.
26. Simpson G. Menstrual anaphylactoid reactions and presumed systemic mast cell activation syndrome. Intern Med J. 2016;46(7):858–9.
27. Stachenfeld NS. Sex hormone effects on body fluid regulation. Exerc Sport Sci Rev. 2008;36(3):152–9.
28. Castori M, Morlino S, Dordoni C, et al. Gynecologic and obstetric implications of the joint hypermobility syndrome (a.k.a. Ehlers-Danlos

syndrome hypermobility type) in 82 Italian patients. Am J Med Genet A. 2012;158A(9):2176–82.
29. Sorokin Y, Johnson MP, Rogowski N, Richardson DA, Evans MI. Obstetric and gynecologic dysfunction in the Ehlers-Danlos syndrome. J Reprod Med. 1994;39(4):281–4.
30. Hurst BS, Lange SS, Kullstam SM, et al. Obstetric and gynecologic challenges in women with Ehlers-Danlos syndrome. Obstet Gynecol. 2014;123(3):506–13.
31. Hugon-Rodin J, Lebègue G, Becourt S, Hamonet C, Gompel A. Gynecologic symptoms and the influence on reproductive life in 386 women with hypermobility type Ehlers-Danlos syndrome: a cohort study. Orphanet J Rare Dis. 2016;11(1):124.
32. Afrin L, Dempsey T, Rosenthal L, Dorff S. Successful mast-cell-targeted treatment of chronic dyspareunia, vaginitis, and dysfunctional uterine bleeding. J Obstet Gynaecol. 2019;39(5):664–9.
33. Jia X, Rana N, Crouss T, Whitmore KE. Gynecological associated disorders and management. Int J Urol. 2019;26(Suppl 1):46–51.
34. Afrin LB, Molderings GJ. A concise, practical guide to diagnostic assessment for mast cell activation disease. World J Hematol. 2014;3:1–17.
35. Sun Y, Harlow BL. The association of vulvar pain and urological urgency and frequency: findings from a community-based case-control study. Int Urogynecol J. 2019;30(11):1871–8.
36. Krapf JM, Goldstein A. Two case presentations of profound labial edema as a presenting symptom of hypermobility-type Ehlers-Danlos syndrome. J Sex Med. 2013;10(9):2347–50.
37. Wells R, Tonkin A. Clinical approach to autonomic dysfunction [published correction appears. [Intern Med J. 2017;47(1):126]. Intern Med J. 2016;46(10):1134–39.
38. Izquierdo-Casas J, Comas-Baste O, Latorre-Moratalla ML, Lorente-Gascon M, Duelo A, Soler-Singla L, Vidal-Carou. Low serum diamine oxidase (DAO) activity levels in patients with migraine. J Physiol Biochem. 2018;74:93–9.
39. Mušič E, Korošec P, Šilar M, Adamič K, Košnik M, Rijavec M. Serum diamine oxidase activity as a diagnostic test for histamine intolerance. Wien Klin Wochenschr. 2013;125:239–43.
40. Manzotti G, Breda D, Di Gioacchino M, Burastero SE. Serum diamine oxidase activity in patients with histamine intolerance. Int J Immunopathol Pharmacol. 2016;29(1):105–11.
41. Nurmatov UB, Rhatigan E, Simons FE, Sheikh A. H1-antihistamines for primary mast cell activation syndromes: a systematic review. Allergy. 2015;70(9):1052–61.
42. Doherty TA, White AA. Postural orthostatic tachycardia syndrome and the potential role of mast cell activation. Auton Neurosci. 2018;215:83–8.
43. https://bnf.nice.org.uk/drug/sodium-cromoglicate.html#indicationsAndDoses.
44. Zhu TH, Zou G, Ding SJ, Li TT, Zhu LB, Wang JZ, et al. Mast cell stabilizer ketotifen reduces hyperalgesia in a rodent model of surgically induced endometriosis. J Pain Res. 2019;29(12):1359–69.
45. Barber MD, Maher C. Epidemiology and outcome assessment of pelvic organ prolapse. Int Urogynecol J. 2013;24(11):1783–90.
46. Veit-Rubin N, Cartwright R, Singh AU, Digesu GA, Fernando R, Khullar V. Association between joint hypermobility and pelvic organ prolapse in women: a systematic review and meta-analysis. Int Urogynecol J. 2016;27(10):1469–78.
47. Mastoroudes H, Giarenis I, Cardozo L, et al. Lower urinary tract symptoms in women with benign joint hypermobility syndrome: a case-control study. Int Urogynecol J. 2013;24(9):1553–8.
48. Chen B, Yeh J. Alterations in connective tissue metabolism in stress incontinence and prolapse. J Urol. 2011;186:1768–72.
49. Knuuti E, Kauppila S, Kotila V, Risteli J, Nissi R. Genitourinary prolapse and joint hypermobility are associated with altered type I and III collagen metabolism. Arch Gynecol Obstet. 2011;283(5):1081–5.

Dizziness—The Audiovestibular Perspective

Louisa Murdin and Katherine Harrop-Griffiths

Introduction

Dizziness is a cardinal symptom in PoTS. It has been reported as a symptom in 90% of PoTS patients, and 43% describe their dizziness as a spinning sensation [1]. However, it is important to consider reported dizziness carefully since there can be multiple different mechanisms for this symptom, and it is not uncommon for patients with PoTS to experience more than one mechanism of dizziness. PoTS may have specific associations with additional conditions that can also cause dizziness, such as migraine, although further research is required to verify this. Dizziness is also a common symptom in the general population and therefore an individual with PoTS may well have dizziness from causes unrelated to PoTS itself [2]. These additional conditions may have specific effective evidence-based treatments. It is important therefore to adopt a systematic approach to the evaluation of dizziness, and where the patient describes more than one type of dizziness symptom, each needs to be evaluated separately.

L. Murdin (✉)
Guy's and St Thomas' NHS Foundation Trust
London, London, UK
e-mail: louisa.murdin@gstt.nhs.uk

K. Harrop-Griffiths
Royal National Throat Nose and Ear Hospital, University College London Hospitals NHS Trust, London, UK

Vestibular Pathology as a Cause for Dizziness

- The vestibular organs function as the body's sensor system for linear and angular acceleration of the head.
- Vestibular disorders can cause disabling symptoms of dizziness or vertigo.
- Many vestibular disorders have specific effective treatments.

Essential Clinical Anatomy and Physiology of the Vestibular System

- The key components of the vestibular organs are:
  - the three semi-circular canals which are orientated in three planes and detect angular acceleration; and
  - the otolith organs (saccule and utricle) which detect linear acceleration.
- Output signals from the vestibular organs are relayed via the eighth cranial nerve to the vestibular nuclei in the brainstem.
- The four key neurological connections of the vestibular system are:
  - to the extra-ocular muscles (the vestibulo-ocular reflex, VOR) for gaze stability.
  - to the muscles of posture (the vestibulo-spinal reflex, VSR) to maintain core stability and upright posture.

N. Gall et al. (eds.), *Postural Tachycardia Syndrome*, https://doi.org/10.1007/978-3-030-54165-1_19

- to the autonomic nervous system to maintain homeostasis.
- to the cerebral cortex for perception of balance.

Clinical Presentation of Acute Unilateral Vestibular Dysfunction

A key clinical presentation in vestibular medicine is acute unilateral loss of vestibular function, for example as seen in vestibular neuritis (see below). The signs and symptoms relate to the four key outputs listed in the previous section.

When the vestibular system is disrupted acutely, individuals may experience:

- seeing surroundings moving, due to disruption of the vestibulo-ocular reflex, seen by clinicians as nystagmus;
- imbalance, due to disruption of the vestibulo-spinal reflex;
- nausea and vomiting, due to disturbance of autonomic reflexes;
- the sensation of being dizzy, due to the cortical projections.

All symptoms tend to be worse during head movement in any plane and persist in any posture. This means that vestibular symptoms, unlike those related to orthostatic intolerance, tend to be persistently problematic when lying down; unless the patient is able to stay completely still while supine. Older patients may not describe vertigo specifically but can describe more non-specific dizziness symptoms.

Clinical Recovery from an Acute Unilateral Loss of Vestibular Function Occurs via Vestibular Compensation

Symptomatic recovery from acute unilateral loss of vestibular function is usually complete, and takes around three months. This is due to the process of cerebral compensation, occurring in the central nervous system [3].

- Factors which promote vestibular compensation
  - early mobilisation
  - good visual function
- Factors which inhibit vestibular compensation
  - prolonged use of vestibular sedative medication (cinnarizine, prochlorperazine, cyclizine)
  - persistent avoidance of movements which provoke dizziness
  - poor mobility
  - poor visual function
  - migraine
  - secondary depression or anxiety.

Common Causes of Vertigo

1. **Acute unilateral vestibular loss (vestibular neuritis and labyrinthitis)**

Vestibular neuritis is a clinical condition in which there is acute unilateral loss of vestibular function, frequently attributed to a viral infection [3]. It occurs fairly commonly.

Much less common and often confused with vestibular neuritis is labyrinthitis which presents as acute vertigo accompanied by sensorineural hearing loss. The cause may be vascular occlusion or bacterial or viral infection, although in clinical practice most are idiopathic. Bacterial labyrinthitis is very rare in adults and is associated with significant systemic upset and maybe meningitis.

Clinical features of vestibular neuritis

- The presentation is of acute vertigo, often incapacitating and associated with vomiting, persisting for days and gradually diminishing.
- There is a positive *head thrust test* (see Box 1).
- There is *vestibular nystagmus* (see Box 2).
- It is treated with short term (less than one week) vestibular sedatives/antiemetic, if needed, followed by mobilisation and vestibular rehabilitation, if needed.
- In some cases, symptoms can persist and develop into a more chronic form of dizziness.

Predictors for chronicity include both physiological variables related to integration of visual and vestibular function, and also psychological factors including anxiety [4].

2. **Benign paroxysmal positional vertigo (BPPV)**

BPPV is the commonest cause of recurrent vertigo in adults. It is caused by calcium carbonate crystal debris from otolith organs becoming trapped in one of the semi-circular canals, usually the posterior semi-circular canal.

Clinical features of BPPV

- There are recurrent episodes of short lived (<1 min) positional vertigo, provoked by movements in the plane of the posterior semi-circular canal such as turning in bed or extending the neck ("top shelf vertigo", for example when in the shower, at the hairdressers).
- There is a positive *Dix Hallpike test* (see Box 3).
- It is treated very effectively with particle repositioning manoeuvres such as the Epley manoeuvre [5].

3. **Vestibular migraine**

Vestibular migraine is the association of episodic vestibular symptoms (such as vertigo or head motion intolerance) with migraine headaches or other migrainous symptoms such as aura, photophobia or phonophobia. It is the commonest cause of recurrent vertigo in children [6].

Clinical features of vestibular migraine

- There are episodes of vertigo or other vestibular symptoms associated with migrainous features such as headache, light or sound sensitivity or aura.
- Examination is usually normal in between episodes.
- Hearing tests such as pure tone audiometry are usually normal.
- Management is along standard lines for migraine with trigger avoidance if possible, migraine prophylaxis for frequent symptoms, with additional short term vestibular sedatives for acute vertigo relief [7].

4. **Meniere's disease**

Meniere's disease is believed to represent the clinical syndrome associated with endolymphatic hydrops (altered pressure regulation within the fluid filled spaces of the inner ear). It is much less common than BPPV or vestibular migraine [2].

Clinical features of Meniere's disease

- There are episodes of vertigo with vomiting lasting 30 min to a few hours.
- There is unilateral tinnitus, aural fullness or hearing disturbance associated with the vertigo episodes.
- Pure tone audiometry characteristically shows a fluctuating low frequency sensorineural hearing loss on the affected side.
- Management options include regular betahistine, or a low salt diet (with a low level of evidence base) and intratympanic steroids or gentamicin that can be provided in ENT clinics.

5. **Stroke**

Stroke in the posterior circulation is a rare cause of isolated acute vertigo, but it is important not to miss this diagnosis because the clinical course can be potentially catastrophic.

Clinical features of vertigo due to stroke

- There are usually other neurological signs/symptoms.
- There is nystagmus which is not of peripheral vestibular type (for example, vertical, bidirectional, unsuppressed by visual fixation).

- The head thrust test is negative.
- There is associated acute unilateral sensorineural hearing loss.

6. **Chronic dizziness and persistent perceptual postural dizziness (PPPD)**

Acute or episodic dizziness of any cause can become chronic in a number of cases. This can result in the functional neurological disorder persistent perceptual postural dizziness (PPPD). Mal de debarquement is a subtype related to maladaptation after a long boat trip.

Clinical features of PPPD

- There are fluctuating symptoms of non-rotational dizziness present most days and lasting three months or more.
- Symptoms tend to be worse in rich visual environments such as supermarkets or railway stations.
- Symptoms tend to be worse in the upright posture.
- Migraine, neck pain and fatigue are common associates.

Treatment is multidisciplinary and can include exercise-based therapy, psychological and medication-based components.

Clinical Assessment of the Dizzy Patient—History

- **What do you mean by dizziness?** Vertigo is a feeling of abnormal subjective movement. This is usually rotatory but does not have to be; the description can be of more subtle disorientation. Light-headedness or feeling as if about to pass out is not vertigo. Losing consciousness is extremely rare when vertigo is due to vestibular disease.
- **Is the feeling continuous or episodic?** Continuous vertigo persisting for months or more can either be PPPD or be central in origin. Most vertigo of peripheral origin is episodic, with vestibular neuritis being the main exception because the vertigo is more continuous.
- **What started your dizziness?**
  - *Head injury/ear surgery.* Consider benign paroxysmal positional vertigo (BPPV) . If associated with a concomitant ipsilateral hearing loss, patients will need to be seen in a neurotology clinic to consider rarer causes such as structural abnormality of the inner ear, temporal bone fracture, perilymph fistula or other disorders.
  - *Stress.* Consider anxiety. Remember though that anxiety is a very common complication of somatic causes of dizziness.
  - *Medication.* A common cause of dizziness, especially centrally acting medications like antidepressants and anxiolytics, and antihypertensives.
  - *Boat, plane or other long trip.* Consider mal de debarquement. Often associated with vestibular migraine this can be a continuous feeling of vertigo.
  - *Upper respiratory tract infection.* Consider vestibular neuritis.
- **What brings on your dizziness?**
  - *Lying down or rolling over in bed, looking up to tall cupboards or reaching up to the washing line?* Consider BPPV in an adult over 30 years of age. If younger, ask about head injury and if not present consider referral for specialist assessment as causes can include intracranial tumour or other central conditions.
  - *Standing up?* Consider postural hypotension or PoTS.
  - *Menstrual cycling, alcohol, food?* Consider vestibular migraine.
  - *Stress?* Consider vestibular migraine or anxiety.
  - *Straining, diving, carrying weights, going down a deep tunnel (e.g. Tube train)?* Consider referring to ENT or Neuro-otology for evaluation of rare causes such as a perilymph fistula.
  - *Loud sounds?* Consider referring to ENT for evaluation of rare causes such as a superior semicircular canal dehiscence.

- **Do you have any associated symptoms?**
  - *Nausea.* This is a common accompaniment of vertigo. Vomiting is less common but denotes that the vertigo is marked.
  - *Headache.* Consider vestibular migraine. Do not forget intracranial tumour, benign intracranial hypertension or other secondary causes of headache. Also ask about light and sound sensitivity.
  - *Hearing loss and/or tinnitus.* Consider Meniere's disease or perilymph fistula or abnormal inner ear anatomy.
  - *Hearing internally generated sounds e.g. heartbeat, eye movements, autophony.* Consider superior semicircular canal dehiscence.
  - *Visual changes.* Consider the aura of migraine, visual changes with multiple sclerosis or the oscillopsia and visual lag that occur with vestibular disorder.
  - *Neurological symptoms.* Consider intracranial pathology, episodic ataxia type 2 or multiple sclerosis.

What Is the Time Course?

- **Sudden Onset**: A sudden onset of severe vertigo lasting a week with resolution can indicate vestibular neuritis or, more rarely, stroke. In posterior inferior cerebellar artery (PICA) strokes there will often be other symptoms and signs of lateral medullary syndrome. In anterior inferior cerebellar artery (AICA) strokes hearing will often be affected.
- **Episodic**: BPPV causes episodes of vertigo with characteristic head position triggers. Vestibular migraine is the most common cause of spontaneous episodic vertigo. Other episodic presentations include Meniere's disease when there is an accompanying fluctuating unilateral hearing loss and tinnitus, vestibular paroxysmia with very short episodes (minutes), Episodic Ataxia type 2 associated with cerebellar symptoms and signs. Positional symptoms can, rarely, have a central cause.
- **Continuous**: Consider PPPD or a central cause.

Other History

- A history of cardiovascular disease, hyperlipidaemia, diabetes mellitus, hypertension or other vascular risk factors may indicate a vascular origin.
- A family history of vertigo may suggest vestibular migraine or, rarely, Meniere's disease or Episodic Ataxia type 2.
- A long standing hearing loss with vertigo as a consequence of minor head trauma raises the possibility of a structural abnormality such as widened vestibular aqueducts. A family history of hearing loss may help.

Examination

1. General observation and blood pressure—lying and standing
   Looking for: postural hypotension, hypertension, tachycardia
2. Otoscopy
   Looking for: signs of middle ear disease, cause of any associated hearing loss
3. Eye movements
   Looking for: nystagmus, cranial nerve palsy, abnormalities of saccades or smooth pursuit movement
4. Head thrust test
   Looking for: impairment of the vestibulo-ocular reflex
5. Cranial nerves and other neurological examination
   Looking for: indicators of neurological disease
6. Stance and gait assessment
   Looking for: ataxia, signs of neurological disease, functional gait disturbance
7. Dix Hallpike test
   Looking for: BPPV, central positional nystagmus.

Who to Refer?

- Any red flag signs for neurological or otological disease.
- Dizziness with any hearing loss or auditory symptoms.

- Positional vertigo which is recurrent or unresponsive to conventional manoeuvres.
- Chronic dizziness lasting three months or more.
- Vestibular migraine impacting quality of life despite standard treatments.

Conclusion

Patients with dizziness due to PoTS can experience other causes of dizziness. In some cases there may be a specific relationship of PoTS and another dizziness condition. Clinical experience suggests there may be an association with vestibular migraine, and possibly also PPPD, but further research is needed to clarify this hypothesis. Individuals with PoTS can also get other common dizziness conditions. A knowledge of common and important causes of dizziness is essential for the systematic assessment of these patients, in order to implement appropriate effective management strategies.

Box 1: How to do the head thrust test

The patient is instructed to fixate on a specific point, usually the bridge of the examiner's nose. The examiner then holds the patient's head as illustrated, and makes rapid but small head movements in the lateral plane of around 20 degrees. The patient should be able to maintain visual fixation during the passive head thrust. If there is a vestibular lesion on one side, this ability is impaired. Slower movements are used to compensate so that a corrective "catch-up" saccade is observed.

Box 2: How to distinguish vestibular from central nystagmus in acute vertigo

	Peripheral (vestibular)	Central
Direction	Horizontal	Vertical[a]
Consistency	Always beats in the same direction, no matter where the gaze is directed	Can change direction, depending on the direction of gaze
Effect of visual fixation	Suppressed in the light, so can be better seen with an ophthalmoscope	Unaffected by visual fixation

[a]The exception is BPPV, in which induced positional nystagmus seen in a Dix Hallpike test has an upbeat component due to the involvement of the posterior semi-circular canal

Box 1 Head thrust test

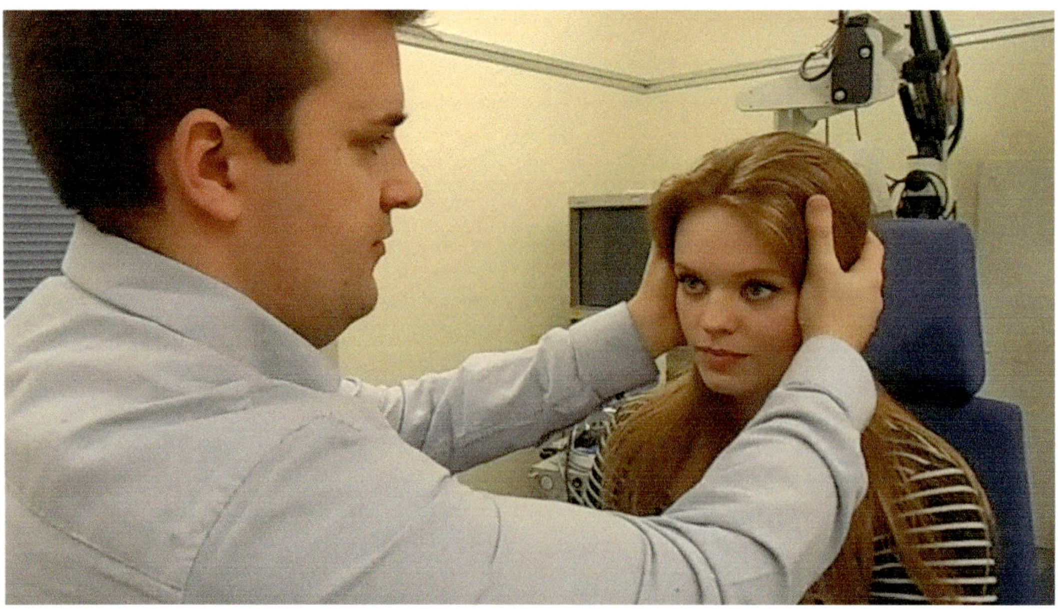

Box 3 Dix Hallpike test

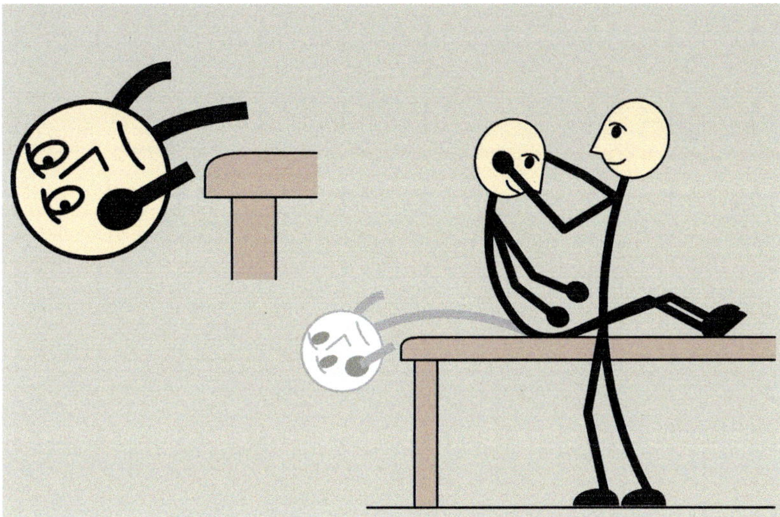

Box 3: How to do the Dix Hallpike test

With the patient seated on the examination couch, the examiner holds the patient's head at an angle of 45° from the midline. The patient is then moved rapidly to a supine position with the neck extended. Posterior canal benign paroxysmal positional vertigo produces a torsional nystagmus when the affected ear is lowermost. Note that the examiner can perform an adequate Hallpike manoeuvre with the head resting on the couch as opposed to hanging the head off the couch.

Figure taken from [8]

References

1. Kavi L, Nuttall N, Low PA, Opie M, Nicholson L, Caldow E, et al. A profile of patients with postural tachycardia syndrome and their experience of healthcare in the UK. Br J Cardiol. 2016;23(33).
2. Murdin L, Schilder AGM. Epidemiology of balance symptoms and disorders in the community: a systematic review. Otol Neurotol. 2014.
3. Bronstein AM, Dieterich M. Long-term clinical outcome in vestibular neuritis. Curr Opin Neurol. 2019;32(1):174–80.
4. Cousins S, Kaski D, Cutfield N, Arshad Q, Ahmad H, Gresty MA, et al. Predictors of clinical recovery from vestibular neuritis: a prospective study. Ann Clin Transl Neurol. 2017;4(5):340–6.
5. Hilton MP, Pinder DK. The Epley (canalith repositioning) manoeuvre for benign paroxysmal positional vertigo. Cochrane Database Syst Rev. 2014(12):Cd003162.
6. Lempert T, Olesen J, Furman J, Waterston J, Seemungal B, Carey J, et al. Vestibular migraine: diagnostic criteria. J Vestib Res Equilib Orientat. 2012;22(4):167–72.
7. Maldonado Fernández M, Birdi Jasminder S, Irving Greg J, Murdin L, Kivekäs I, Strupp M. Pharmacological agents for the prevention of vestibular migraine. Cochrane Database Syst Rev. 2015;(6). http://onlinelibrary.wiley.com/doi/10.1002/14651858.CD010600.pub2/abstract.
8. Murdin L, Seemungal BM, Bronstein AM. Assessment of Dizziness in Neurology. Medicine. 2020;48(8):517–521.

Other Conditions Linked to PoTS

Is PoTS an Autoimmune Condition?

Gurvinder Rull and Melvin D. Lobo

Key Abbreviations

AAG	Autoimmune Autonomic Gangliopathy
ANA	Antinuclear antibody
APLS	Antiphospholipid syndrome
ASIA	Autoimmune/autoinflammatory syndrome induced by adjuvant
gAChR	Ganglionic acetylcholine receptor
HPV	Human papillomavirus
NMDA	N-methyl-d-aspartate
PoTS	Postural tachycardia syndrome
WHO	World Health Organisation

Introduction

The underlying aetiology of PoTS remains unknown. An autoimmune basis has been postulated and there is increasing evidence to support this, but it remains inconclusive. One difficulty is the lack of a clear definition of an autoimmune condition. Moreover, many of the autoimmune findings in PoTS are widely varying, nonspecific, and lacking consistency. Nevertheless, there are clear features of PoTS, which do suggest underlying autoimmunity. This chapter reviews the current evidence supporting PoTS as an autoimmune condition. The chapter will be divided into four main themes of evidence:

1. The clinical features
2. Presence of triggering event
3. Presence of autoantibodies
4. Response to immunomodulatory treatments.

1. The Clinical Features

A key hallmark of autoimmune conditions is the preponderance in females, which is also seen in PoTS [1]. The incidence of PoTS in females has been estimated at 80–94%, with females being five times more likely than males to develop PoTS [2, 3]. Compared with males, females produce more antibodies from B cells and exhibit a T helper-2 predominant immune response. The T helper-2 responses are often associated with heightened antibody facilitated pathology. These sex differences may relate to oestrogen, and oestrogen is known to promote inflammation, which can lead to the development of autoimmunity [4]. Oestrogen has been shown to directly bind to hormone receptors on immune cells and cytokine receptors are present on oestrogen

G. Rull · M. D. Lobo
Barts BP Centre of Excellence, Barts Heart Centre, St Bartholomew's Hospital, West Smithfield, London EC1A 7BE, UK

G. Rull (✉) · M. D. Lobo
Barts NIHR Cardiovascular Biomedical Research Unit, Charterhouse Square, William Harvey Research Institute, Queen Mary University London, London EC1M 6BQ, UK
e-mail: gurvinder.rull@nhs.net

N. Gall et al. (eds.), *Postural Tachycardia Syndrome*, https://doi.org/10.1007/978-3-030-54165-1_20

producing tissues [5]. Oestrogen has also been shown to facilitate the production of various interleukins and cluster differentiating cells that promote immune responses [6–8]. Females with PoTS also have a higher incidence of oestrogen-related gynaecological disorders [9].

There are clinical features in PoTS common to those in chronic immune dysfunction [10]. Although classically PoTS lead to tachycardia and dizzy spells, many patients describe other non-specific symptoms such as tiredness, poor concentration, and sleep disorders. These symptoms are often encountered in autoimmune conditions. In addition, PoTS leads to significant morbidity occurring at the prime of life, which is again seen in many autoimmune diseases. Autoimmune disorders rarely affect a single organ and in PoTS there is also evidence of multiple organ pathology for example, gastrointestinal tract dysmotility and mast cell related allergic features.

PoTS patients often report a personal history or family history of autoimmune disorders, estimated at around 20% [11]. A family history of PoTS suggests the possibility of a genetic predisposition, similar to other autoimmune diseases [3, 12, 13]. Penny et al. reported a higher incidence of biopsy proven Coeliac's disease in PoTS compared with the general population (4% compared with 1% respectively), and self-reported gluten sensitivity was also higher than controls [14]. The bowel symptoms may occur either before or after a diagnosis of PoTS. Sjögrens syndrome is closely associated with PoTS and the initial presentation of Sjögrens syndrome is very similar to PoTS [10]. In one case series of 55 patients with Sjögrens syndrome, 13 had autonomic dysfunction of which eight would fit the diagnosis of PoTS [15]. In cases with neurological manifestations, these were noted to precede the Sicca syndrome by up to 10 years. Furthermore, those with neurological manifestations may have negative autoantibody tests although positive salivary gland histology. In another study, 8 out of 15 patients with antiphospholipid syndrome (APLS) and symptoms of autonomic dysfunction met the criteria for PoTS [16]. Other reported associated autoimmune conditions include Hashimoto's thyroiditis and Rheumatoid arthritis (both adult and juvenile) [10]. Table 1 lists various conditions associated with PoTS.

2. **Presence of a Triggering Event**

Autoimmune conditions are the result of the interplay between genetic and environmental factors [17]. A number of autoimmune diseases begin with a triggering event. This may be infection, trauma, vaccines, or surgery for example [18]. Many of these events are known to activate the immune system [10]. Indeed the initial reports of PoTS by Da Costa in 1871 described episodes of postural tachycardia following intestinal infection and war wounds [19]. PoTS after concussion has also been described, with an incidence of 11.4% in the first 3 months in one cohort [20]. Fatigue is common in PoTS as is exercise intolerance, features also seen in viral infections such as coxsackie B and Epstein-Barr virus and some chronic bacterial infections including Lyme disease.

Vaccination and its role in the aetiology of PoTS has led to much controversy. Three vaccines are available towards Human papillomavirus (HPV) type 16 and 18, produced by recombinant technology. HPV vaccination has been associated with new onset PoTS supported by a number of case reports [21–26]. The time to development

Table 1 Some of the reported co-morbid conditions seen in PoTS patients

Co-morbid conditions associated with PoTS
Sjögrens syndrome [52, 65, 66]
Hashimotos thyroiditis [38]
Coeliac's disease [14]
Antiphospholipid syndrome [16]
SLE [38, 67]
Rheumatoid arthritis [3]
Raynauds syndrome [68]
Multiple sclerosis [69]
Chronic fatigue syndrome [70]
Ehlers Danlos syndrome [71]

is days or months after vaccination, the majority occurring after the second vaccination. In the United States, post-marketing surveillance of 100,000 reports revealed approximately 120 cases of PoTS after HPV vaccine in the age range of 6–29 years [27]. PoTS is not the only possible autoimmune condition described after HPV vaccine, one case report of a 14-year-old patient discusses the development of PoTS and chronic fatigue syndrome two months after a second HPV vaccination (Gardasil type) [22]. This patient tested positive for antinuclear (ANA; titre 1:1280), lupus anticoagulant, and antiphospholipid antibodies. A large post-licensure, safety study has looked at the interaction between HPV vaccine and autoimmune conditions and failed to find any clear associations [28]. Unfortunately, PoTS was not one of the defined conditions in this observational study although, syncope remains one of the commonest adverse events following HPV vaccine [29]. Currently, WHO 2017 has not reported any safety concerns [30].

Vaccines result in protection through stimulation of the immune system; an effect much greater than that expected through infection, and thus it would be expected that other vaccines should also lead to PoTS type conditions. Certainly, PoTS has been reported after treatment with the H1N1 influenza vaccine, meningococcal vaccination, and varicella vaccine [31]. Nevertheless, the incidence is 3–5 times higher with HPV vaccines suggesting either presence of greater immune change with HPV or other as yet, unknown factors [31]. Further, these effects may be intensified for vaccines where multiple doses are given within a short space of time [22]. This may explain the differing frequency of PoTS and various vaccinations. Excipients must also be considered when determining causality. The Gardasil type HPV vaccine contains aluminium and this can elicit immune changes [ASIA—autoimmune/autoinflammatory syndrome induced by adjuvant) [32, 33]. HPV may have a preferential effect on the circulation and the vaccine shares a number of peptides with human proteins shown to produce a number cardiac manifestations [34]. Table 2 lists the different types of events that have been described as triggering PoTS.

3. **Presence of Autoantibodies and Other Immunological Findings**

Autoimmune conditions have circulating autoantibodies in some or the majority of cases. Much work has been done to try to identify the autoantibodies in PoTS if it is indeed an autoimmune condition. Autoimmune autonomic gangliopathy (AAG), is a rare condition with severe diffuse autonomic failure in which 50% of patients have presence of (nicotinic) ganglionic acetylcholine receptor (gAChR) autoantibodies. AAG has many similarities with PoTS in terms of being associated with a precipitating event at onset and overlap of symptoms. PoTS may represent one phenotype of AAG and gAChR antibodies have been detected in PoTS patients [35]. Depending on the cut-off values and assays used, a prevalence of 10–20% has been reported in PoTS with serum levels of gAChR correlating with disease severity [36–38]. However gAChR autoantibodies are present in 4–5% of controls and improved assays mean low-positive results are being seen more readily and appear to be less clinically significant [37, 39]. None-the-less gAChR autoantibodies are associated with autonomic dysfunction and autoimmune rheumatic disease. Vernino and colleagues also

Table 2 The different types of events that have been described as triggering PoTS

Triggering event
Infection (viral and bacterial) [36, 70, 72–77]
Vaccination [26, 31, 78, 79]
Trauma [13]
Pregnancy [36, 72]
Surgery [34]
EDS/JHS [71, 80]
Psychosocial stress [36]
Mast cell activation disorder [81]
Lyme disease [82]
Other autoimmune disease [83]
Medications e.g., antihypertensives, antipsychotics [12]

found lower levels of gAChR autoantibodies in milder forms of dysautonomia including PoTS [35]. The gAChR α-3 subunit has been more frequently associated with PoTS [37]. In this study, those who were seropositive for the gAChR α-3 subunit had more autoimmune complications. Some of the major criticisms of the studies of gAChR include the use of different methods of detection, differing cut-off levels, and no defined levels of specificity or sensitivity [10]. Vernino also postulated some patients may have their gAChR antibodies stored in organs making them inaccessible to the current measurement methods [35].

Other autoantibodies that have been detected in PoTS include G-protein coupled receptor autoantibodies that activate α1 and β-adrenergic receptors and muscarinic cholinergic receptor autoantibodies [40–42]. Fedorowski showed that adrenergic receptor autoantibodies from PoTS patients act as both direct activators of adrenergic receptors as well as demonstrating allosterically-mediated positive modulatory effects on β1 adrenergic receptors and a negative modulatory effect on α1 adrenergic receptors leading to enhanced effects of the sympathetic nervous system on posture [43]. These findings might explain why there is a change in heart rate but not much significant change in blood pressure in PoTS. In a recent report involving 55 patients with PoTS, it was observed that 89% of PoTS patients had elevated levels of antibodies to the α1-adrenergic receptors and that 51% had elevated antibodies to the M4 muscarinic cholinergic receptor. Intriguingly muscarinic cholinergic receptor antibody titres were only elevated in those patients who had antibodies to the α-adrenoceptor [44]. Evidence therefore exists to support autoimmune involvement of both the sympathetic and parasympathetic nervous systems in PoTS although further research to clarify the role of these autoantibodies is needed.

Angiotensin II receptor type I receptor autoantibodies have also been reported and may have a role in orthostatic circulatory homeostasis [45, 46]. Blitshteyn reported ANA positivity in 1:4 patients with PoTS, mostly with low tires (1:40 to 1:320), which is still higher than the general population [11]. They also found that 7% of the patient group had APLS antibodies. Five of the patients had more than one comorbid autoimmune condition. Of the specific autoimmune conditions, 11% had a history of Hashimotos thyroiditis, 5% antiphospholipid syndrome, and 2% systemic lupus erythematosus and 2% Sjögrens syndrome, all of which supports autoimmunity in PoTS. One case report found serum anti-NMDA receptor antibodies following HPV vaccination with PoTS but no encephalitis [41, 47]. Non-specific autoantibodies towards various cardiac proteins have also been detected including towards proteins implicated in cardiac hypertrophy, cardiac remodelling, and cardiomyopathy [25]. Table 3 summarises the autoantibodies detected in PoTS to date.

It is not just autoantibodies that have been investigated in PoTS but also other immunological changes have been reported that lend credence to the role of chronic immune activation. Cytokines like interleukin 6 are associated with increased sympathetic nervous system activity [48]. This can also result in circulatory changes including vasodilatation and increased vascular permeability [49].

4. Response to Immunomodulatory Treatments

Given the potential for an underlying autoimmune disorder, there have been a number of case reports in patients with PoTS using immunomodulatory treatments. The treatments used include intravenous immunoglobulins, immunosuoppressant agents, monoclonal antibodies, plasmapheresis, and stem cell infusion [47, 50–56]. The outcomes must be viewed with caution as they are reported in patients with widespread dysautonomia and not always PoTS. More specific to PoTS, one report of two patients with APLS and PoTS showed symptom improvement with intravenous immunoglobulin, when treatment for APLS failed [16]. PoTS after HPV vaccination has been treated with immunotherapies, plasmapheresis and prednisolone with varying results [47, 57, 58]. Vagus nerve stimulation (which is known to induce an anti-inflammatory

Table 3 Autoantibodies detected in PoTS

Autoantibody family
Antinuclear antibodies [11]
Antiphospholipid antibodies [11]
Sjögren syndrome A antibodies [56]
Carbonic anhydrase-6, parotid secretory protein; salivary protein-1 [56]
Anti-ganglionic acetylcholine receptor [2, 10, 35]
Voltage- gated potassium channel complex [84]
Cardiac lipid raft-associated proteins [25, 85]
α1-adrenergic receptors [40]
α1 and β2 adrenergic receptors [42]
M2 and M3 muscarinic receptors [42]
N-type acetylcholine receptors [35, 36]
Angiotensin II type 1 receptor [45]
Anti-NMDA receptor [47]
Thyroid stimulating hormone antibodies; thyroglobulin antibodies; thyroid peroxidase antibodies [11]

response) has been tested in a few autoimmune conditions including rheumatoid arthritis and Sjögrens syndrome [59, 60]. Vagal tone can be increased using conservative measures like exercise, meditation and acupuncture and these have been used in PoTS [61]. In one report of a patient with PoTS and presence of serum anti-NMDA receptor antibodies response was seen with immunomodulatory treatment [47]. Weinstock describes a case of PoTS in a patient with mast cell activation disorder which was treated successfully with low dose naltrexone followed by intravenous immunoglobulin and methylprednisolone [62]. Many of these reports only include patients with detectable autoantibodies (the commonest being APLS autoantibodies) and often multiple treatments are required and benefits short-lived [53]. However intravenous immunoglobulins have shown benefits even when antibody testing is negative [63, 64]. These case reports do however suggest repeated treatments are safe and add to the potential autoimmune causality of PoTS.

Conclusion

There is ample evidence of an association of PoTS with autoimmunity, but causality remains unclear. The major difficulties arise from the description of a wide variety of autoantibodies, which may just be innocent bystanders. Much of the information is based around case reports and there is a paucity of randomised trials. The selection criteria for many of the studies have often been biased, with some centres using only the most symptomatic of patients or only those with detectable autoantibodies. Assays and cut-off points are often different between studies making a comparison of the current literature difficult. Further work must include larger numbers of patients, more consistent autoantibody detection methods, and a greater focus on PoTS. An additional understanding of the mechanisms behind the predominance of autoimmune conditions in females may lead to the detection of further biomarkers and antibodies in PoTS. Similarities with AAG can also not be ignored and better gAChR and G-protein coupled antibody assays which are inexpensive and more widely available are needed.

References

1. Fairweather D, Frisancho-Kiss S, Rose NR. Sex differences in autoimmune disease from a pathological perspective. Am J Pathol. 2008;173(3):600–9.
2. Stiles L, Shaw BH, Green EA, et al. Sensory neuropathic symptoms in postural tachycardia syndrome: insights from a cross-sectional community-based

survey. In: Poster presented at: The 69th annual American academy of neurology meeting; 2017.
3. Raj SR. The postural tachycardia syndrome (POTS): pathophysiology, diagnosis and management. Indian Pacing Electrophysiol J. 2006;6(2):84–99.
4. Grimaldi CM, Cleary J, Dagtas AS, Moussai D, Diamond B. Estrogen alters thresholds for B cell apoptosis and activation. J Clin Invest. 2002;109(12):1625–33.
5. Wilder RL. Neuroendocrine-immune system interactions and autoimmunity. Annu Rev Immunol. 1995;13:307–38.
6. Straub RH. The complex role of estrogens in inflammation. Endocrine Rev. 2007;28:521–74.
7. Verthelyi D, Kilinman DM. Sex hormone levels correlate with the activity of cytokine-secreting cells in vivo. Immunology. 2000;100:384–90.
8. Karpuzoglu-Sahin E, Hissong BD, Ahmed SA. Interferon-γ levels are upregulated by 17-β-estradiol and diethylstilbestrol. J Reprod Immunol. 2001;52:113–27.
9. Peggs KJ, Nguyen H, Enayat D, et al. Gynecologic disorders and menstrual cycle lightheadedness in postural tachycardia syndrome. Int J Gynaecol Obstet. 2012;118(3):242–6.
10. Vernino S, Stiles LE. Autoimmunity in postural orthostatic tachycardia syndrome: current understanding. Auton Neurosci Basic Clin. 2018;215:78–82.
11. Blitshteyn S. Autoimmune markers and autoimmune disorders in patients with postural tachycardia syndrome (POTS). Lupus. 2015;24:1364–9.
12. Grubb BP, Kanjwal Y, Kosinski DJ. The postural tachycardia syndrome: a concise guide to diagnosis and management. J Cardiovasc Electrophysiol. 2006;17:108–12.
13. Kanjwal K, Karabin B, Kanjwal Y, Grubb BP. Autonomic dysfunction presenting as postural tachycardia syndrome following traumatic brain injury. Cardiol J. 2010;17:482–7.
14. Penny HA, Aziz I, Ferrar M, et al. Is there a relationship between gluten sensitivity and postural tachycardia syndrome? Eur J Gastroenterol Hepatol. 2016;28(12):1383–7.
15. Goodman BP, Crepeau A, Dhawan PS, Khoury JA, Harris LA. Spectrum of autonomic nervous system impairment in Sjögrens syndrome. Neurologist. 2017;22(4):127–30.
16. Schofield JR, Blitshteyn S, Shoenfeld Y, Hughes GRV. Postural tachycardia syndrome (POTS) and other autonomic disorders in antiphospholipid (Hughes) syndrome (APS). Lupus. 2014;23:697–702.
17. Rosenblum MD, Remedios KA, Abbas AK. Mechanisms of human autoimmunity. J Clin Invest. 2015;125(6):2228–33.
18. Theofilopoulos AN, Konon DH, Baccala R. The multiple pathways to autoimmunity. Nat Immunol. 2017;18(7):716–24.
19. Da Costa J. On irritable heart: a clinical study of a form of a functional cardiac disorder and its consequences. Am J Med Sci. 1871;61:17–52.
20. Miranda NA, Boris JR, Kouvel KM, Stiles L. Activity and exercise intolerance after concussion: identification and management of postural orthostatic tachycardia syndrome. JNPT. 2018;42:163–71.
21. Blitshteyn S. Postural tachycardia syndrome after vaccination with Gardasil. Eur J Neurol. 2010;17:e52.
22. Tomljenovic L, Colafrancesco S, Perricone C, Shoenfeld Y. Postural orthostatic tachycardia with chronic fatigue after HPV vaccination as part of the "autoimmune/auto-inflammatory syndrome induced by adjuvants": case report and literature review. J Investig Med High Impact Case Rep. 2014;2.
23. Kinoshita T, Abe RT, Hineno A, Tsunekawa K, Nakane S, Ikeda S. Peripheral sympathetic nerve dysfunction in adolescent Japanese girls following immunization with the human papillomavirus vaccine. Intern Med. 2014;53:2185–200.
24. Brinth LS, Pors K, Theibel AC, Mehlsen J. Orthostatic intolerance and postural tachycardia syndrome as suspected adverse effects of vaccination against human papilloma virus. Vaccine. 2015;33:2602–5.
25. Wang X-L, Chai Q, Charlesworth MC, Figueroa JJ, Low P, Shen W-K, et al. Autoimmunoreactive IgGs from patients with postural orthostatic tachycardia syndrome. Proteomics Clin Appl. 2012;6(0):615–25.
26. Blitshteyn S. Postural tachycardia syndrome following human papillomavirus vaccination. Eur J Neurol. 2014;21(1):135–9.
27. Butts BN, Fischer PR, Mack KJ. Human papillomavirus vaccine and postural orthostatic tachycardia syndrome: a review of current literature. J Child Neurol. 2017;32(11):956–65.
28. Chao C, Klein NP, Velicer CM, et al. Surveillance of autoimmune conditions following routine use of quadrivalent human papillomavirus vaccine. J Intern Med. 2012;271:193–203.
29. Slade BA, Leidel L, Vellozzi C, et al. Postlicensure safety surveillance for quadrivalent human papillomavirus recombinant vaccine. JAMA. 2009;302:750–7.
30. Observed rate of vaccine reactions: human papilloma virus vaccine. World Health Organization; 2017.
31. Tsai CK, Chu H, Cheng CA. Novel H1N1 influenze vaccine the cause of postural orthostatic tachycardia syndrome followed by cerebral hypoperfusion. J Med Sci. 2011;31:91–3.
32. Lujan L, Perez M, Salazar E, et al. Autoimmune/autoinflammatory syndrome induced by adjuvants (ASIA syndrome) in commercial sheep. Immunol Res. 2013;56:317–24.
33. Exley C, Swarbrick L, Gherardi RK, Authier FJ. A role for the body burden of aluminium in vaccine-associated macrophagic myofasciitis

and chronic fatigue syndrome. Med Hypotheses. 2009;72:135–9.
34. Dahan S, Tomljenovic L, Shoenfeld Y. Postural orthostatic tachycardia syndrome (POTS)—a novel member of the autoimmune family. Lupus. 2016;25:339–42.
35. Vernino S, Sandroni P, Singer W, Low PA. Invited article: autonomic ganglia: target and novel therapeutic tool. Neurology. 2008;70(20):1926–32.
36. Thieben MJ, Sandroni P, Sletten DM, Benrud-Larson LM, Fealey RD, Vemino S, et al. Postural orthostatic tachycardia syndrome: the Mayo clinic experience. Mayo Clin Proc. 2007;82(3):308–13.
37. Watari M, Nakane S, Mukaino A, et al. Autoimmune postural orthostatic tachycardia syndrome. Ann Clin Transl Neurol. 2018;5(4):486–92.
38. Ruzieh M, Batizy L, Dasa O, Oostra C, Grubb B. The role of autoantibodies in the syndromes of orthostatic intolerance: a systematic review. Scand Cardiovasc J. 2017;51(5).
39. Li Y, Jammoul A, Mente K, et al. Clinical experience of seropositive ganglionic acetylcholine receptor antibody in a tertiary referral centre. Muscle Nerve. 2015;52(3):386–91.
40. Li H, Yu X, Lilese C, Khan M, Vanderlinde-Wood M, Galloway A, et al. Autoimmune basis for postural tachycardia syndrome. JAHA. 2014;3:e000755.
41. Jones PK, Shaw BH, Raj SR. Clinical challenges in the diagnosis and management of postural tachycardia syndrome. Pract Neurol. 2016;16:431–8.
42. Yu X, Stavrakis S, Hill MA, et al. Autoantibody activation of beta-adrenergic and muscurinic receptors contributes to an "autoimmune" orthostatic hypotension. J Am Soc Hypertens. 2012;6:40–7.
43. Fedorowski A, Li HL, Yu XL, et al. Antiadrenergic autoimmunity in postural tachycardia syndrome. Europace. 2017;19:1211–9.
44. Gunning WT, Kvale H, Kramer PM, Karabin BL, Grubb BP. Postural orthostatic tachycardia syndrome is associated with elevated G-protein coupled receptorautoantibodies. J Am Heart Assoc. 2019;8:e013602.
45. Yu X, Li H, Murphy TA, et al. Angiotensin II type 1 receptor autoantibodies in postural tachycardia syndrome. J Am Heart Assoc. 2018; e008351.
46. Mustafa HI, Raj SR, Diedrich A, et al. Altered systemic heemodyanmic and baroreflex response to angiotensin II in postural tachycardia syndrome. Circ Arrhythm Electrophysiol. 2012;5:173–80.
47. Blitshteyn S, Brook J. Postural tachycardia syndrome (POTS) with anti-NMDA receptor antibodies after human papillomavirus vaccination. Immunol Res. 2017;65:282–4.
48. Okamoto LE, Raj SR, Gamboa A, et al. Sympathetic activation is associated with increased IL-6, but not CRP in the absence of obesity: lessons from postural tachycardia syndrome and obesity. Am J Physiol Heart Circ Physiol. 2015;309(12):H2098–107.
49. Pavlov VA, Tracey KJ. The vagus nerve and the inflammatory reflex–linking immunity and metabolism. Nat Rev Endocrinol. 2012;8(12):743–54.
50. Schroeder C, Vernion S, Birkenfeld AL, et al. Plasma exchange for primary autoimmune autonomic failure. N Engl J Med. 2005;353:1585–90.
51. Adamec I, Bilić E, Lovrić M, Habek M. Postural orthostatic tachycardia syndrome (POTS) as presenting symptom of CIDP. Neurol Sci. 2016;37(7):1163–6.
52. Goodman BP. Immunoresponsive Autonomic Neuropathy in Sjögren Syndrome-case series and literature review. Am J Ther. 2017;26(1):e66–71.
53. Hendrickson JE, Hendrickson ET, Gehrie EA, et al. Complex regional pain syndrome and dysautonomia in a 14-year-old girl responsive to therapeutic plasma exchange. J Clin Apher. 2016;13:368–74.
54. Numan MT, Kamdar A, Young J, et al. Autologous adipose stem cell therapy for autonomic nervous system dysfunction in two young patients. Stem Cell Dev. 2017;26:391–3.
55. Gibbons CH, Vernino SA, Freeman R. Combined immunomodulatory therapy in autoimmune autonomic gangliopathy. Arch Neur. 2008;65(2):213–7.
56. Schofield SR, Chemali KR. Intravenous immunoglobulintherapy in refractory autoimmune dysautonomias: a restrospective analysis of 38 patients. Am J Ther. 2018.
57. Hendricksen JE, Tormey CA. Human papilloma virus vaccination and dysautonomia: considerations for autoantibody evaluation and HLA typing. Vaccine. 2015;34:4468.
58. Brinth L, Theibel AC, Pors K, Mehlsen J. Suspected side effects to the quarivalent human papilloma vaccine. Dan Med J. 2015;62:A5064.
59. Koopman FA, Chavan SS, Miljko S, et al. Vagus nerve stimulation inhibits cytokine production and attenuates disease severity in rheumatoid arthritis. Proc Natl Acad Sci USA. 2016;113(29):8284–9.
60. Tarn J, Legg S, Mitchell S, Simon B, Ng WF. The effects of noninvasive vagus nerve stimulation on fatigue and immune responses in patients with primary Sjögren's syndrome. Neuromodulation. 2018.
61. Andersson U, Tracey KJ. Neural reflexes in inflammation and immunity. J Exp Med. 2012;209:1057–68.
62. Weinstock LB, Brook JB, Myers TL, Goodman B. Successful treatment of postural orthostatic tachycardia and mast cell activation syndromes using naltrexone, immunoglobulin and antibiotic treatment. BMJ Case Rep. 2018.
63. Mreicle RA, Triggs WJ. Treatment of acute pandysautonomia with IV immunoglobulin. J Neurol Neurosurg Psychiatry. 1997;62:529–31.
64. Heafield MT, Gammage MD, Nightingale S, Williams AC. Idiopathic dysautonomia treated with intravenous gammaglobulin. Lancet. 1996;347:28–9.
65. Calbrese LH, Davis ME, Wilke WS. Chronic fatigue syndrome and a condition resembling Sjogren's

syndrome: preliminary report. Clin Infect Dis. 1994;18(Suppl 1):S28–31.
66. Birnbaum J. Peripheral nervous system manifestations of Sjogrens syndrome: clinical patterns, diagnostic paradigms, etiopathogenesis, and therapeutic strategies. Neurologist. 16:287–97.
67. Tang S, Calkins H, Petri M. Neurally mediated hypotension in systemic lupus erythematosus patients with fibromyalgia. Rheumatology. 2004;43:609–14.
68. Mallipeddi R, Mathias CJ. Raynaud's phenomenon after sympathetic denervation in patients with primary autonomic failure: questionnaire survey. BMJ. 1998;316:438–9.
69. Kanjwal K, Karabin B, Kanjwal Y, Grubb BP. Autonomic dysfunction presenting as postural orthostatic tachycardia syndrome in patients with multiple sclerosis. Int J Med Sci. 2010;7:62–7.
70. Sheldon RS, Grubb BP, Olshansky B, et al. Heart rhythm society expert consensus statement on the diagnosis and treatment of postural tachycardia syndrome, inappropriate sinus tachycardia, and vasovagal syncope. Heart Rhythm. 2015;12:e41–63.
71. Mathias CJ, Low DA, Iodice V, Owens AP, Kirbis M, Grahame R. Postural tachycardia syndrome—current experience and concepts. Nat Rev Neurol. 2012;8:22–43.
72. Low PA, Opfer-Gehrking TL, Textor SC, et al. Postural tachycardia syndrome (POTS). Neurology. 1995;45:S19–25.
73. Robertson D. The epidemic of orthostatic tachycardia and orthostatic intolerance. Am J Med Sci. 1999;317:75–7.
74. Brinth L, Pors K, Spahic JM, Sutton R, Fedorowski A, Mehlsen J. Postural orthostatic tachycardia syndrome (POTS) in Denmark: increasingly recognized or new epidemic? Auton Neurosci. 2018;213:92–5.
75. Stewart JM, Boris JR, Chelimsky G, et al. Pediatric disorders of orthostatic intolerance. Pediatrics. 2018;141(pii):e20171673.
76. Sandroni P, Opfer-Gehrking TL, McPhee BR, Low PA. Postural tachycardia syndrome: clinical features and follow-up study. Mayo Clin Proc. 1999;82:1106–10.
77. Arnold AC, Ng J, Raj SR. Postural tachycardia syndrome—diagnosis, physiology, and prognosis. Auton Neurosci. 2018.
78. Agmon-Levin N, Schoenfeld Y. Chronic fatigue syndrome with autoantibodies: the result of an augmented adjuvant effect of hepatitis-B vaccine and silicone implant. Autoimmun Rev. 2008;8:52–5.
79. Schofield JR, Hendrickson JE. Autoimmunity, autonomic neuropathy, and the HPV vaccination: a vulnerable subpopulation. Clin Pediatr (Phila). 2018;57:603–6.
80. Kanjwal K, Saeed B, Karabin B, Kanjwal Y, Grubb B. Comparative clinical profile of postural orthostatic tachycardia patients with and without joint hypermobility syndrome. Indian Pacing Electrophysiol J. 2010;10:173–8.
81. Shibao C, Arzubiaga C, Roberts LJ. Hyperadrenergic postural tachycardia syndrome in mast cell activation disorders. Hypertension. 2005;45:385–90.
82. Kanjwal K, Karabin B, Kanjwal Y, Grubb BP. Postural orthostatic tachycardia syndrome following Lyme disease. Cardiol J. 2011;18:63–6.
83. Stojanovich L. Autonomic dysfunction in auoimmune rheumatic disease. Autoimmun Rev. 2009;8:569–72.
84. Bp G. Evaluation of postural tachycardia syndrome (POTS). Auton Neurosci Basic Clin. 2018;215:12–9.
85. Wang XL, Ling TY, Charlesworth MC, et al. Autoimmunoreactive IgGs against cardiac lipid raft-associated proteins in patients with postural orthostatic tacycardia syndrome. Transl Res. 2013;162:34–44.

Mast Cell Activation Syndrome (MCAS)

Clive E. H. Grattan

Introduction

The mast cell has become a focus of increased interest in health and disease. It is ubiquitous in humans and widely represented in the animal kingdom. It forms part of the innate immune system with ramifications for health that are often hidden until activation results in illness symptoms. It is best known as a cause of immediate hypersensitivity reactions that may be confined to a single organ, such as the skin, eye or nose or a more generalized reaction involving multiple body systems, culminating in anaphylactic shock. The physiology of the mast cell is complex with both pre-formed and newly formed mediators being released on activation to cause acute effects on blood vessels, sensory nerve endings and smooth muscle cells that may lead to illness if activation is sufficiently intense and widespread. Subclinical activation no doubt occurs since mediators, like histamine, can be detected in blood and other tissues of healthy individuals and may be important in day-to-day physiological health. It is simplistic to think of mast cells being activated in isolation from other inflammatory and immunological events. Biopsies of tissues involved in immediate allergic reactions show ingress of other cell types including eosinophils, neutrophils, basophils and lymphocytes that take days to disperse even when disease symptoms have improved. Mast cells numbers may increase in chronic inflammation and this may offer evidence of benefit as much as harm.

Mast cells originate in the bone marrow from pluripotent precursor cells and migrate in the blood to tissues where they mature into stable populations with specific characteristics under the influence of local cytokines. They are probably fixed once they have matured with prolonged survival but natural involution (apoptosis) will be influenced by factors including expression of gain-of-function mutations in the membrane receptor for stem cell factor known as KIT. There is an element of plasticity in respect of mast cell surface receptors that may be expressed or hidden, depending on the degree of maturation or activation so there is a degree of dynamism to an individual cell that will influence whether, in highly simplistic terms, it is 'sleepy' or 'awake'. A key membrane receptor in addition to KIT is FcεRI, the high affinity receptor for IgE. Activation results in a cascade of calcium-dependent signalling events resulting in degranulation with externalization of granules containing histamine, heparin and tryptase and other preformed mediators with generation of leukotrienes (including LTC_4, D_4, E_4) and prostaglandin D_2 from arachidonic acid metabolism. Cross-linking of

C. E. H. Grattan (✉)
Consultant Dermatologist, St John's Institute of Dermatology, Guy's Hospital, SE1 9RT London, UK
e-mail: Clive.E.Grattan@gstt.nhs.uk

N. Gall et al. (eds.), *Postural Tachycardia Syndrome*, https://doi.org/10.1007/978-3-030-54165-1_21

specific IgE on FcεRI by allergen is the classic stimulus for an immediate allergic event that may be localized (e.g. immunological contact urticaria) or generalized (e.g. anaphylaxis). Other mechanisms, such as binding of IgG anti-IgE to the heavy chain of cell bound IgE (in chronic spontaneous urticaria and as a standard laboratory stimulus) or autoantibodies against the α-subunit of FcεRI may lead to cutaneous mast cell and basophil degranulation but do not appear to activate mast cells systemically. There is increasing indirect, and some direct evidence, that IgE directed against specific autoantigens is relevant to some patients with chronic spontaneous urticaria through FcεRI activation. Other receptors expressed on mast cells of potential relevance to activation include the C5a receptor, toll-like receptors (TLR) stimulated by infections and Mas-related G-protein-coupled receptor (MRGPRX2) that has recently been proposed as an important signalling receptor for the neuropeptide, substance P, and drug-induced degranulation. Signalling receptors are different to markers of activation that include the membrane expressed cluster differentiation antigens, CD63, 69 and 203c. In short, the origin, distribution and physiology of mast cells is complex, dynamic and interactive with other inflammatory cells, extracellular proteins, neural and vascular tissues and this might, perhaps, be relevant to possible overlap between mast cell activation and the autonomic nervous system. Detailed information on mast cell physiology is available in standard texts of Allergy [1] and Immunology [2].

Background

Anaphylaxis is a potentially life-threatening event characterised by the sudden onset of severe hypotension, difficulty with breathing or both. It is often accompanied by skin manifestations with or without bowel symptoms [3]. It may have an allergic or a non-allergic cause. A single cause may not be identifiable if more than one stimulus has to be present at the same time to induce mast cell activation, as in food and exercise-induced anaphylaxis. Anaphylaxis that has no apparent cause or combination of causes is called idiopathic. This systemic reaction is usually accompanied by a rise and fall in blood tryptase over 6 hours, peaking at 1 hour, which can be diagnostic. By contrast, localized mast cell degranulation in single organ systems, including skin, eye, nose and lung would not be expected to cause a significant rise in tryptase. The best example of a cutaneous mast cell activation disorder is urticaria. This can be localized or generalized, mild or severe. It may be accompanied by deep swellings of the skin or oral mucosa called angio-oedema. Spontaneous and inducible subtypes may co-exist.

Allergic rhinitis and conjunctivitis are also mast cell activation disorders. They may occur together or separately. Allergic rhinitis is often associated with asthma with exacerbations involving mast cell activation. There are no disease states characterised exclusively by mast cell degranulation of bowel, bladder, or brain although mast cells are present in these tissues and may be activated. Increased numbers of mast cells may be present in chronic inflammation involving skin, bowel and bladder. It is likely that they are reactive to the inflammation rather than a cause of it. By contrast, accumulation of clonal mast cells in mastocytosis ('too many mast cells') in different tissues is independent of inflammation. The mutated KIT transmembrane receptor promotes mast cell survival and expression of aberrant markers including CD2 and CD25. These are not present in reactive (non-clonal) mast cells. Clonal mast cells expressing CD2 and CD25 may be more 'twitchy' than normal resident mast cells, thereby presenting an increased risk of anaphylaxis, after multifactorial activation or activation after a specific stimulus, such as an allergen.

Mast Cell Activation Disorders (MCAD)

A unifying concept of mast cell disorders was proposed by Akin et al. in 2010 to provide a structured approach for the assessment of patients with illness related to mast cell activation [4]. The authors confined the concept to patients with episodic and severe symptoms involving one or more tissues. They broadly classified mast cell disorders into primary (activation with evidence of underlying clonality, namely patients meeting all or some criteria for mastocytosis), secondary (activation due to a known cause, including IgE mediated anaphylaxis and autoimmune or physical urticarias) and idiopathic (no cause identifiable). They separated idiopathic anaphylaxis from idiopathic mast cell activation syndrome (MCAS), which was a diagnosis of exclusion. They also proposed three fundamental criteria for making a diagnosis of MCAS (Table 1). The patient must present with episodic severe symptoms suggestive of mast cell activation in at least two body systems concurrently, the patient must respond to appropriate anti-mast cell mediator treatments and there must be objective evidence of mast cell degranulation in blood or urine assays on at least two occasions. These criteria have remained unchanged over several revisions of the original proposal and should be regarded as a necessary burden of proof for a confirmed diagnosis of MCAS. Akin later proposed including idiopathic anaphylaxis within MCAS [5].

Publications from different authors since the original article have taken different viewpoints. Valent et al. included patients with primary, secondary and idiopathic causes of episodic mast cell activation under the umbrella term of mast cell activation syndromes (confusingly in the plural) [6] and Afrin et al. have broadened the concept even further to include illness that may relate to mast cell activation in patients with chronic disease as diverse as obesity, atherosclerosis, hypertension, chronic kidney disease, inflammatory bowel disease, fibromyalgia, neuropsychiatric disease and autoimmune disease with a very wide range of possible clinical features [7]. All authors emphasise the wide differential diagnosis of illnesses that present with overlapping symptoms but are unrelated to mast cell activation. There is now increasing convergence of opinion in Europe and the US [8, 9] on a restricted definition of MCAS as an illness (now referred to as primary, secondary or idiopathic syndromes) where mast cell activation plays a pivotal role, presenting with recurrent mast cell activation with systemic consequences of known or unknown cause. This evolution over the last decade embraces the mast cell activation disorders originally proposed by Akin et al. [4] but not urticaria because it does not usually present in at least 2 body systems. By moving away from a concept of MCAS being an uncommon and unexplained clinical syndrome when other recognisable causes of mast cell activation have been excluded, it has almost become a surrogate group term for recurrent anaphylaxis or near-anaphylaxis of any cause and this may or may not represent an advance in daily clinical practice. Opinion is however hardening against inclusion of chronic illness with other diagnostic labels that may have some overlapping symptoms and incomplete or absent evidence of episodic mast cell activation. This contrasts with non-specialist opinion that mast cell activation

Table 1 Criteria for mast cell activation syndrome

1. **Episodic clinical features consistent with mast cell mediator release affecting ≥ 2 organ systems,**
(a) Cutaneous: wheals, angio-oedema, itching, flushing
(b) Gastrointestinal: nausea, vomiting, diarrhoea, abdominal cramping
(c) Cardiovascular: hypotensive syncope or near syncope, tachycardia
(d) Respiratory: wheezing or angio-oedema of the oropharynx with shortness of breath
(e) Naso-ocular: conjunctival redness, chemosis, pruritus, nasal stuffiness
2. **A decrease in frequency or severity or resolution of symptoms with anti-mast cell mediator therapies**: H1 and H2 antihistamines, antileukotrienes or mast cell stabilizers (sodium cromoglicate)
3. **Evidence of an increase in a validated urinary or serum marker of mast cell activation**: documentation of an increase of the marker to greater than the patient's baseline value during a symptomatic period on ≥ 2 occasions

may be a key feature of complex chronic illness, including postural tachycardia syndrome (PoTS) and hypermobile-type Ehlers-Danlos syndrome (hEDS). Clinical experience shows that mast cell disease and PoTS, hEDS or both may sometimes coincide, but coincidence is not proof of MCAS. The full diagnostic criteria in Table 1 still have to be met. The importance of being as correct as possible is to give the most appropriate treatment and to avoid a risk of mislabelling other illness with overlapping symptomatology (such as ischaemic heart disease, endocrine disorders or malignancy) that may otherwise be missed with serious consequences for health. Correct diagnosis is also important to minimise unnecessary or inappropriate investigations incurring risk, anxiety and costs.

Terminology around mast cell-related illness:

- **Mastocytosis**: an expansion of mast cell numbers, for which a clonal origin can usually be demonstrated, presenting in skin, systemically or both. The increase in mast cells above normal may or may not cause symptoms. Systemic mastocytosis (as defined by the updated 2016 WHO criteria [10]) is diagnosed by biopsy of bone marrow or any tissue *other than skin*. Mastocytosis is usually indolent but may rarely present with, or progress to, advanced disease (aggressive systemic or mast cell leukaemia). Mastocytosis may also be complicated by anaphylaxis that may be due to allergen exposure, non-allergic triggers or be multifactorial and remain unexplained. Recurrent anaphylaxis in patients with mastocytosis due to any cause is now accepted as a presentation of MCAS.
- **Monoclonal mast cell activation syndrome (MMAS)**: is uncommon but could typically present with recurrent symptoms of mast cell activation, including anaphylaxis at the severe end of the spectrum, in patients with some features of mastocytosis but who do not fulfil the full WHO criteria. For example, a patient presenting with one or two minor criteria of clonality found in systemic mastocytosis including the common KIT mutation or expression of CD25 on extracutaneous mast cells.
- **Single organ mast cell activation disorders**: urticaria is understood to be due to mast cell activation in nearly every instance with the exception of non-immunological contact urticaria and the mechanistically unrelated hereditary angio-oedema. Rhinitis, conjunctivitis and asthma are often, but not exclusively, due to mast cell activation following allergen exposure. Single-organ symptoms due to mast cell activation are very important in their own right but do not define a syndrome.
- **Reactive mast cell hyperplasia**: mast cell numbers can increase in chronic inflammation. Their role in the inflammatory process is unclear. A reactive increase will diminish as the inflammation resolves. Reactive mast cells are mature and not clonal.
- **Alpha tryptasaemia**: patients with persistently raised blood tryptase may have an inherited copy gene multiplication in TPSAB1. Symptoms described with the mutation include urticaria, irritable bowel syndrome symptoms and autonomic dysfunction, including PoTS [11]. More needs to be known about the spectrum of clinical features in symptomatic and asymptomatic individuals and any enhanced risk of mast cell activation in addition to constitutively increased tryptase levels. It is not a subset of MCAS.
- **Mast cell activation syndrome (MCAS)**: the currently accepted definition of MCAS is a recurrent intermittent severe illness affecting at least two body systems (skin, gastrointestinal, cardiovascular, respiratory or naso-ocular) concurrently with laboratory evidence of mast cell activation from any cause on at least two occasions and responding to anti-mast cell mediator therapies [8, 9]. A wider definition of chronic illness with mast cell involvement is a different concept where some patients may benefit from anti-mast cell mediator therapies as indirect evidence of mast cell activation. However, therapeutic gains alone do not equate to an

MCAS label. Clinical experience supports the adoption of the acronym CHARISMA (chronic antihistamine-responsive illness as an indirect sign of mast cell activation) as a practical surrogate for better scientific understanding of the physiological events underlying complex illness symptoms. More information from careful retrospective data collection, audit and prospective studies is needed.

Epidemiology of MCAS and Complex Illness with Suspected Mast Cell Activation

Patients with primary or secondary MCAS share the epidemiology of their underlying condition. There is no gender difference for those with mastocytosis, allergic or idiopathic anaphylaxis.

By contrast, evidence from large studies on patients presenting with complex illness symptoms (including those with PoTS and hEDS) and suspected mast cell activation is lacking but clinical experience shows that females predominate [9]. Patients with this may present after puberty or later with increasing health issues requiring time off school or work and rarely in childhood. Other patients present acutely after an identifiable illness in adult life but onset in the elderly is rare.

Clinical Presentations of MCAS

Symptoms and signs of acute mast cell activation may present in cutaneous, respiratory, cardiovascular, gastrointestinal and urogenital systems.

Cutaneous features of acute mast cell activation

The most constant and troublesome feature is **itch**. Other descriptors include burning, prickling, biting or pricking sensations. It tends to be maximal within minutes of the onset of an event and subsides within an hour if histamine is the major mediator but other mediators, including leukotrienes and prostaglandins, are almost certainly relevant. Transient flushing will usually accompany itch and may be generalized. Weals may be small or large, confluent, localized or generalized in anaphylaxis. They are often symmetrical in distribution. Itchy linear weals after light skin stroking or scratching is called symptomatic dermographism (a type of inducible urticaria). Angio-oedema of deeper mucocutaneous surfaces may occur anywhere on the body, including the oropharynx but favours the soft tissues of the face and, sometimes, genitalia. By contrast with weals, angio-oedema may present asymmetrically and extend over hours to become bilateral. Mild angio-oedema may be difficult to distinguish from other causes of tissue oedema including positional oedema, pregnancy, the acute phase of allergic contact dermatitis, some drugs (e.g. calcium antagonists) and less common general medical causes including heart failure, superior vena cava obstruction and hypoalbuminaemia.

Respiratory features of acute mast cell activation

Difficulty with breathing may be due to upper airways obstruction from angio-oedema or lower airway obstruction due to bronchial spasm, oedema and mucus plugging. Oedema of the larynx may present with a scratching or tickling sensation in the throat followed by a sensation of tightness, coughing and loss of voice. Feeling unable to draw in sufficient breath will often lead to panic with rapid inspiratory effort. Swelling of the lips can be very unsightly but is not a cause of respiratory obstruction, whereas bilateral tongue swelling or laryngeal oedema can cause respiratory obstruction with a risk of suffocation when extreme. Wheezing is a feature of expiratory difficulty due to bronchospasm. Sneezing and congestion of the upper respiratory tract may be an early sign of an impending anaphylactic reaction.

Cardiovascular features of acute mast cell activation

A rapid drop in blood pressure (systolic below 90 mm Hg) is a key feature of anaphylactic shock. It is accompanied by tachycardia and faintness. Hypotension may progress to loss of consciousness if measures are not taken to reverse it, such as lying down with leg raising and administration of intramuscular adrenaline with or without administration of additional measures, including intravenous fluids. Symptoms of profound hypotension may include blackness of vision, loss of hearing, a feeling of doom and chest pain if there is myocardial ischaemia. The initial symptoms of tachycardia and faintness due to anaphylaxis may be similar to an episode of PoTS but this is not associated with other symptoms of anaphylaxis, such as pruritus and urticaria, and generally recovers more quickly on lying or sitting and without adrenaline.

Gastrointestinal features of acute mast cell activation

Acute nausea and vomiting may be features of anaphylaxis followed by diarrhoea, especially with food allergic reactions. Symptoms of bloating and hyperacidity are not expected features of anaphylaxis but may be described in patients with systemic mastocytosis. Hyperacidity is described by a small proportion of patients with chronic spontaneous urticaria.

Urogenital features of acute mast cell activation

Angio-oedema of the genitalia can occur in urticaria but is not an expected feature of anaphylaxis. Increased frequency of urination may be described in some patients with systemic mastocytosis and urinary incontinence could be a consequence of profound shock following anaphylaxis.

Investigation

There are no tests that are one hundred percent specific and sensitive for mast cell activation. This is partly due to the lack of highly sensitive detection markers for events that occur in tissue initially with 'spill over' into blood followed by elimination in urine and partly because detectable mediators of inflammation, including histamine, are not specific to mast cells. Furthermore, biochemical assays that are currently available have not been validated in the context of mast cell activation cut-off's shown to be clinically relevant in large and carefully controlled studies of healthy controls and populations of interest. Blood tryptase is considered to be the best marker of anaphylaxis and less severe systemic mast cell activation events. Beta tryptase peaks in the blood around 1 hour after anaphylaxis and returns to baseline in 6 hours. A rise of 20% from baseline with + 2 ng/ml has been agreed by an international panel to be relevant to mast cell activation in mastocytosis [12]. A rise of at least 30% in urinary methyl histamine above the upper limit of normal has been proposed as an arbitrary threshold for clinical relevance in a recent publication on MCAS [13]. Timing of collection of acute samples is also relevant and handling of samples to minimize degradation before and during assays has been highlighted.

Histamine and histamine degradation products

Histamine is produced from histidine by histidine decarboxylase in several cell types but only stored in granules of mast cells and basophils, which are therefore the major source. Endogenous histamine is broken down in vivo by N-methyl transferase to N-methyl histamine, which is eliminated in urine and is much more stable to degradation but undergoes a further oxidation step to methyl imidazole acetic acid (MIMA). Diamine oxidase is said to be the main metabolic enzyme for dietary histamine which is broken down to inactive imidazole acetic acid. Although histamine can be measured in blood and urine, the specimens need rapid freezing or acidification to minimize degradation and this is a practical disadvantage. By contrast, N-methyl histamine is relatively stable to degradation and can be stored cool for transport to the collection point before freezing on receipt by the laboratory prior to assay. Both 24 hour urine collections and random urine sampling can be performed to detect N-methyl histamine as evidence of mast cell activation. A potential advantage of 24 hour collections is having a wider window for capturing a histamine peak but a potential disadvantage is dilution of the peak by lower levels of basal histamine excretion either side of it. A more logical approach is to collect a baseline 'spot' urine methyl histamine followed by another sample 1–3 hours after the onset of symptoms. Patients should be asked to void at the onset of symptoms and to collect a random 10 ml sample one to three hours afterwards to capture N-methyl histamine elimination over the peak.

Although histamine is present in all mast cells and is accepted to be a major mediator of symptoms following systemic degranulation, the latest US guidelines report that it has a relatively low sensitivity for detecting mast cell activation events. This emphasises the importance of standard operating procedures for collection and sampling. It may also reflect the difficulty in knowing whether mast cell activation had occurred or not.

Prostaglandin D2

Prostaglandin D_2 is a vasoactive mediator formed by cyclooxygenase on arachidonic acid in phospholipid membranes. It is generated at the time of mast cell degranulation but is not specific to mast cells. It may cause burning erythema but not itch or wealing in the skin. It is broken down to 11 β PGF2α and then PGDM, both of which can be assayed in urine. The peak time for collection is between 1–3 hours with PGDM peaking later. The US guidelines state that 11 β PGF2α is detected more frequently after mast cell activation events than N-methyl histamine but has the twin disadvantages of not being specific to mast cells and cut-off thresholds have not been validated for MCAS. The assays are available in the UK but not widely used in clinical practice and are relatively expensive.

Cysteinyl leukotrienes

$LTC_4D_4E_4$ (also historically known as slow release substance of anaphylaxis) is generated by the action of 5-lipoxygenase on arachidonic acid. It is generated by basophils and eosinophils as well as mast cells. Anti-leukotrienes are approved for asthma but are widely used in other diseases in which mast cells are involved, including chronic urticaria and allergic rhinitis. LTE_4 (the most stable metabolite of the cysteinyl leukotrienes) can be measured in urine but is not assayed routinely in most centres.

Clinical Assessment of Patients with Suspected MCAS

The history is an essential first step in assessment of suspected mast cell disorders. If the story is wrong, the diagnosis should be in doubt and enquiry should be widened to include other possible medical explanations (Table 2).

History

All aspects of the illness should be explored, including timing of onset, description of symptoms, aggravating and relieving factors, medications, known allergies, family and occupational history. Specific enquiry should be made for leading symptoms in all body systems and any previous conditions, including hypermobility and postural tachycardia. An open mind should be maintained for illness mimics that share similar symptoms. Screening questions for uncommon causes of illness include foreign travel (intestinal parasitosis), tick bites (borreliosis),

Table 2 History checklist

Background
Antecedent events e.g. surgery, illness, allergies
Systems enquiry
1. Skin
a. Itch (transient-persistent; localized-generalized)
b. Urticaria (weals or angio-oedema, spontaneous; inducible; overlap)
c. Flush (transient-persistent; localized-generalized)
d. Sweating
e. Bruising, paper-thin scars, hernias
f. Markers of cutaneous or systemic disease (e.g. eczema, livedo reticularis, erythema chronicum migrans)
2. Cardiovascular
a. Dizziness, light-headedness, fainting, collapse on standing up or prolonged standing
b. Palpitations (tachycardia, bradycardia; extra beats; forceful beats)
c. Orthostatic cyanosis
3. General
a. Fatigue
b. Loss of concentration ('brain-fog')
c. Intolerance of smells, fumes, smoke, drugs
d. Sleep health
4. Gastro-intestinal
a. Weight loss
b. Bloating, constipation, diarrhoea, dyspepsia, nausea
5. Urogenital
a. Dysuria
b. Frequency
6. Musculoskeletal
a. Hypermobility
b. Back pain
c. Spontaneous subluxation-dislocation of joints
7. Neurological
a. Headache
b. Depression
8. Respiratory
a. 'tight' chest or shortness of breath, throat symptoms but not wheeze
9. Medications
a. Anti-mast cell mediator treatments (e.g. antihistamines, antileukotrienes, sodium cromoglicate)
b. Anti-arrythmics (e.g. ivabradine, bisoprolol)
c. Vasocontrictors (e.g. midodrine)
10. Lifestyle
a. Food, exercise and employment restrictions
b. Alcohol intolerance

Table 3 Examination checklist

Examination
• Urticaria or rash (patient's photos)
• Maculo-papular cutaneous mastocytosis
• Skin flexibility, scarring, bruising (but not loss of recoil)
• Autoimmune disease, including lupus or rheumatoid
• Acro- and orthostatic cyanosis, cool peripheries
• Hepatosplenomegaly, lymphadenopathy
• Supine blood pressure and pulse (active stand test); repeat within 10 min of standing (rise in pulse > 30 bpm, PoTS; orthostatic hypotension, autonomic failure)
• Joint hyperextensibility (e.g. 5th finger and elbow hyperextension, thumb to forearm, prayer sign behind back, hands flat on floor with straight leg bending over)
• Marfanoid habitus (height to span and high palate)
• Scoliosis

diet (haematinic deficiencies), periodic fever (autoinflammatory syndromes), cold intolerance (Raynaud's) and weight loss (lymphoma or other neoplasia). Documentation of events and other consultations should be sought whenever possible since patients often see multiple specialists. Subtleties around a diagnosis from another specialist can easily be overlooked or misunderstood. Recording an incorrect or skewed diagnosis relating to another specialty can indirectly lead to incorrect conclusions being perpetuated down the line. Similarly, original test results should be shared to avoid unnecessary repetition or misinterpretation. Photographs can be useful but changes may be subtle, especially in the context of oedema that may be obvious to a patient because of associated discomfort but not obvious to an outside observer. Extravagant description of symptoms may be used to convey the frustration felt by patients who feel that they are not being understood or believed since conventional examination for abnormal physical signs and routine investigations are often normal. Patients will often attend with a relative or close friend who may be able to offer additional insights into the practical aspects of caring, degree of disability, impairment in quality of life and social background.

Examination

A whole-body examination for cutaneous mastocytosis, lymphadenopathy or organomegaly should be undertaken (Table 3). Cutaneous mastocytosis has a range of presentations from extensive confluent or discrete erythematous pigmented macules (urticaria pigmentosa) that usually weal easily with light stroking (positive Darier's sign) to minimal change, sometimes seen with more advanced disease. The term maculopapular cutaneous mastocytosis is now preferred to urticaria pigmentosa and also embraces telangiectasia macularis eruptiva perstans (TMEP). Diffuse cutaneous mastocytosis (DCM) and solitary mastocytomas present in early childhood. DCM is rare and may persist into adulthood but mastocytomas regress. They are associated with flushing and swelling but anaphylaxis is uncommon.

Testing normal skin for dermographism with a calibrated dermographometer is useful to distinguish simple (physiological) dermographism (a non-itchy red weal response to skin stroking seen at pressures of 60 g/mm^2 or above (Fig. 1a) that is a common finding in healthy individuals) from symptomatic dermographism, which is characterised by an immediate itchy red weal response at 36 g/

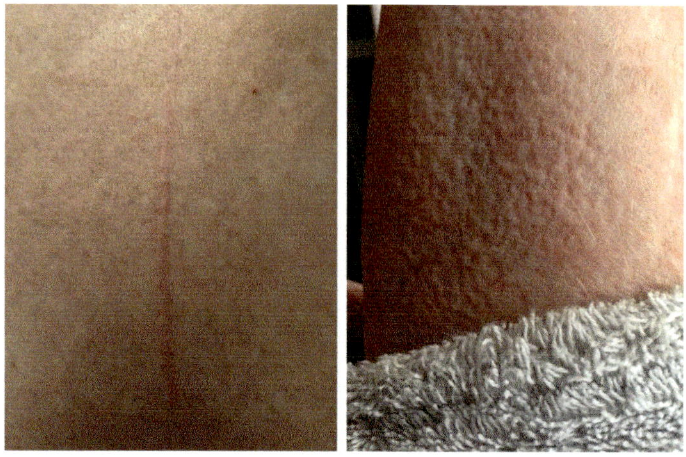

Fig. 1 Representative physiological events in healthy individuals that may be interpreted as skin features of MCAS but are, in fact, normal events. For example, (**a**) non-itchy wealing of the skin after stroking with a firm stimulus (simple or physiological dermographism), here illustrated by a weal response to a calibrated dermographometer set at 60 g/mm2 but not below this (**b**) indentation in the skin after prolonged pressure against a rough surface or fabric in normal skin

mm^2 or below. Dry or broken skin suggests eczema or an atopic background as a predisposing reason for pruritus. Indentation of the skin from sustained clothing fabric pressure (Fig. 1b), seams or buckles is normal but can be exaggerated by persistent skin oedema. Fixed livedo should raise the possibility of an underlying connective tissue disease, including lupus, mixed connective tissue disease and anti-phospholipid antibody syndrome. Dusky discoloration of the lower legs and feet on standing (orthostatic cyanosis) may suggest dysautonomia or cryoglobulinaemia. Spontaneous bruising may be a feature of classical Ehlers-Danlos syndrome and less commonly with hypermobile Ehlers-Danlos syndrome. Assessing joints for hypermobility requires experience since there is a spectrum of normality for different ages. Similarly, assessment of dysautonomia requires expert input although a history of postural symptoms may suggest it and an active stand test by the bedside may provide useful evidence of postural pulse rate changes.

Patient Related Outcome Measures (PROMS)

These validated assessment tools allow patients to communicate symptom severity, life quality impairment, depression and anxiety. They may be generic or disease-specific. The most useful measures in the dermatological assessment of patients with suspected MCAS are the Dermatology Life Quality Index (DLQI), Hospital Anxiety and Depression Scale (HADS) and Generalized Anxiety Disorder-2 item screening tool (GAD-2). Other illness specific PROMS are available.

Investigations

Baseline Investigation

Standard investigations should be targeted at the likely cause of the patient's symptoms to support the initial clinical assessment rather than a standard order set. Some routine screening tests are appropriate in nearly every new patient including haematology and biochemical profiles, C reactive protein or erythrocyte sedimentation rate (as non-specific markers of inflammation or chronic infection), tryptase (as a screen for systemic mastocytosis without skin lesions and α tryptasaemia), total IgE as a guide to an underlying atopic diathesis (accepting that it may be normal in around 20% of atopics) and spot urinary N-methyl histamine collected at baseline and 1–3 hours after an episode of severe symptoms (to look for a relationship between mast cell activation and symptomatology), which can be collected at home rather than relying on acute medical services.

Additional tests that may be requested in the context of suspected mast cell activation include 24 hours urinary assays for PGD_2 and its metabolites, cysteinyl leukotrienes and N-methyl histamine, depending on their availability, but isolated abnormalities without a careful supporting clinical assessment and a response to anti-mast cell mediator treatments do not define MCAS.

Extended Investigations

Further investigation to follow up specific leads from the history might include tests for infection (borrelia, human immunodeficiency virus, Epstein Barr virus, bowel parasites), connective tissue disease (anti-nuclear antibodies and extractable nuclear antibodies, anti-phospholipids), autoimmune disease (thyroid antibodies, coeliac screen and the basophil histamine release assay in patients with chronic spontaneous urticaria), haematinics (iron, folate, vitamin B12) in patients with very restricted diets and vitamin D, endocrine (thyroid function, glucose tolerance test for reactive hypoglycaemia, HbA1c for sustained glucose intolerance), specific IgE (whole allergen and allergen components), inflammatory markers (ferritin for adult-onset Still's disease, serum amyloidosis A protein for auto-inflammatory syndromes) and immunoglobulins (with electrophoresis for paraproteins) cryoglobulins (for cryoglobubinaemia), neuroendocrine tumours (urinary metanephrines and 5 hydroxy indole acetic acid), diamine oxidase for dietary histamine intolerance, electrocardiography and appropriate imaging. Investigation of peripheral blood for *KIT* mutations and increased *TPSAB1* copy numbers may be appropriate if systemic mastocytosis and alpha tryptasaemia are suspected respectively where these tests are available.

Management

Avoidance

Avoiding known triggers of anaphylaxis is essential for good care when they can be identified. This particularly applies to immediate hypersensitivity reactions but may be relevant to life-style changes in the context of exercise or cold-induced anaphylaxis. Patients with dysautonomia are often sensitive to smells and fumes. Those who react to non-steroidal anti-inflammatories and opiates due to intolerance rather than allergy may be able to tolerate small exposures since adverse effects tend to relate to pharmacological potency and dose.

Pharmacological Treatments

There is no specific protocol for introducing anti-mast cell mediator drugs but all patients with suspected MCAS deserve a trial of anti-mast cell mediator drugs. As a rule, antihistamines and other anti-mast cell mediator treatments are safe and usually well tolerated to the point where it is good practice to offer a trial of treatment whether mast cell activation seems likely or not. A good response is always welcome and provides indirect evidence that the symptoms may have been due to mast cell activation (or histamine if anti-histamines alone are helpful). It is important to recognize though that all treatments may have a placebo effect. It is therefore good practice to down-dose or

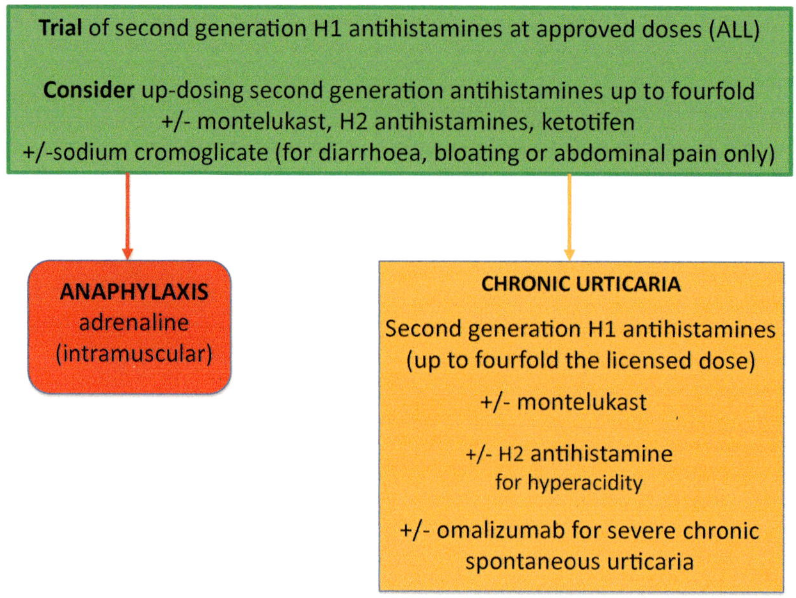

Fig. 2 Some pharmacological options for patients with mast cell activation disorders. All patients should be offered a second generation H1 antihistamine (sg H1 antihistamine) at approved (licensed) doses before escalating treatments according to the clinical scenario and response to treatment

withdraw treatment temporarily for symptom responders and then re-introduce medication to be more sure whether it should be maintained for a longer period or not. Some options for treating anaphylaxis, symptomatic mastocytosis and chronic urticaria are illustrated in Fig. 2.

H1 antihistamines

A trial of second generation H1 antihistamines should be offered to all patients with suspected MCAS or those in whom mast cells may be contributing to a more complex multisystem illness spectrum whether tests support mast cell activation as a cause of it or not. This approach is justifiable because second generation H1 antihistamines as a class are very safe and tests for increased histamine excretion after mast cell activation episodes may be negative [9]. Up-dosing H1 antihistamines up to fourfold above licence is now standard practice in symptomatic chronic urticaria and this approach can be offered for patients with CHARISMA subject to any cautions based on drug elimination, interactions, pregnancy, age restrictions or intolerance. However, it must be emphasised at the outset that a trial means just that. Introduction of a second generation H1 antihistamine should be followed by its withdrawal within a month if there is no benefit or a further trial of up-dosing to double then fourfold at fortnightly intervals. Second generation H1 antihistamines are absorbed and eliminated rapidly with the exception of desloratadine that takes 27 h to reach maximum plasma concentration and up to 6 days after a single oral dose to be eliminated in healthy volunteers. Clinical (Table 4) and pharmacokinetic (Table 5) properties of the most widely available second generation H1 antihistamines should be taken into account when prescribing. H1 antihistamines can be discontinued and restarted with no loss of effectiveness, withdrawal symptoms or other long term physiological changes (such as adrenal suppression; a risk of long term oral corticosteroids). Because there are no tests for efficacy that can be applied simply in the clinic and benefits are often subjective with chronic disease symptoms (such as fatigue

Table 4 Second generation (non-sedating) H1 antihistamines: some relevant clinical properties—Age* relates to UK licence for chronic urticaria. Grapefruit juice reduces absorption of fexofenadine and bilastine but increases absorption of rupatadine. Mizolastine concentrations may increase when erythromycin is taken at the same time

Drug	Daily dose	Age*	Sedation	Metabolism	Drug/food interaction
Acrivastine	24 mg	> 12y	-	-	-
Cetirizine	5-10 mg	≥ 6 y	+	-	-
Levocetirizine	2.5-5 mg	≥ 2 y	+	-	-
Fexofenadine	180 mg	≥ 12 y	-	-	+
Loratadine	5-10 mg	≥ 2 y	-	+	+
Desloratadine	1.25-5 mg	≥ 1 y	-	+	-
Mizolastine	10 mg	≥ 12 y	-	+	+
Rupatadine	10 mg	≥ 12 y	-	+	+
Bilastine	10-20 mg	≥ 6y	-	-	+

Table 5 Second generation (non-sedating) H1 antihistamines: pharmacokinetic properties—*loratadine is metabolised to desloratadine

Name	T_{max} (h)	T1/2 (h) elimination		5 × T1/2 (days)	Principal elimination	Renal impairment GFR < 10 ml/min
		Adults	Children			
Acrivastine	1.5	1.5		<1	Renal	Avoid
Cetirizine	0.5–1	10	6	2	Renal	Half dose
Levocetirizine	0.9	8		2	Renal	Reduced dose
Loratadine	1 (2 h after food)	(8.4)*		(2)	Hepatic (CYP 3A4)	Caution
Desloratadine	3	27		6	Hepatic	Caution
Fexofenadine	1–3	11–15		3	BIliary	Same dose
Mizolastine	1.5	13		3	Hepatic	Same dose
Rupatadine	0.75	5.9		1.25	Hepatic	Same dose
Bilastine	1.3	14.5		3.0	Renal	Same dose

or intolerance of food), patients need to be as objective as possible and the possibility of a placebo response should be discussed. Even when benefit is convincing, the principle that 'what goes up must come down' should be discussed at review to avoid taking unnecessary medication if the need lessens and to minimize the risk of drug interactions with multiple prescribing. First generation 'classical' antihistamines (such as chlorphenamine, diphenhydramine and promethazine) should generally be avoided because of their long half-lives, sedating potential and additional anti-cholinergic properties that may compound constipation or urinary retention. Diphenhydramine and promethazine are sold in the UK as sleep aids. Ketotifen has a special place in mast cell disorder management as a sedating H1 antihistamine that is credited with additional mast cell stabilizing and anti-inflammatory properties and may be popular with some patients. It is approved for the symptomatic treatment of allergic conditions, including rhinitis and conjunctivitis.

Sodium cromoglicate

Sodium cromoglicate is a chromone that reduces influx of calcium into mast cells thereby reducing mast cell activation. However, it is poorly absorbed from the gastro-intestinal tract and is primarily used for allergic conjunctivitis as an eye drop to stabilise submucosal mast cells in the prevention of hay fever. It is also available as a nasal spray for allergic rhinitis, an inhaler for asthma and a capsule for food allergy. It is generally well-tolerated by the oral route but may cause nausea or arthralgia. Patients with bowel symptoms of diarrhoea, constipation or bloating may benefit but there is unlikely to be any significant systemic benefit due to its poor absorption from the bowel.

H2 antihistamines

These are approved for treatment of gastric ulceration and hyperacidity. There is pharmacological evidence of H2 receptors in the skin as well as the stomach and this is the logic for adding them to second generation H1 antihistamines to treat refractory chronic urticaria. There is some evidence of benefit from combined treatment of acute urticaria but there have been no large, well-designed controlled double-blind studies in chronic urticaria so they are not recommended in current guidelines. Some patients with chronic urticaria benefit nevertheless and this may be true for MCAS.

Montelukast

At the time of writing montelukast is the only marketed antileukotriene in Europe for prophylaxis of asthma. It is widely used as a prophylactic for allergic conditions in combination with an H1 antihistamine, including chronic urticaria, rhinosinusitis and anaphylaxis and may be a useful add-on. It should not be prescribed as monotherapy. It is a logical treatment for MCAS patients with increased urinary cysteinyl leukotriene excretion but leukotrienes are generated by eosinophils and basophils as well as mast cells so are not specific for mast cell activation. Nevertheless, they may be beneficial indirectly by controlling inflammation linked with mast cell activation rather than mast cell activation itself. Montelukast is generally well tolerated at approved doses and does not require blood monitoring but does carry a number of adverse effects including abdominal discomfort, nausea, diarrhoea and neuropsychiatric effects (especially in children) so it may be difficult to separate any benefit from ongoing bowel symptoms attributed to mast cell activation.

Non steroidal anti-inflammatories

Non-steroidal anti-inflammatory drugs (NSAIDs) are generally avoided in illness due to suspected mast cell activation because of concern that they might aggravate or cause it. However, a few MCAS patients with increased 11 β PGF2α elimination over 24 hours in their urine may benefit symptomatically from the careful introduction of small doses of aspirin [14].

Omalizumab

Omalizumab is an IgG humanised monoclonal antibody directed against the Cε3 domain of free IgE without anaphylactogenic potential. It was originally licensed for asthma but is now more widely used for chronic spontaneous urticaria, its other approved indication. Its mechanism of action in urticaria involves a rapid reduction in free IgE, followed by dissociation of IgE from its receptor on mast cells and basophils, and then a much slower reduction in the number of expressed high affinity IgE receptors (FcεRI) although it does not appear to alter the natural history of the illness. The consequence of reducing FcεRI density is to stabilise the mast cell to immunological stimulation and this has been utilized to reduce adverse reactions during hymenoptera venom immunotherapy in mastocytosis, in symptomatic systemic mastocytosis and as a treatment of idiopathic anaphylaxis but the experience with it for these indications is limited and there is little or no evidence to support its

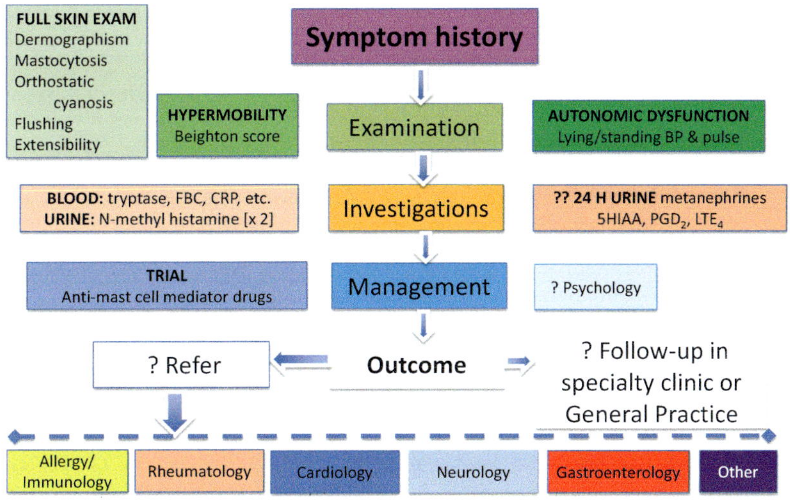

Fig. 3 Algorithm illustrating a possible pathway for the assessment and investigation of patients presenting with complex illness symptoms in whom MCAS is suspected

use in CHARISMA patients with co-morbidities of dysautonomia and hEDS unless there is co-incidental severe chronic spontaneous urticaria or recurrent anaphylaxis (used off-label).

MCAS: A Multidisciplinary Approach

Those patient with established MCAS should be managed by specialists with experience of mast cell disease. Patients with suspected MCAS in whom MCAS is unlikely should be referred to the relevant specialist(s) to address the predominant clinical problem (Fig. 3). Clinical Psychology may be useful for some individuals to promote positive thinking about the value of life-style adjustments and the benefits and limitations of available conventional medications.

Prognosis

There is little literature on the prognosis for recovery from illness to health but anecdotal experience suggests that this is achievable in some individuals, through the natural history of their illness, medical support and combined physical and mental reconditioning.

Relationship of MCAS to HEDS and PoTs

Because of overlapping symptomatology between hypermobility, dysautonomia and mast cell activation symptoms, it is often assumed that MCAS is related to hEDS and PoTS. A recent review of the literature showed no current evidence for the existence of an association between MCAS, PoTS or hEDS [15]. The authors concluded that studies proposing a relationship between the three clinical entities are either biased or based on outdated criteria. Anecdotally, some patients with PoTS, hEDS or both do find some benefit from anti-mast cell mediator drugs and mast cell activation disorders may occur in patients with PoTS and hEDS so further studies are needed to allow conclusions to be drawn with more confidence.

References

1. Holgate ST, Church MK, Broide DH, Martinez FD, editors. Allergy, 4th edn. Elsevier Saunders, Edinburgh; 2012.
2. Rich RR, Fleischer TA, Shearer WT, Schroeder HW, Frew AJ, Weyland CM, editors. Clinical Immunology: Principles and Practice, 5th edn. Elsevier; 2019.

3. Simons FER, Ebisawa M, Sanchez-Borges M, Thong BY, Worm M, et al. 2015 update of the evidence base: World allergy organization anaphylaxis guidelines. World Allergy Organization Journal. 2015;8:32.
4. Akin C, Valent P, Metcalfe DD. Mast cell activation syndrome: Proposed diagnostic criteria. J Allergy Clin Immunol. 2010;126(6):1099–104.
5. Akin C. Mast cell activation syndromes. J Allergy Clin Immunol. 2017;140(2):349–55.
6. Valent P. Mast cell activation syndromes: definition and classification. Allergy. 2013;68(4):417–24.
7. Afrin LB. Mast cell activation disease and the modern epidemic of chronic inflammatory disease. Transl Res. 2016;174:33–59.
8. Valent P, Akin C, Bonadonna P, Hartmann K, Brockow K, Niedoszytko M, Nedoszytko B, Siebenhaar F, Sperr WR, Oude Elberink JNG, Butterfield JH, Alvarez-Twose I, Sotlar K, Reiter A, Kluin-Nelemans HC, Hermine O, Gotlib J, Broesby-Olsen S, Orfao A, Horny HP, Triggiani M, Arock M, Schwartz LB, Metcalfe DD. Proposed diagnostic algorithm for patients with suspected mast cell activation syndrome. J Allergy Clin Immunol Pract. 2019;7(4):1125–33.
9. Weiler CR, Austen KF, Akin C, Barkoff MS, Bernstein JA, Bonadonna P, Butterfield JH, Carter M, Fox CC, Maitland A, Pongdee T, Mustafa SS, Ravi A, Tobin MC, Vliagoftis H, Schwartz LB. AAAAI mast cell disorders committee work group report: mast cell activation syndrome (MCAS) diagnosis and management. J Allergy Clin Immunol. 2019;144(4):883–96.
10. Horny HP, Akin C, Arber DA Peterson LC, Tefferi A, Metcalfe DD, Bennett JM, Bain BJ, Escribano L, Valent P. Mastocytosis. In: Swerdlow SH, Campo E, Harris NL, et al. editors. World Health Organization (WHO) classification of tumours. Pathology & Genetics. Tumours of haematopoietic and lymphoid tissues. Lyon, France: IARC Press; 2016.
11. Lyons JJ, Yu X, Hughes JD, Le QT, Jamil A, Bai Y, Ho N, Zhao M, Liu Y, O'Connell MP, Trivedi NN, Nelson C, DiMaggio T, Jones N, Matthews H, Lewis KL, Oler AJ, Carlson RJ, Arkwright PD, Hong C, Agama S, Wilson TM, Tucker S, Zhang Y, McElwee JJ, Pao M, Glover SC, Rothenberg ME, Hohman RJ, Stone KD, Caughey GH, Heller T, Metcalfe DD, Biesecker LG, Schwartz LB, Milner JD. Elevated basal serum tryptase identifies a multisystem disorder associated with increased TPSAB1 copy number. Nat Genet. 2016;48(12):1564–9.
12. Valent P, Bonadonna P, Hartmann K, Broesby-Olsen S, Brockow K, Butterfield JH, Triggiani M, Lyons JJ, Oude Elberink JNG, Arock M, Metcalfe DD, Akin C. Why the 20%+2 Tryptase formula is a diagnostic gold standard for severe systemic mast cell activation and mast cell activation syndrome. Int Arch Allergy Immunol. 2019;180(1):44–51.
13. Weiler CR. Mast cell activation syndrome: Tools for diagnosis and differential diagnosis. J Allergy Clin Immunol Pract. 2020;8(2):498–506.
14. Ravi A, Butterfield J, Weiler CR. Mast cell activation syndrome: improved identification by combined determinations of serum tryptase and 24-hours urine 11 & #x03B2;-PGF2α. J Allergy Clin Immunol Pract. 2014;2:775–8.
15. Kohn A, Chang C. The relationship between hypermobile Ehlers-Danlos Syndrome (hEDS), Postural Orthostatic Tachycardia Syndrome (POTS), and Mast Cell Activation Syndrome (MCAS). Clin Rev Allergy Immunol. 2020;58(3):273–297.

Inherited Metabolic Diseases

Radha Ramachandran

Inherited Metabolic Diseases (IMD) (or inborn errors of metabolism) are a group of monogenic disorders that occur as a result of impairment in enzyme activity in one or more metabolic pathways. Although individually rare, collectively they are not that uncommon, with reported prevalence ranging from 1 in 800 to 1/2500 live births. Prevalence may be even higher in populations where consanguinity is common or in relatively isolated societies with a small ancestral pool.

Hundreds of disorders exist, with the number of known individual disorders reported to be increasing yearly. Whilst the majority of IMDs present in childhood, there is an increasing recognition that they may present for the first time in adulthood, and that presenting features may differ from those seen in the paediatric setting.

IMDs can present for the first time in adulthood as a metabolic emergency. A diagnosis of an IMD should therefore be considered in patients presenting with atypical seizure or stroke, encephalopathy, acid–base disturbance, neuropsychiatric symptoms, rhabdomyolysis, if a more common alternative diagnosis is not forthcoming. Presentation is however, often chronic, with non-specific symptoms and with multisystem involvement. A diagnosis of IMD should therefore also be considered in patients with multisystem involvement where more common aetiologies have been excluded.

Autonomic dysfunction and impaired glucose homeostasis, leading to features suggestive of PoTS may be a feature of some IMDs. In these patients, a diagnosis of an IMD should be considered if

(i) There is documented hypoglycaemia where insulin excess has been excluded
(ii) Apparently unrelated multisystem involvement including one or more of the following: cardiomyopathy, myopathy, renal disease, liver disease
(iii) Central nervous system (CNS) manifestations—particularly neurodegenerative/neuropathic disorders and abnormalities on brain imaging
(iv) Dysmorphia
(v) Family history of similar complaints/consanguinity/death.

R. Ramachandran (✉)
Departments of Chemical Pathology/Metabolic Medicine, Guy's and St Thomas' Hospitals NHS Foundation Trust, London SE1 7EH, UK
e-mail: radha.ramachandran@gstt.nhs.uk

R. Ramachandran Adult Inherited Metabolic Diseases, Centre for Inherited Metabolic Diseases, Guy's and St Thomas' Hospitals NHS Foundation Trust, Lambeth Palace Road, London SE1 7EH, UK

N. Gall et al. (eds.), *Postural Tachycardia Syndrome*, https://doi.org/10.1007/978-3-030-54165-1_22

Some IMDs Where Orthostatic Hypotension Is a Common Feature Are Described Below

Dopamine Beta-Hydroxylase Deficiency (DBH Deficiency)

DBH deficiency is an autosomal recessive condition occurring as a result of mutations in the *DBH* gene. Very few cases have been reported in the literature, and prevalence is very rare, reported to be less than 1 in 1,000,000. In the CNS, dopamine is hydroxylated to noradrenaline by DBH. Noradrenaline is subsequently methylated to form adrenaline. Therefore deficiency of DBH enzyme leads to very high levels of dopamine and very low levels of adrenaline and noradrenaline.

The disease is characterised by a lack of sympathetic noradrenergic function but intact parasympathetic and sympathetic cholinergic function. Presentation is usually at birth with temperature dysregulation, hypotonia, ptosis, dehydration and hypoglycaemia. However, diagnosis is often delayed until late childhood or adolescence when patients present with severe orthostatic hypotension (systolic blood pressure falling to less than 80 mmHg and compensatory tachycardia on standing); nasal stuffiness is reported in 100% of patients. There is often a history of a complicated peri-natal course. Ptosis, high arched palate, joint hypermobility and profoundly reduced exercise tolerance are other commonly reported features in this group of patients. Sweating is normal in these patients and pupils are small but reactive to light and accommodation.

Diagnosis

- Plasma catecholamine measurement—minimal or absent adrenaline and noradrenaline with 5–tenfold increase in dopamine levels.
- Molecular genetic testing for pathogenic mutations in the *DBH* gene.

Treatment

Treatment is mainly supportive. Standard therapies for autonomic failure are not very helpful. Drug of choice is L-threo-3,4-dihydroxyphenylserine (Droxidopa), a synthetic precursor of noradrenaline.

Prognosis

Prognosis is largely unknown, although survival beyond 60 years in some individuals has been previously reported.

Menkes Disease

Menkes disease is a rare X-linked disorder caused by mutations in the *ATP7A* gene. The incidence of Menke's disease has been reported to range between 1:40,000 to 1:350,000. The clinical features are due to severe copper deficiency. DBH is a copper dependent enzyme and therefore patients often have partial DBH deficiency. Plasma catecholamine analysis shows high levels of dopamine with low levels of dihydroxyphenylglycol.

Clinical features are characteristic. Patients with classical Menke's present with severe neurological and marked connective tissue dysfunction, often leading to death in early childhood. Patients often present with sparse, hypopigmented, kinky hair. A less severe form presenting in adulthood, is characterised mainly by connective tissue dysfunction including skin laxity and hyperelasticity, and characteristic occipital horns on imaging resulting from calcification of the trapezius and sternocleidomastoid joints. Neurological manifestations in adult presenting patients may be mild or even absent.

Cytochrome B561 Deficiency (CYB561)

4 patients in 2 families with severe orthostatic hypotension, due to CYB561 protein defect have recently been described. The diagnosis was made following exome sequencing,

homozygosity mapping and subsequent Sanger sequencing.

The CYB561 protein defect leads to a disruption in ascorbate-hydroxyascorbate recycling within the catecholamine secretory vesicles. This in turn results is impaired conversion of dopamine to epinephrine, in effect, leading to a functional DBH deficiency.

Patients presented with severe life-threatening orthostatic hypotension. In contrast to patients with DBH deficiency, compensatory tachycardia, ptosis and generalised hypotonia were not noted to be present.

Patients responded to treatment with L-threo-3,4-dihydroxyphenylserine.

Other Disorders Associated with Orthostatic Hypotension

Other disorders that present with orthostatic hypotension as a feature include.

1. Familial dysautonomia (Riley-Day syndrome), an autosomal recessive condition due to pathogenic mutations in the *ELP1* gene.
2. Familial transthyretin amyloidosis, resulting from autosomal dominant mutations in the *TTR* gene.
3. Shy-Drager syndrome due to mutations in the *COQ2* gene.

The following references provide further details on clinical features, investigations and management [1–3].

References

1. Garland EM, Biaggioni I. Dopamine Beta-Hydroxylase Deficiency. In: Adam MP, Ardinger HH, Pagon RA, Wallace SE, Bean LJH, Stephens K, et al, editors. GeneReviews (R) Seattle (WA): University of Washington, Seattle. GeneReviews is a registered trademark of the University of Washington, Seattle; 1993.
2. Tumer Z, Moller LB. Menkes disease. Eur J Hum Genet. 2010;18(5):511–8.
3. van den Berg MP, Almomani R, Biaggioni I, van Faassen M, van der Harst P, Sillje HHW, et al. Mutations in CYB561 causing a novel orthostatic hypotension syndrome. Circ Res. 2018;122(6):846–54.

Chronic Fatigue Syndrome

Julia Newton

Chronic fatigue syndrome (CFS) is a chronic debilitating condition that is thought to affect between 0.2 and 0.4% of the UK population. In order to make the diagnosis of chronic fatigue syndrome patients need to experience a cluster of associated symptoms. Fatigue usually has been present for longer than 6 months and alternative diagnoses consistent with fatigue need to have been ruled out. Typical symptoms are sore throat, autonomic symptoms, post-exertional myalgia, cognitive problems, etc. More details about the epidemiology and pathophysiology of CFS are available in the UK National Institute for Clinical Excellence (NICE [1]).

There are a number of different diagnostic criteria for chronic fatigue syndrome which are all subjective. The most commonly used in clinical services in the UK is the Fukuda Criteria [2].

The demographic of those affected by PoTS is very similar to that of a group with a diagnosis of CFS. As a result, historically, there has been overlap and studies suggest that significant numbers of those with a diagnosis of postural tachycardia syndrome may have been diagnosed with CFS. Studies from our group and others suggest that up to 30% of those with a diagnosis of chronic fatigue syndrome when tested objectively in an autonomic lab will have a diagnosis of postural tachycardia syndrome [3]. Using a low estimate of approximately 20% considering the stated prevalence of CFS at 0.2 to 0.4%, this suggests that up to 0.1% of the UK population may have PoTS with an estimated annual prevalence of 1000 per million population.

J. Newton (✉)
Population Health Sciences Institute, Faculty of Medical Sciences, Newcastle University, Newcastle N2 4HH, UKe-mail: julia.newton@ncl.ac.uk

Investigation

Currently in the UK, chronic fatigue syndrome services are configured in multiple different ways with some services being led by physicians and others by psychologists or psychiatrists. It is not currently part of the NICE guidelines [1] to formally test for PoTS despite studies confirming the high prevalence of orthostatic intolerance [4].

Management

The NICE guidelines recommend graded exercise therapy and cognitive behavioural therapy as the core elements of their management strategy for chronic fatigue syndrome. Neither have been formally tested in the subgroup of CFS patients who may have positional tachycardia syndrome. In our experience patients with PoTS tend to have worse symptoms of orthostatic

N. Gall et al. (eds.), *Postural Tachycardia Syndrome*, https://doi.org/10.1007/978-3-030-54165-1_23

intolerance and as a result find it extremely difficult to participate in graded exercise therapy in its current recommended form. It is therefore felt that these patients would benefit from a pacing regime with strengthening of core muscle strength to allow better postural control before progressing on to therapies such as graded exercise therapy.

As knowledge of PoTS increases, this has highlighted potential phenotypic variability in chronic fatigue syndrome groups and as such a potential opportunity for therapeutic intervention. To date there have not been randomised control trials of therapies that may be applicable to CFS patients with a PoTS phenotype in order to determine whether, not only does tachycardia improve but whether this is associated with any symptomatic benefit. In contrast many of the treatments that show symptomatic improvements for patients with PoTS have applicability in chronic fatigue syndrome and may provide insights into the pathophysiology of this condition.

The finding of up to 30% of CFS patients formally tested as having PoTS and the recognition of the high prevalence of orthostatic intolerance, does begin to point towards autonomic dysfunction as a potential underpinning pathophysiological mechanism in some with chronic fatigue syndrome that certainly warrants further investigation [5].

References

1. NICE Guidelines. https://www.nice.org.uk/guidance/cg53.
2. Fukuda K, Straus SE, Hickie I, Sharpe MC, Dobbins JG. Komaroff AL & the international chronic fatigue study group the chronic fatigue syndrome: a comprehensive approach to its definition and study. Ann Intern Med. 1994;121:953–9.
3. Hollingsworth KG, Hodgson T, Macgowan GA, Blamire AM, Newton JL. Impaired cardiac function in chronic fatigue syndrome measured using magnetic resonance cardiac tagging. J Intern Med. 2012;271(3):264–70.
4. Newton JL, Okonkwo O, Sutcliffe K, Seth A, Shin J, Jones DE. Symptoms of autonomic dysfunction in chronic fatigue syndrome. QJM. 2007;100(8):519–26.
5. Hoad A, Spickett G, Elliott J, Newton J. Postural orthostatic tachycardia syndrome is an under-recognized condition in chronic fatigue syndrome. QJM. 2008;101:961–5.

Lyme Disease

John Lambert and Anne Cruikshank

Orthostatic intolerance and postural tachycardia syndrome (PoTS) have been recognised in some patients following a diagnosis of Lyme disease [1, 2].

Lyme disease, or Lyme borreliosis, is named after the town of Old Lyme in Connecticut, USA, where a large number of children developed symptoms similar to juvenile arthritis in the 1970s. However, its dermatological and neurological manifestations have been recognised in Europe since the late 1800s. Bannwarth's syndrome, lymphocytic meningo-radiculitis, was described in 1941. A variant of *Borrelia burgdorferi* DNA has since been identified in the ice-age mummy, Ötzi [3].

Lyme disease is a zoonotic bacterial infection caused by the spirochaete *Borrelia burgdorferi*, transmitted by the bite of an infected tick. There are many species of Borrelia worldwide, and those which cause Lyme disease are referred to as *Borrelia burgdorferi* sensu lato (Bbsl). In the UK, there are three main genospecies known to cause Lyme disease and symptoms may vary depending on the species:

- *Borrelia garinii* (Bg) is associated with neurological conditions
- *Borrelia afzelii* (Ba) is associated with skin and atypical neurological presentations
- *Borrelia burgdorferi* sensu stricto (Bbss), may cause Lyme arthritis, especially of large joints such as the knee.

Borrelia burgdorferi sensu stricto is the main cause of Lyme disease in the USA. The American strains of Bbsl are thought to cause a more severe inflammatory reaction and have been associated with fatal Lyme carditis.

Lyme disease is increasing in incidence throughout the world. Whilst early recognition and treatment lead to resolution of the illness for many patients, late or missed diagnosis may result in persistent, debilitating symptoms. It has been described by some as "The New Great Imitator".

Cases of Lyme disease have been reported throughout the UK, with a higher incidence in Southern England and the Scottish Highlands. Ticks are carried on deer, small mammals and birds, are most active between late spring and early autumn and most commonly found in wooded or grassy areas in both rural and urban areas. Other tick-borne pathogens include Anaplasma, Babesia, Bartonella, *Coxiella burnetii* and Rickettsia, as well as a number of viruses.

J. Lambert
UCD School of Medicine, Consultant in Infectious Diseases, Mater Misericordiae University Hospital, Dublin, Ireland

A. Cruikshank (✉)
Oxfordshire, UK
e-mail: anne.cruikshank@nhs.net

N. Gall et al. (eds.), *Postural Tachycardia Syndrome*, https://doi.org/10.1007/978-3-030-54165-1_24

Diagnosing Lyme disease

The symptoms of Lyme disease, whether early or late stage, may be non-specific and are easily missed or misdiagnosed. Diagnosis should be clinical, taking into account medical history, signs, symptoms and tick-exposure risk. Since patients may not recall or may omit to mention a tick bite or unusual skin rash, a detailed clinical history is essential. Lyme serology may be supportive, though a negative test result does not necessarily exclude the diagnosis.

The Royal College of General Practitioners has produced a Lyme Disease Toolkit and a Lyme disease e-learning module as a guide for general practitioners and other health care professionals [4, 5].

Testing

The accuracy of Lyme serology testing has a number of known limitations. The immunoblot may be positive despite a negative Elisa result [6, 7]. Possible reasons for a false negative result may include:

(a) Test carried out too early
(b) Early antibiotics may abrogate the immune response
(c) Test does not cover all strains of borrelia.

False positive results may also occur, mainly due to cross reactions or persistent serological scar post-treatment.

PCR testing of samples is also available (skin, synovial membrane and CSF), but sensitivity is limited due to the low numbers of Borrelia present.

Early Lyme disease

Early symptoms in adults may include: an erythema migrans (EM) rash, flu-like symptoms of aching, fever, headache, fatigue, sweating, joint pain, neck pain, migratory myalgia, brain fog and paraesthesiae. These may be non-specific and easily missed.

An EM rash is diagnostic of Lyme disease and a blood test is not required or recommended in this instance. However, in approximately 30% of UK cases of Lyme disease there is no EM rash.

Facial palsy in children with headache and fever has been shown to predict early Lyme neuroborreliosis during peak Lyme season in endemic areas (April–October) [8].

Late Lyme disease

If not diagnosed in the early stages, Lyme disease may present with acute or chronic multi-systemic signs and symptoms, weeks, months or even years later. These may include facial palsy, meningitis, dizziness, unexplained radiculopathy, encephalitis, neuropsychiatric presentations, inflammatory arthritis, neurological conditions, cardiac problems, ME/CFS, fibromyalgia, uveitis or keratitis and skin rashes.

Diagnosis at this stage may be difficult. Negative serology does not exclude the diagnosis.

Life-threatening and even fatal outcomes such as sudden cardiac arrest and suicide have been reported. These are considered to be rare occurrences, though their true incidence is unknown.

Treatment Guidelines

The optimal treatment regimes for early or disseminated Lyme disease have not yet been determined. Some protocols advocate limited courses of antibiotic treatment. Others consider that persistent symptoms are the result of persistent infection and require individualised treatment regimes.

The NICE Guideline on Lyme disease (NG95) recommends a minimum of 21 days of antibiotics with specific antibiotic regimes for adults and children depending on symptoms.

However, the guideline committee acknowledged the limited evidence upon which their recommendations were based and made research recommendations.

Guidelines from the International Lyme and Associated Diseases Society (ILADS) recommend longer courses of antibiotics and a more individualised approach to treatment.

However, many uncertainties remain regarding the diagnosis and treatment. There is an acknowledged lack of European treatment studies or controlled trials on the most effective antibiotics and length of treatment for late stage Lyme disease. Research data, together with a significant number of case studies provide evidence that spirochetes may persist after standard treatment regimes [9–11].

Persistent Symptoms

It is now well-recognised that a significant number of patients appear to fail standard antibiotic treatment regimens and go on to develop chronic illness. There is no international consensus of opinion on the cause or management of these persistent symptoms. Possible explanations for persistent symptoms following a diagnosis of Lyme disease include treatment failure, immune dysfunction, non-adherence, re-infection or tissue damage.

This condition is variously described as either "Post treatment Lyme disease syndrome" (PTLDS), Post treatment Lyme disease (PTLD) or Chronic Lyme disease.

Research from John Hopkin's University in 2017 reported the following conclusion:

> Although physical exam and clinical laboratory tests showed few objective abnormalities, standardized symptom questionnaires revealed that patients with PTLDS are highly and clinically significantly symptomatic, with poor health-related quality of life. PTLDS patients exhibited levels of fatigue, musculoskeletal pain, sleep disturbance, and depression which were both clinically relevant and statistically significantly higher than controls. Our study shows that PTLDS can be successfully identified using a systematic approach to diagnosis and symptom measurement. As the prevalence of PTLDS continues to rise, there will be an increased need for physician education to more effectively identify and manage PTLDS as part of integrated patient care [12].

In 2018 the USA Tick-Borne Diseases group, a federal advisory committee, recognised the need to provide increases in federal resources to meet urgent research and patient care needs [13].

Lyme Disease and PoTS

Some USA and European clinicians with extensive experience of treating Lyme disease have observed an apparent correlation between chronic tick-borne infection and postural tachycardia syndrome (PoTS). They estimate that PoTS may occur in up to 10% of cases, with another 20% of patients appearing to have other disorders of the autonomic nervous system. These symptoms seem to develop months or years after the initial infection—when the Lyme disease diagnosis may have been forgotten or never considered.

Borrelia burgdorferi is known to have an affinity for nervous tissue. In a USA study from 1993, anti-ganglioside IgM antibodies were found to be significantly more frequent in some patients with neurological Lyme disease [14].

It has been reported that autonomic symptoms often improve and sometimes resolve following treatment of the underlying condition. There is however, at present, no research data to support these observations.

In patients diagnosed with PoTS or dysautonomia, it may be appropriate to consider the possibility of a co-existent Lyme borreliosis infection.

Patients presenting with PoTS or other dysautonomia associated with Lyme disease may benefit from a multi-disciplinary approach to their clinical care.

References

1. Kanjwal K, Karabin B, Kanjwal Y, Grubb BP. Postural orthostatic tachycardia syndrome following Lyme disease. Cardiol J. 2011;18(1):63–6. https://www.ncbi.nlm.nih.gov/pubmed/21305487.
2. Noyes AM, Kluger J. A tale of two syndromes: Lyme disease preceding postural orthostatic tachycardia syndrome. Ann Noninvasive Electrocardiol. 2015;20(1):82–6. https://www.ncbi.nlm.nih.gov/pubmed/24830783.
3. Keller A, Graefen A, Ball M, et al. New insights into the Tyrolean Iceman's origin and phenotype as inferred by whole-genome sequencing. Nat Commun. 2012;3:698. https://doi.org/10.1038/ncomms1701.
4. https://www.rcgp.org.uk/clinical-and-research/resources/toolkits/lyme-disease-toolkit.aspx.
5. https://elearning.rcgp.org.uk/course/info.php?popup=0&id=164.
6. https://bmcinfectdis.biomedcentral.com/articles/10.1186/s12879-016-1468-4.
7. Ang CW, et al. Large differences between test strategies for the detection of anti-Borrelia antibodies are revealed by comparing eight ELISAs and five immunoblots. Eur J Clin Microbiol Infect Dis. 2011. https://www.ncbi.nlm.nih.gov/pubmed/21271270.
8. Nigrovic, et al. Clinical predictors of Lyme disease among children with a peripheral facial palsy at an emergency department in a Lyme disease-endemic area. Pediatrics. 2008;122(5):e1080–5.
9. Oksi J, Marjamäki M, Nikoskelainen J, Viljanen MK. *Borrelia burgdorferi* detected by culture and PCR in clinical relapse of disseminated Lyme borreliosis. Ann Med. 1999;31(3):225–32. https://doi.org/10.3109/07853899909115982. https://www.ncbi.nlm.nih.gov/pubmed/10442678.
10. Preac-Mursic V, Weber K, Pfister HW, et al. Survival of *Borrelia burgdorferi* in antibiotically treated patients with Lyme borreliosis. Infection. 1989;17(6):355–59. doi:https://doi.org/10.1007/bf01645543. https://www.ncbi.nlm.nih.gov/pubmed/2613324.
11. Marques A, Telford SR 3rd, Turk SP, et al. Xenodiagnosis to detect *Borrelia burgdorferi* infection: a first-in-human study. Clin Infect Dis. 2014;58(7):937–45. https://doi.org/10.1093/cid/cit939. https://www.ncbi.nlm.nih.gov/pubmed/24523212.
12. Rebman AW, Bechtold KT, Yang T, et al. The clinical, symptom, and quality-of-life characterization of a well-defined group of patients with posttreatment Lyme disease syndrome. Front Med (Lausanne). 2017;4:224. https://doi.org/10.3389/fmed.2017.00224.
13. Press Release: Tick-Borne Disease Working Group Calls for More Resources for Research, Prevention, Diagnostics and Treatment, U.S. Department of Health & Human Services. 2018. https://www.hhs.gov/about/news/2018/11/14/tick-borne-disease-working-group-calls-more-resources.html.
14. García Moncó JC, Wheeler CM, Benach JL, et al. Reactivity of neuroborreliosis patients (Lyme disease) to cardiolipin and gangliosides. J Neurol Sci. 1993;117(1–2):206–14. https://doi.org/10.1016/0022-510x(93)90175-x. https://www.ncbi.nlm.nih.gov/pubmed/8410057.

Therapy

Non-pharmacological Management (Hydration, Diet and Compression)

Helen Eftekhari and Diane L. Bruce

Introduction

The lifestyle management of PoTS is the cornerstone of current treatment. It is important for health care professionals to understand the issues which are specific to people with PoTS and need to be addressed. The evidence base, as with all management in PoTS, is limited and recommendations are framed around the available research and rationale practiced by PoTS clinicians.

Key Points

- Take a detailed diet and fluid intake history.
- Fluid intake needs to be minimally 2 Litres per day aiming for up to 3 Litres daily in adults.
- Fluids should be front loaded in the morning.
- Increase salt intake (unless contraindicated) aiming for 10 grams total in one day.
- Eat small meals and often.
- Low refined carbohydrate intake.
- Check for gluten sensitivity and Coeliac disease.
- Compression garments can be effective.

At an initial consultation a detailed history of a typical days food and fluid intake should be taken and documented. This enables the clinician to identify areas in diet and fluid intake which need improving, and support people with POTS in the areas discussed in this chapter.

Good Hydration

The cornerstone of initial PoTS management is aimed at expansion of blood volume through the simple activity of increasing fluid intake, aiming to take in greater than 2 Litres of fluid per day in adults. People with PoTS (n = 15) have been found to have a 13% reduction in blood volume compared with healthy controls (n = 14) [1]. In the small PoTS studies, water ingestion of 480 millilitres has been found to reduce the heart rate response to standing by 15 beats per minute (n = 9) [2]. Neuropathic PoTS is thought to result from reduced peripheral vasoconstriction and venous pooling [3]. Increasing oral fluid intake is thought to enhance vasoconstriction in addition to increasing plasma volume [4]—See Table 1.

Dehydration is reported by 86% of people with PoTS as a trigger for a number of symptoms, including mental clouding, also known

H. Eftekhari (✉)
University Hospitals Coventry & Warwickshire, NHS Trust, Coventry, UK
e-mail: helen.eftekhari@uhcw.nhs.uk

D. L. Bruce
Consultant Cardiologist Royal Bournemouth Hospital, Bournemouth, UK

N. Gall et al. (eds.), *Postural Tachycardia Syndrome*, https://doi.org/10.1007/978-3-030-54165-1_25

Table 1 Studies of water ingestion to improve orthostatic intolerance

4 studies of water ingestion	Design	Sample	Outcome
The effect of drinking 480 mls of water on heart rate within 5 minutes [2]	A protocolised, unblinded cohort study	n = 9	Water ingestion had a significant effect on standing heart rate similar to the effect of IV saline therapy or midodrine
The effect of drinking water on heart rate and blood pressure [8]	A protocolised unblinded cohort study	n = 20	Water drinking decreased heart rate and increased blood pressure
The effect of 480 mls of room temperature water compared with clear soup on heart rate [9]	A protocolised unblinded cohort study	n = 7	Water and clear soup had a pronounced effect on heart rate. 6 out of 7 participants reported improved toleration of a tilt table test following water and clear soup
The effect of drinking rapidly 500 mls of mineral water on cognitive function and heart rate [10]	A protocolised non-randomised control study	n = 8	Rapid water drinking improved cognitive function and decreased delta heart rate on tilt table test

as "brain fog" (n = 138) [5]. There have been small studies (n ~ 20) that have found rapid ingestion of 480mls of fluid (within 5 minutes), improved subjective symptoms, orthostatic tolerance, ability to tolerate tilt table testing, ability to maintain blood pressure and reduced delta heart rate (heart rate rise on standing), from 123 beats per minute (bpm) to 108 bpm [2, 6–8]. In neuropathic PoTS there is blood pooling in the extremities, with resultant baroreceptor unloading entraining a feedback loop which increases heart rate and aims to restore blood pressure. One study (n = 7) found a positive effect on delta heart rate in PoTS by ingesting soup [9]. A recent study (n = 8) found rapidly ingesting 500mls of mineral water improved orthostatic cognitive function, with a reduction of delta heart rate of 18 bpm [10].

In older people with normal physiology, water ingestion of 480 millilitres has been found to increase blood pressure (the pressor effect) when studied [4]. In conditions of autonomic failure, for instance orthostatic hypotension, increasing fluid consumption has been shown to have a pressor effect [4]. Studies in these population groups on water drinking have suggested the pressor effect of water is through vasoconstriction in addition to increasing blood volume [4]. The effect of drinking water on heart rate reduction in PoTS is not fully understood, however in clinical practice people with PoTS report fewer symptoms when maintaining adequate oral fluid intake. This supports the findings of the small studies. People with PoTS should aim for a minimum of 2 Litres of fluid and close to 3 Litres across the day. On hot days or when exercising, additional fluids need to be consumed.

Front Loading Fluid in the Morning

Although there are no studies, in clinical practice we recommend drinking water prior to getting out of bed in the morning, and within the first hour of waking up to aim for 1 Litre oral fluid intake. This can be achieved with a glass of water before getting out of bed, taking a large cup of fluid with breakfast, and having a cereal-based breakfast with milk. Orthostatic symptoms are often worse when first waking and rising, and fluid loading has been found to reduce both delta heart rate, and blood pressure drops [2, 4, 7, 11]. Anecdotally, people with PoTS report an improvement in morning orthostatic intolerance with front-loading fluids.

Types of Fluid

The types of oral fluid consumed needs to be varied. Fluids should include those with a similar osmotic pressure as body fluids, for example cordials, squash, fruit juices, isotonic drinks (avoiding those high in sugar), milk and Bovril.

Fluids to Avoid/Limit

When taking a detailed fluid intake history, there are considerations around specific types of fluids. There is no clear evidence on the benefits or not of drinking tea and coffee, with people reporting variable responses. Tea and coffee can exacerbate dehydration. In hyperadrenergic PoTS caffeine should be avoided as levels of natural stimulants are already high. Generally, people can trial tea and coffee assessing their responses, whilst limiting their overall intake. Highly caffeinated energy drinks should be completely avoided. Some drinks contain twice the caffeine content of coffee and there is one report of Red Bull causing PoTS, resolving after stopping consumption of this highly caffeinated beverage [12]. Carbonated drinks should be minimized/avoided as they contain processed sugars, which are associated with obesity, and artificial flavours.

Alcohol should be avoided or minimized with PoTS. In normal healthy people, alcohol causes fainting. In one study alcohol was found to blunt normal muscle and blood vessel responses to standing, dropping blood pressure and increasing heart rate [13]. Additionally, alcohol is a strong diuretic, leading to dehydration and therefore further exacerbating the symptoms of PoTS. Alcohol is best kept to a minimum and, when consuming alcohol, we recommend supplementation with non-alcoholic fluids to maintain hydration. Ideally if drinking alcohol, a person with PoTS should sit down. If PoTS symptoms become worse, sitting minimizes the risk of syncope, and helps avoid injury if they proceed to have a full syncopal episode.

Increase Salt consumption*—Aim for 10–12 grams daily (1 teaspoon estimated to contain 5 grams)*

To further increase blood volume, salt intake needs to be increased unless contraindicated. Conditions where salt should be avoided include primary hypertension, heart or kidney disease. Through increasing salt, fluid is retained, thereby increasing blood volume. Studies have shown that a high salt intake in PoTS expands blood plasma volume, lowers adrenaline, improving symptoms & reducing standing heart rate (9–13 beats per minute) [14, 15].

Migraine is common in people with PoTS [16–19]. High salt intake has been associated with a reduction in migraines [16, 20]. In one study, orthostatic headache occurred during daily activity in 14 patients (58.3%) and during tilt table testing in 15 patients (62.5%). Age under 30 years and increasing duration of tilt were predictive of an orthostatic headache. Of the 24 patients in one study, 23 (95.8%) had non-orthostatic headache fitting the criteria of migraine or probable migraine [18].

Our recommendations to increase salt intake include carrying a salt shaker for the person with PoTS to enable salt addition at all meal times. Also consumption of foods high in salt which include canned soups, stock cubes, salted nuts, crisps, and canned beans with salt. A useful guide is to read food labels and use foods with a high salt intake. Others find it preferable to include salt or naturally salt containing vegetables such as celery, in smoothies/juices, which can be varied and include other ingredients to provide a longer lasting snack.

It is important to emphasize that some of the medications used to treat PoTS can only work effectively with an adequate salt and fluid intake. In clinical experience, many people are concerned about increasing salt in their diet. Therefore, a careful explanation is warranted as to why a high salt diet is recommended in people with PoTS (who have no contraindication). The discussion should emphasise that whilst there are important recommendations around lowering salt in the general population, these do not however apply to the person being counselled.

Diet

It is vital to take a detailed food and drink history, particularly at presentation. Many people with PoTS appear to have relative "thirstlessness" and need prompting to eat and drink. Keeping a food diary can be useful as can having prompts to eat and drink on mobile phone apps.

People with PoTS frequently report gastrointestinal symptoms [21] (see also chapter "Postural Tachycardia Syndrome and the Gut"). The splanchnic vascular bed receives up to 25% of the resting cardiac output in a healthy person. There is approximately a 300% increase in the mesenteric blood volume following a standard meal. In people with severe autonomic instability there is an observed severe post-prandial hypotension [21, 22]. One study in people with PoTS found an increase in resting mesenteric blood flow which could partly explain the worsening orthostatic tolerance following meals [23]. In this context, dietary modifications are recommended (see chapter "Postural Tachycardia Syndrome and the Gut". This includes reducing the size and increasing frequency of meals (for instance five small meals per day), whilst keeping refined carbohydrates, which can exacerbate post prandial hypotension, to a minimum. Foods high in fat and fibre tend to prolong gastric emptying and therefore it may be useful to reduce these in the diet [21]. One small study in people with severe post prandial hypotension (n = 7), found drinking 480mls of water rapidly before a meal improved orthostatic blood pressure 35 min following ingestion (systolic drop of 43 ± 36 mm Hg without pre meal water, compared to a systolic drop of 22 ± 10 mm Hg with drinking water pre meal) [2]. It is useful to try this with people who have postprandial symptoms. Raising legs and resting following a meal will also help.

Gluten Free Diet for Gluten Intolerance and Coeliac Disease

Coeliac disease is an immune mediated small bowel disease affecting 1% of the general population. Symptoms of coeliac disease include abdominal pain, bloating and diarrhoea. There has been an association with coeliac disease and general autonomic dysfunction, although this is not well understood [24]. People with PoTS experience a range of gastrointestinal symptoms including chronic nausea, vomiting, bloating, diarrhoea and/or constipation [21]. One study found 4% prevalence of coeliac disease in a PoTS cohort (4:100) compared to 1% prevalence in the general population (12/1200). This study found a higher prevalence of self-reported gluten sensitivity amongst people with PoTS (42% vs. 19%) [25]. It is therefore recommended to test for coeliac disease (total immunoglobulin (IgA) and IgA tissue transglutaminase antibody (tTG), and, if negative to consider screening for gluten sensitivity with Immunoglobulin G (IgG) EMA, IgG deamidated gliadin peptide (DGP) and IgG tTG, [21, 25].

Ideally a low FODMAP diet under a dietician's supervision is recommended. FODMAP stands for fermentable oligo-,di,mono-saccharides and polyols. These are the classifications for the groups of carbohydrates which are notorious for generating digestive symptoms such as bloating, gas and stomach pain, with a low FODMAP diet being associated with improved symptoms [26]. In a randomised controlled trial in people with coeliac disease there was a significant improvement in symptoms and psychological health in people who followed a FODMAP diet [27]. A low FODMAP diet includes vegetables, fresh fruits, lactose free dairy, hard cheeses, beef, pork, chicken, fish, eggs.

Flavonoids and Low Histamine Diet

"Brain fog" is a symptom described in various conditions, including people with PoTS [28]. There is evidence of an association with PoTS and mast cell activation disorder [29]. It has been proposed that natural flavonoids, specifically the flavone luteolin, may improve, and potentially be a treatment for "brain fog", particularly in people with possible mast cell disorder [28]. Flavonoids are found mostly in green plants and seeds, and luteolin in olive fruit extract (for example, olive oil). There may a benefit in increasing dietary flavonoids and following a low histamine diet.

Weight

Weight should be within normal ranges as a general principle of good health. There are specific issues for those with PoTS and care should be taken when assessing people with PoTS; severe gastric symptoms can result in difficulties maintaining a healthy weight. In these people there are specific gastrointestinal issues, including the need for a soft/liquid diet as, discussed in chapter "Postural Tachycardia Syndrome and the Gut".

Being overweight can impact on PoTS, and it is reasonable to recommend a healthy weight maintenance which could positively impact on PoTS symptoms. There are no PoTS specific studies into the effects of weight loss, however it is well recognized that there is an increased sympathetic drive in PoTS [30]. Sympathetic activation is augmented in overweight people and is associated with an inflammatory process [31]. Excessive weight has been found to contribute to sympathetic discharge in women and body weight reduction in women has been shown to reduce muscle sympathetic nerve activity [32]. There is one case report of PoTS improving following weight loss [33]. A study of obesity in polycystic ovary syndrome found those who were overweight (n = 64) had a higher rate of autonomic dysfunction reflected in a higher delta heart rate and higher plasma adrenalin than the healthy weight, control group (n = 40) [34]. Finally, excess body weight is associated with neuroinflammation and mast cells, potentially exacerbating "brain fog" [28]. Incidentally, dramatic weight reduction treatment with bariatric surgery is associated with post-surgery induced orthostatic intolerance, autonomic dysfunction and severe orthostatic hypotension [35, 36]. The emphasis should be on a healthy weight, achieving and maintaining this with a healthy lifestyle adapted around the PoTS person's specific needs.

Tips

When preparing food and planning a healthy balance with the above recommendations, people with PoTS may find the following tips helpful. These suggestions can help minimize fatigue and orthostatic intolerance associated with food preparation when maintaining a healthy diet.

- *Sit down whilst preparing food—a perch stool can help*
- *On a good day cook larger batches and freeze food*
- *Use energy saving devices (i.e: slow cookers/ electric chopper)*
- *Plan & Pace to minimize fatigue*
- *Stick to a routine*
- *Get someone else to do the washing up!*

Compression Garments

Finally, in addition to the fluid and diet strategy for lifestyle management of PoTS, compression hosiery has demonstrated efficacy in small studies. In the PoTS UK charity survey, 58% of PoTS respondents reported syncope [37]. Compression of the lower limbs has been shown to be "very effective" in rendering tilt table testing negative in people with vasovagal syncope (n = 20) [38]. Compression of the lower limbs causes an increased blood return from the superficial leg veins to the heart. Although there are no adult studies in PoTS and compression (published at time of writing), one study in adolescent PoTS patients (n = 20), found abdominal and extremity compression decreased orthostatic symptoms and tachycardia during repeat tilt table testing [39].

Research using an antigravity suit in a small number of patients with chronic symptomatic orthostatic hypotension (n = 14) demonstrated that compression of both lower abdomen and lower limbs was the most efficacious method to improve symptoms and BP levels [40]. Furthermore abdominal compression alone was superior to compression of both lower limbs (legs and thighs) in this study. In clinical practice however, although waist high lower limb compression hosiery is the best option, we mostly recommend full length grade II compression stockings due to the impracticalities of obtaining/using abdominal compression which can be difficult to put on or cause difficulty with overwarming of the lower body.

People often report compression stockings to be helpful, particularly if having to stand for long periods or on long days out. Compression stockings/tights are available on prescription, with the focus being on both full length and strong compression. The strength of the compression garment should be as follows; the European standard (RAL), class II provides recommended pressure (23–32 mmHg at the ankle); other standards include British standard (class 3—providing 25–35 mmHg), and French standard (class 3 21–36 mmHg). There are a variety of companies offering a wide range of fashionable compression tights/stockings, and sports recovery leggings can also be an option. Garments should be replaced every 3–6 months. Correct measurements need to be taken to ensure the right size and appliance aids are available to purchase to aid putting hosiery on. Detailed information regarding procurement of compression hosiery is available on the PoTS UK website (https://www.potsuk.org/compression_clothing).

Conclusion

PoTS encompasses a wide spectrum of cardiovascular symptoms and universally in clinical practice the cornerstone of lifestyle management is centred around a high daily fluid intake and increased consumption of salt. After this there are a number of other considerations to take into account, including compression hosiery. A detailed history of diet and fluid is important to ensure people are maintaining an appropriate diet and fluid intake. Everyone is different and what improves symptoms for one person may not help another person with PoTS. The above are therefore recommendations. Paying careful attention to lifestyle is essential to improving symptoms. This requires trial and error to help find specific triggers in individuals, and guide lifestyle management.

References

1. Raj SR, Biaggioni I, Yamhure PC, Black BK, Paranjape SY, Byrne DW, et al. Renin-aldosterone paradox and perturbed blood volume regulation underlying postural tachycardia syndrome. Circulation. 2005;111(13):1574–82.
2. Shannon JR, Diedrich A, Biaggioni I, Tank J, Robertson RM, Robertson D, et al. Water drinking as a treatment for orthostatic syndromes. Am J Med. 2002;112(5):355.
3. Sheldon RS, Grubb BP 2nd, Olshansky B, Shen WK, Calkins H, Brignole M, et al. 2015 Heart rhythm society expert consensus statement on the diagnosis and treatment of postural tachycardia syndrome, inappropriate sinus tachycardia, and vasovagal syncope. Heart Rhythm. 2015;12(6):e41-63.
4. Mathias CJ, Young TM. Water drinking in the management of orthostatic intolerance due to orthostatic hypotension, vasovagal syncope and the postural tachycardia syndrome. Eur J Neurol. 2004;11(9):613–9.
5. Ross AJ, Medow MS, Rowe PC, Stewart JM. What is brain fog? An evaluation of the symptom in postural tachycardia syndrome. Clin Autonom Res. 2013;23(6):305–11.
6. Gordon VM, Opfer-Gehrking TL, Novak V, Low PA. Hemodynamic and symptomatic effects of acute interventions on tilt in patients with postural tachycardia syndrome. Clin Autonom Res. 2000;10(1):29–33.
7. Jacob G, Shannon JR, Black B, Biaggioni I, Mosqueda-Garcia R, Robertson RM, et al. Effects of volume loading and pressor agents in idiopathic orthostatic tachycardia. Circulation. 1997;96(2):575–80.
8. Taneja I, Raj SR, Harris P, Byrne D, Jordan J, Robertson D. Autonomic effect of water ingestion in postural tachycardia syndrome. FASEB J. 2007;21(5):A512-A.
9. Z'Graggen WJ, Hess CW, Humm AM. Acute fluid ingestion in the treatment of orthostatic intolerance - important implications for daily practice. Eur J Neurol. 2010;17(11):1370–6.
10. Rodriguez B, Zimmermann R, Gutbrod K, Heinemann D, Z'Graggen WJ. Orthostatic cognitive dysfunction in postural tachycardia syndrome after rapid water drinking. Front Neurosci. 2019;13:327.
11. Jordan J. Effect of water drinking on sympathetic nervous activity and blood pressure. Curr Hypertens Rep. 2005;7(1):17–20.
12. Terlizzi R, Rocchi C, Serra M, Solieri L, Cortelli P. Reversible postural tachycardia syndrome due to inadvertent overuse of red bull. Clin Autonom Res. 2008;18(4):221–3.

13. Carter J, Stream S, Durocher J, Larson R. Influence of acute alcohol ingestion on sympathetic neural responses to rothostatic stress in humans. Am J Physiol ENdocrinol Metab. 2011;300(5):77108.
14. Celedonio J, Garland E, Nwazue V, Paranjape S, Black B, Okamoto L, et al. Effects of high sodium intake on blood volume and catecholamines in patients with postural tachycardia syndrome and healthy females. Clin Autonom Res. 2014;24(5):211. https://doi.org/10.1007/s10286-014-0251-0. Available at https://onlinelibrary.wiley.com/o/cochrane/clcentral/articles/869/CN-01099869/frame.html.
15. Nwazue V, Garland E, Black B, Okamoto L, Paranjape S, Shibao C. Differential effects of dietary salt on blood volume regulation in postural tachycardia syndrome and healthy subjects. Clin Autonom Res. 2013;23(5):269. https://doi.org/10.1007/s10286-013-0211-0. Available from: https://onlinelibrary.wiley.com/o/cochrane/clcentral/articles/903/CN-00999903/frame.html.
16. Greb E. Postural tachycardia syndrome is common among migraineurs. Neurol Rev. 2015;23(4):8.
17. Khurana RK. Syncope and headache. Curr Pain Headache Rep. 2018;22(8):54.
18. Khurana RK, Eisenberg L. Orthostatic and nonorthostatic headache in postural tachycardia syndrome. Cephalalgia. 2011;31(4):409–15.
19. Thijs RD, Kruit MC, van Buchem MA, Ferrari MD, Launer LJ, van Dijk JG. Syncope in migraine: the population-based camera study. Neurology. 2006;66(7):1034–7.
20. Blitshteyn S. Dietary sodium intake and migraine: is salt the answer? Headache J Head Face Pain. 2016;56(7):1210–1.
21. Mehr SE, Barbul A, Shibao CA. Gastrointestinal symptoms in postural tachycardia syndrome: a systematic review. Clin Autonom Res. 2018.
22. Seligman WH, Low DA, Asahina M, Mathias CJ. Abnormal gastric myoelectrical activity in postural tachycardia syndrome. Clin Autonom Res. 2013;23(2):73–80.
23. Tani H, Singer W, McPhee BR, Opfer-Gehrking TL, Haruma K, Kajiyama G, et al. Splanchnic-mesenteric capacitance bed in the postural tachycardia syndrome (POTS). Autonom Neurosci. 2000;86(1–2):107–13.
24. Gibbons CH, Freeman R. Autonomic neuropathy and coeliac disease. J Neurol Neurosurg Psychiat. 2005;76:579–81.
25. Penny HA, Aziz I, Ferrar M, Atkinson J, Hoggard N, Hadjivassiliou M, et al. Is there a relationship between gluten sensitivity and postural tachycardia syndrome? Eur J Gastroenterol Hepatol. 2016;28(12):1383–7.
26. Dieterich W, Schuppan D, Schink M, Schwappacher R, Wirtz S, Agaimy A, et al. Influence of low FODMAP and gluten-free diets on disease activity and intestinal microbiota in patients with non-celiac gluten sensitivity. Clin Nutr. 2018.
27. Roncoroni L, Bascunan KA, Doneda L, Scricciolo A, Lombardo V, Branchi F, et al. A low FODMAP gluten-free diet improves functional gastrointestinal disorders and overall mental health of celiac disease patients: a randomized controlled trial. Nutrients. 2018;10(8).
28. Theoharides TC, Stewart JM, Hatziagelaki E, Kolaitis G. Brain, "fog," inflammation and obesity: key aspects of neuropsychiatric disorders improved by luteolin. Front Neurosci. 2015;9:225.
29. Doherty T, White A. Postural orthostatic tachycardia syndrome and the potential role of mast cell activation. Autonom Neurosci. 2018.
30. Lambert E, Lambert GW. Sympathetic dysfunction in vasovagal syncope and the postural orthostatic tachycardia syndrome. Front Physiol. 2014;5:280.
31. Okamoto LE, Raj SR, Gamboa A, Shibao CA, Arnold AC, Garland EM, et al. Sympathetic activation is associated with increased IL-6, but not CRP in the absence of obesity: lessons from postural tachycardia syndrome and obesity. Am J Physiol Heart Circul Physiol. 2015;309(12):H2098–107.
32. Fu Q. Microneurographic research in women. Front Physiol. 2012;3:278.
33. Sullivan D. Losing weight saved our lives. Woman's Day. 2011;74(9):114–8.
34. Hashim ZH, Hamdan FB, Al-Salihi AR. Autonomic dysfunction in women with polycystic ovary syndrome. Iran J Reproduct Med. 2015;13(1):27–34.
35. Romen R, Ciubotaru M, Hadar E, Bitterman H. Severe orthostatic hypotension following weight reduction surgery. Arch Intern Med. 2001;161(17):2145–7.
36. Ponnusamy V, Owens AP, Purkayastha S, Iodice V, Mathias CJ. Orthostatic intolerance and autonomic dysfunction following bariatric surgery: a retrospective study and review of the literature. Autonom Neurosci Basic Clin. 2016;198:1–7.
37. Kavi L. A profile of patients with postural tachycardia syndrome and their experience of healthcare in the UK. Br J Cardiol. 2016.
38. Dos Santos RQ, Smidt L, Suzigan BH, De Souza LV, Barbisan JN. Efficacy of lower limb compression in the management of vasovagal syncope–randomized, crossover study. Pacing Clin Electrophysiol. 2013;36(4):451–5.
39. Heyer GL. Abdominal and lower-extremity compression decreases symptoms of postural tachycardia syndrome in youth during tilt table testing. J Pediatr. 2014;165(2):395–7.
40. Denq JC, Opfer-Gehrking TL, Giuliani M, Felten J, Convertino VA, Low PA. Efficacy of compression of different capacitance beds in the amelioration of orthostatic hypotension. Clin Auton Res. 1997;7(6):321–6.

Exercise Guidelines for Postural Tachycardia Syndrome

I. De Wandele, D. Low, P. Rowe and J. V. Simmonds

Introduction

The Postural Tachycardia Syndrome (PoTS, in which patients are unable to stand or remain upright for prolonged periods of time due to intolerable palpitations, dizziness, or near-syncope) is a major form of chronic orthostatic intolerance in young people, with few definitive therapies [1]. The underlying pathophysiology is not well understood, but recent research has suggested that physical deconditioning and reduced standing stroke volume may be important to the pathogenesis of PoTS and the severity of its disability [2–8].

Treatment of PoTS is challenging; and achieving a tangible effect on symptoms requires a treatment approach on multiple levels which may include: (1) revision of the current medication, (2) education regarding underlying mechanisms of PoTS and the possible non-pharmacological measures, (3) physical training, and (4) pharmacological treatment. This paper reviews the recent literature and discusses the rationale and approach to designing and implementing exercise rehabilitation programmes.

PoTS and Deconditioning

In the current literature, orthostatic intolerance, and PoTS in specific, have been related to deconditioning [3, 8, 9]. However, no consensus yet exists on the exact nature of this relationship. Some authors label deconditioning as the cause of PoTS [6] and believe that it may be cured with reconditioning alone [3, 4]. The combination of a small heart and reduced blood volume, both of which are signs typically seen in deconditioning, lead to a reduced stroke volume and are therefore regarded as the primary abnormalities underlying PoTS [3, 7]. By contrast, others believe that deconditioning is not the primary

I. De Wandele
Center for Medical Genetics, Ghent University Hospital, Ghent, Belgium

D. Low
School of Sport and Exercise Sciences, Liverpool John Moores University, Coventry, UK

P. Rowe
Johns Hopkins Pediatrics, Baltimore, USA

J. V. Simmonds (✉)
Great Ormond Institute of Child Health, University College London, London, UK
e-mail: Jane.simmonds@ucl.ac.uk

J. V. Simmonds
University College London Hospital, London, UK

J. V. Simmonds
The London Hypermobility Unit, Wellington Hospital, London, UK

N. Gall et al. (eds.), *Postural Tachycardia Syndrome*, https://doi.org/10.1007/978-3-030-54165-1_26

cause of PoTS, but rather a secondary factor that contributes to PoTS. Furthermore, recent studies suggest that deconditioning may even be a consequence of PoTS, as the reduced stroke volume seen in patients with PoTS has been related to exercise intolerance [7, 10]. Patients report malaise during exercise [7, 10] and are therefore unable to adhere to conventional exercise programs. These authors report that the reduced stroke volume seen in PoTS is caused by an insufficient preload of the heart, very probably due to peripheral blood pooling [7, 10–12], a phenomenon that can exist without relation to deconditioning.

Regardless of the nature of the relationship—cause or consequence—deconditioning is thought to negatively influence cardiovascular function [13, 14, 15, 16]. The long-term beneficial effects of increased physical fitness that are thought to counteract orthostatic intolerance consist of a larger blood volume, a larger heart and cardiac output, enhanced vascular compression by increased muscle tissue, improved endothelial function, and possibly also improved baroreflex function [17–19]. The research group of Fu et al. showed that moderate gradual endurance and strength training can increase orthostatic tolerance in PoTS, decrease upright heart rate, improve baroreflex sensitivity and heart rate variability, and improve quality of life. After the 3-month training program the majority of the patients included in their study no longer fulfilled the criteria for PoTS [3, 5, 20]. Consequently, exercise training can be regarded as a type of non-pharmacological therapy, with several advantages over pharmacological treatment. Firstly, most of the currently available pharmacological options for treating PoTS are only moderately effective. Secondly, it can take substantial trial and error before the most efficacious treatment is found. And finally, side effects, such as fatigue (betablockers), the development of hypertension (alpha-adrenergic agonists), or hypokalaemia (fludrocortisone), are often cited as the main reason for cessation of pharmacological treatment [5]. Exercise training offers the possibility to enlarge the heart and expand blood volume, while improving baroreflex sensitivity and increasing peak oxygen uptake [3, 5, 20], without any of the side effects of pharmacological treatment.

Clinicians however need to be aware that some individuals cannot tolerate or benefit from exercise until after they have achieved better medication control of their PoTS. As a result, we regard it as improper and punitive to insist that patients always prove they have been adherent to an exercise regimen before medications are introduced. As an example, one young adult had a heart rate in the 104–140 bpm range at rest. When she would attempt exercise, as she often did in an attempt to improve her function, she developed a prompt and marked tachycardic response. Within 2–3 min of initiating treadmill exercise, her heart rate would increase to 180 bpm, and this would provoke a migraine headache that would then last two days. She was prescribed ivabradine, which was associated with the following improvements in HR and exercise tolerance with each dose increase (See Table 1).

Other medications have had similar effects on the ability to tolerate exercise in other patients, and we do not intend to suggest that this

Table 1 Case example of exercise tolerance with Ivabradine

Ivabradine dose	Resting heart rate	Exercise heart rate
0 mg	115	170–180 in 2 mins, w/HA
2.5 mg BID	110	170–180 in 2 mins, w/HA
5 mg BID	90	155, no HA
7.5 mg BID	80	140, no HA
10 mg MID	72	130 with 3–40 minutes on elliptical trainer; no HA

Key BID—Bi daily dose, HA—Headache

response is specific to ivabradine. This example emphasizes the importance of an individualized mix of exercise and medication management, not a rigid adherence to an "exercise first" philosophy.

Exercise Training Guidelines for PoTS

The information below is based on clinical experience and evidence in several overlapping pathologies, such as hypermobility spectrum disorders, Ehlers Danlos syndrome, fibromyalgia, chronic fatigue syndrome, and overtraining. These guidelines are meant as a starting point for clinicians in setting up a training program, and to guide future research.

When prescribing exercise, clinicians should be aware that physical activity is a demanding task for the circulatory system, which is already functioning at its upper limit in patients with orthostatic intolerance. In this population, a restricted tolerance for exercise is prevalent, with reports of post-exertional malaise and symptom aggravation due to exercise [10]. Each acute bout of exercise induces cardiovascular and respiratory changes that affect the regulation of systemic and cerebral blood flow and persist for some time after the activity has ended [21]. After exercise, there is a sustained reduction in blood pressure, the magnitude of which is dependent on the previously recruited muscle mass [22] and the exercise intensity [23]. In addition, the hyperventilatory response during moderate-higher intensity exercise can cause hypocapnia, which leads to vasoconstriction of the cerebral vasculature [24], possibly contributing to symptoms of cerebral hypoperfusion. Adherence to exercise programs is often low in PoTS, because patients perceive physical activity as adversely affecting their condition in the short term. The training program should therefore aim to improve physical fitness, while avoiding excessive stress on the circulatory system. Several aspects of training should be adapted when orthostatic intolerance is present, including the exercise modality (aerobic/resistance training), type of exercise (isometric/dynamic), body position (supine or upright), intensity and frequency, and active muscle mass.

Setting up the Exercise Program

Research regarding exercise in PoTS is still scarce. The reconditioning program developed by the research group of Fu and George et al. could be used as a basis, as it has been studied both in small and large patient populations with PoTS and has yielded beneficial results [3, 5, 20]. Exercise training in orthostatic intolerance is focused on improving aerobic fitness, as well as strengthening the lower limbs to improve the 'muscle pump' function [20, 9]. It should start with exercise that imposes a mild stress on the cardiovascular system, and progress very gradually to more circulatory challenging physical activities. Developing shared realistic goals with patients is an important starting point and these can be reviewed on a regular basis as a form of outcome measure and to help with motivation.

This can be done by taking the following aspects into account:

Exercise modality: In general, aerobic activities with a local resistive component for the lower limbs are preferred, such as reclined cycling, swimming and rowing. This type of activity constitutes the largest part of the training program [5, 20]. Resistance training can be added to the program, but therapists should be aware that this type of training tends to be more demanding for the circulatory system [25]. Strength training elicits larger blood pressure changes than aerobic exercise, in part because generating large forces with the limbs requires stabilization by the trunk muscles [26]. This often causes a Valsalva manoeuvre, that first increases intrathoracic pressure and is followed by a drop in systemic blood pressure. Correction requires sympathetic activation to create sufficient peripheral vasoconstriction [27]. Fu and George and their colleagues advise to exercise 3–4 times per week, of which initially only one training session includes some resistance exercises. This can gradually be increased to two resistance sessions per week [3, 20].

Type of exercise: Dynamic exercise may be better tolerated than isometric exercise, because the latter is thought to constitute a larger circulatory stressor. A sustained muscle contraction causes larger increases in heart rate, systolic and diastolic blood pressure [28]. Even when performing strengthening exercises dynamically, it is advised to breathe out during the generation of force and breathe in during the returning motion to avoid Valsalva maneuvers.

Position: Recent studies demonstrate that patients with PoTS respond to exercise with an insufficient increase in stroke volume [7, 10], which can lead to symptoms of circulatory distress (dyspnea, feeling faint, lightheadedness, weakness). Therefore, exercising in the horizontal position (e.g. rowing, reclined cycling, swimming, supine leg press) is preferred in the first stages of training [3, 20, 9] (See Figs. 1 and 2). Supine activity is better tolerated than upright activity, because a recumbent position increases cardiac filling, since venous return is facilitated when gravity is excluded. Fu and George et al. advise to only add upright activities by the end of the second or beginning of the third month of the training program [3, 20]. The upright position is significantly more stressful for the sympathetic nervous system, because active vasoconstriction is required to compensate for the gravity induced downward displacement of blood.

Intensity and frequency: Choosing a training load in balance with the individual's cardiovascular capacity is a challenging task. Individualized training and progress is vital. Fu and George et al suggest performing a submaximal exercise test [3, 20], such as the Astrand-Saltin incremental treadmill protocol, to estimate the patient's maximum heart rate. However, upright treadmill tests may not be possible in clinical settings. In these cases other submaximal tests can be considered, such as the incremental shuttle walk test [29] or cycle ergometry [30], although these tests have not yet been validated in this patient population. Pragmatically using 220—age to estimate maximum heart rate is recommended [31]. For patients using medication that controls heart rate, including β-blocking agents or ivabradine, the Borg scale for the rating of perceived exertion (RPE) can be used to estimate exercise intensity during the training sessions, since heart rate is not a valid parameter in this group.

Table 2 provides an overview of the training intensity in the program by George et al. [20]. In this example the majority of the training

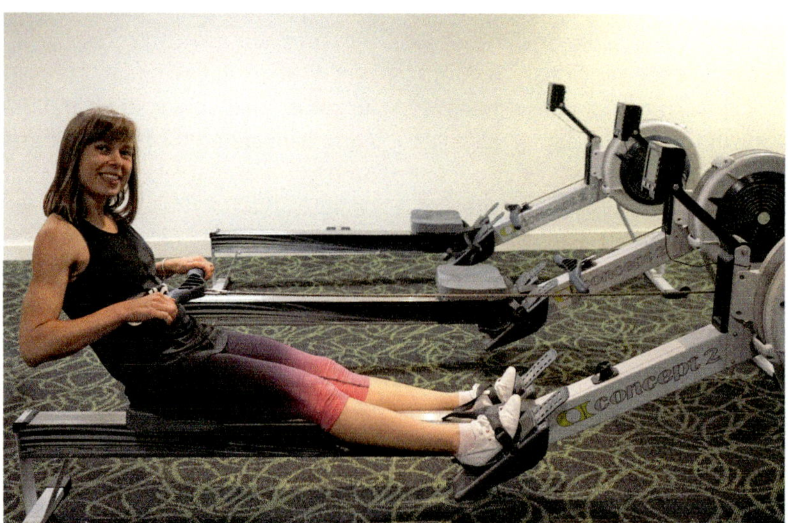

Fig. 1 Rowing is a good example of a recumbent cardiovascular exercise. Care should be taken with posture to avoid hinging on the lumbar spine and flicking into hyperextension of the knee if hypermobile

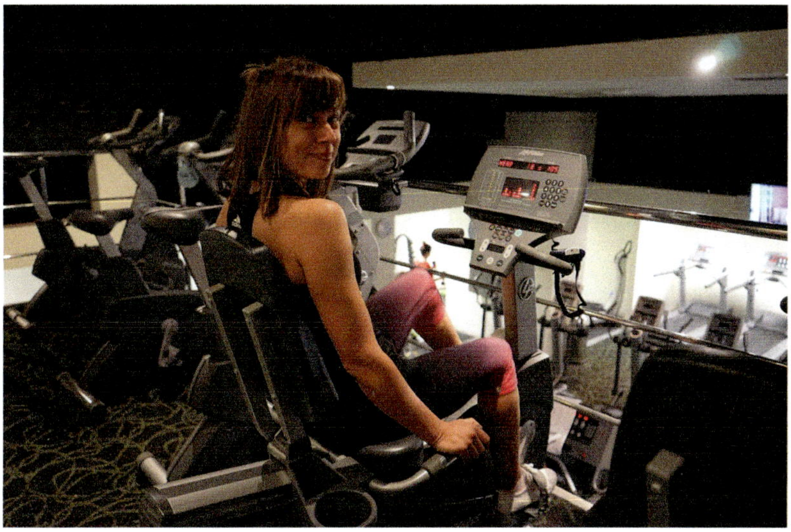

Fig. 2 Recumbent cycling can also be used as a cardiovascular exercise. Ideally knees high to assist blood flow to the heart

Table 2 Example of a 3 month exercise program for PoTS [20] adapted from George et al.

Training type	Month 1	Month 2	Month 3
Base pace (RPE 13–15)	2–3 × 30 min per week	2–3 × 30 min per week	1 × 35 min per week
Max steady state (RPE 16–18)	1 × 20 min per week	1 × 25 min per week	2–3 × 30 min per week
Recovery (RPE 6–12)	1 × 30–40 min per week	1 × 40 min per week	2 × 40 min per week
Resistance training	1 × 15–20 min per week	2 × 2–25 min	2 × 30 min
Cardiovascular modes	Recumbent bike Swimming Rowing	The modes of month 1 + upright cycling	The modes of month 1 and 2 + elliptical and treadmill walking

sessions during the first are considered 'base pace sessions', with a target heart rate of 75% of the estimated maximal heart rate (RPE: 13–15), for 30–40 min per session [3, 20]. These are alternated with 'recovery sessions' below the anaerobic threshold (RPE: 6–12) and a few 'maximal steady state' sessions (RPE: 16–18). For very disabled patients these authors advise to use the same training intensities, but suggest shortening the durations of the sessions. Over the course of three months, the training frequency is increased from 3–4 times per week to 5–6 times per week.

Of note, where patients with PoTS have Hypermobility Spectrum Disorder or Hypermobile Ehlers-Danlos Syndrome, which may augment pain and fatigue exercise, training protocols need to be adapted for individuals with fragile tissues and additional issues of pain and fatigue [32]. The overall rehabilitation timeframe and recovery from exercise is likely to be protracted due to complexity and multi-system involvement. For these patients, aerobic exercise may start with as little as 1–5 min of recumbent exercise at an RPE of 6–12 twice per day on a daily basis, increasing by 10–20% each week (clinical expert opinion). Low impact exercise modes (cycling, leg press, aquatic therapy, etc.) are better suited than exercise that involves a high impact component on the joints of the lower limbs (e.g. running); and exercise that causes joint approximation is preferred over distraction (e.g. rowing may not be tolerated by some patients due to shoulder laxity).

Physiotherapy treatment to address joint stability, muscle strength and motor control will need to be incorporated into the prescription, this often entails closed chain exercises (See Figs. 3 and 4). Once 30 min of low intensity exercise is achieved per day the intensity can be increased to the recommended 13–15 RPE and patients may embark on the prescription recommended by George et al. [20].

Active muscle mass: The larger the active muscle mass, the larger the effort imposed on the circulatory system to counteract the vasodilation in working muscles [22]. Clinical experience demonstrates that most patients with PoTS

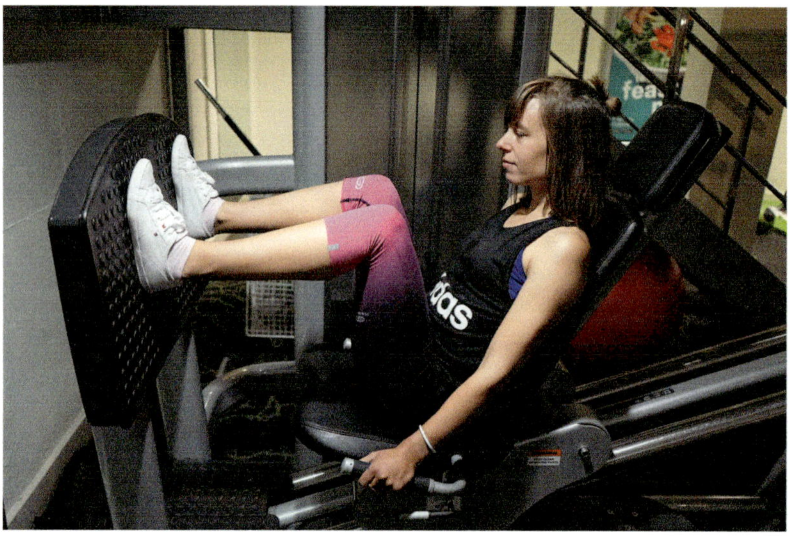

Fig. 3 Leg press is an example of a closed chain exercise to strengthen quadriceps and gluteal muscles. Positioning the knees high, will aid venous return

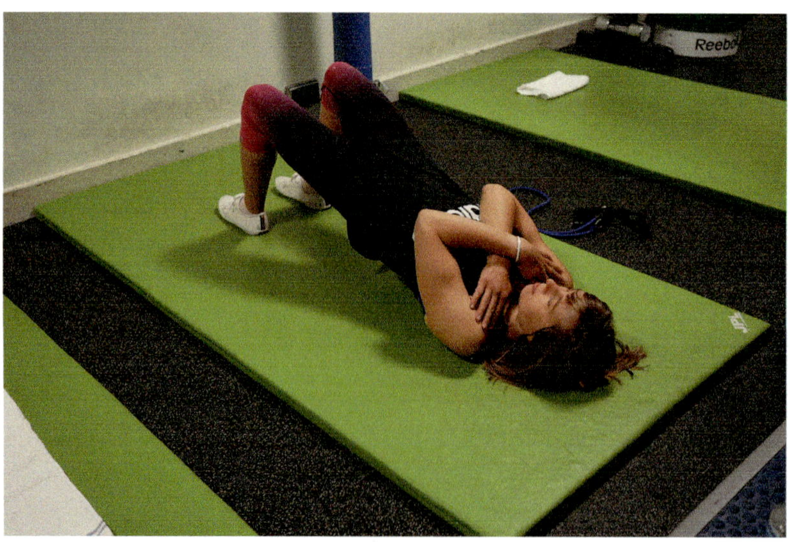

Fig. 4 Bridging is another example of a closed chain exercise for improving gluteal and trunk strength and motor control

tolerate using large muscle groups, for instance for swimming, rowing and cycling, when the activity is performed in a recumbent position. In severely disabled patients who even report symptom aggravation after supine training, exercises that target single muscles can be used as a starting point for training (e.g. calf muscles only, or quadriceps only). The goal is to progress to whole-body exercises.

Peripheral blood pooling: Additional measures that reduce pooling can be used during training. Examples are wearing compressive stockings or an abdominal band during the exercise sessions, or exercising in water [33]. Hydrotherapy is often well tolerated, because of the shift in blood volume from the periphery to the thoracic/abdominal cavity, as a result of the increased hydrostatic pressure. The water temperature is of importance: water that is too warm is anecdotally reported to provoke malaise in patients with orthostatic intolerance due to the increased likelihood of heat stress adding to peripheral blood pooling.

Additional Tips

Prior to a training session, patients are advised to drink about two glasses of water, preferably with a tablet of water-solvable electrolytes or an isotonic sports drink. The pressor response to fluid ingestion can elevate the blood pressure acutely and helps prevent hypotension during and after exercise [34]. Furthermore, patients are instructed to avoid exercising within one hour of the previous meal, since vasodilatation in the gastrointestinal tract lowers the capacity of the circulatory system to cope with another stressor. Patients taking vasoconstrictive medicines, such as midodrine, could take an extra dose about 15 to 20 min prior to exercising, or immediately after, depending on what they perceive as most helpful to prevent symptoms. Oldham et al. suggest that for some patients with PoTS vasoconstrictors may even have a larger effect than volume loading [10].

During a training session, we advise to measure blood pressure and heart rate before, repeatedly during, and after exercise, especially in patients who use medication that affects the cardiovascular system. In addition to being a safety measure, comparison of the heart rate responses to submaximal efforts at different times during the training program can yield an understanding of the patient's progress. Furthermore, during training, sufficient intake of water and electrolytes is important to prevent disturbance of the electrolyte/fluid balance due to sweating. Measurements of body mass before and after each session can provide an index of sweat loss via the reduction in body mass and therefore appropriate amounts of fluids to consume. Avoid exercising in warm environments.

After a training session, a low-intensity cyclical cooling-down activity may prevent a sudden blood pressure drop. For example, low-intensity cycling causes repeated contraction and relaxation of large muscle groups in the lower limbs. This engages the muscle pump and increases venous return without stressing the cardiovascular system excessively. Patients are advised to avoid prolonged standing immediately after a training session, because during the first 5–10 min after exercise the muscle pump is no longer active while vasodilatation is still present in the exercised muscles [35]. Other options are using the pressor effect of water ingestion and wearing compression garments after the bout of exercise [35]. Resting in a supine or seated position with the knees higher than the hips can be advised. This position leads to a passive shift of blood volume towards the center of the body and increases stroke volume, decreasing the demands on the circulatory system.

Finally, to optimize the capacity of the cardiovascular system to cope with circulatory stressors, several non-pharmacological **daily life measures** can be of some benefit. For instance, sleeping with the head of the bed elevated by 4–6 inches, progressively increasing salt intake to 10–12 g per day, and fluid intake to 2 Litres per day can help increase plasma volume [36, 9]. Patients also often benefit from doing simple circulatory exercises in the morning to help move blood from the periphery. For example, heel raises (graduating to about 3 0 repetitions), triceps curls (graduating to about 30 repetitions with a light weight 1–2 kg) and squats or wall slides (graduating to about 15 repetitions) can be performed to reduce peripheral blood pooling.

Return to Work and Maintenance

Where individuals have been off work due to PoTS, a graduated return to school, University or work is recommended. Exercise will be best incorporated into daily routines. This may involve walking or cycling as part of a daily commute and/or undertaking physical activity in the lunchtime. If work is primarily sedentary, it will be important to get up from the desk and move each 30 minutes to prevent peripheral venous pooling. The aim for exercise training/physical activity for PoTS after return to work are in line with the national physical activity guidelines (NHS choices) [37] and not dissimilar from the recommendations of Month 3 of [20], see Table 1; 30–40 minutes of moderate exercise five days a week. This should include two sessions per week of resistance training.

References

1. Schondorf R, Low PA. diopathic postural orthostatic tachycardia syndrome: An attenuated form of acute pandysautonomia? Neurology. 1993;43 (Part 1):132. https://doi.org/10.1212/WNL.43.1_Part_1.132.
2. Benarroch EE. Postural tachycardia syndrome: a heterogeneous and multifactorial disorder. Mayo Clin Proc. 2012;87:1214–25.
3. Fu Q, Vangundy TB, Galbreath MM, Shibata S, Jain M, Hastings JL, Bhella PS, Levine BD. Cardiac origins of the postural orthostatic tachycardia syndrome. J Am Coll Cardiol. 2010;55:2858–68.
4. Fu Q, Vangundy TB, Shibata S, Auchus RJ, Williams GH, Levine BD. Exercise training versus propranolol in the treatment of the postural orthostatic tachycardia syndrome. Hypertension. 2011;58:167–75.
5. Galbreath MM, Shibata S, Vangundy TB, Okazaki K, Fu Q, Levine BD. Effects of exercise training on arterial-cardiac baroreflex function in PoTS. Clin Auton Res. 2011;21:73–80.
6. Joyner MJ, Masuki S. PoTS versus deconditioning: the same or different? Clin Auton Res. 2008;18:300–7.
7. Masuki S, Eisenach JH, Schrage WG, Johnson CP, Dietz NM, Wilkins BW, Sandroni P, Low PA, Joyner MJ. Reduced stroke volume during exercise in postural tachycardia syndrome. J Appl Physiol. 2007;1985(103):1128–35.
8. Parsaik A, Allison TG, Singer W, Sletten DM, Joyner MJ, Benarroch EE, Low PA, Sandroni P. Deconditioning in patients with orthostatic intolerance. Neurology. 2012;79:1435–9.
9. Sheldon RS, Grubb BP, 2nd, Olshansky B, Shen WK, Calkins H, Brignole M, Raj SR, Krahn AD, Morillo CA, Stewart JM, Sutton R, Sandroni P, Friday KJ, Hachul DT, Cohen MI, Lau DH, Mayuga KA, Moak JP, Sandhu RK, Kanjwal K. 2015 heart rhythm society expert consensus statement on the diagnosis and treatment of postural tachycardia syndrome, inappropriate sinus tachycardia, and vasovagal syncope. Heart Rhythm. 1. 2015;2:e41–63.
10. Oldham WM, Lewis GD, Opotowsky AR, Waxman AB, Systrom DM. Unexplained exertional dyspnea caused by low ventricular filling pressures: results from clinical invasive cardiopulmonary exercise testing. Pulm Circ. 2016;6:55–62.
11. Stewart JM, Montgomery LD. Regional blood volume and peripheral blood flow in postural tachycardia syndrome. Am J Physiol Heart Circ Physiol. 2004;287:H1319–27.
12. Streeten DH, Anderson GH, Jr, Richardson R, Thomas FD. Abnormal orthostatic changes in blood pressure and heart rate in subjects with intact sympathetic nervous function: evidence for excessive venous pooling. J Lab Clin Med. 1988;111:326–35.
13. Coupe M, Fortrat JO, Larina I, Gauquelin-Koch G, Gharib C, Custaud MA. Cardiovascular deconditioning: from autonomic nervous system to microvascular dysfunctions. Respir Physiol Neurobiol. 2009;169(Suppl 1):S10–2.
14. Hughson RL, Shoemaker JK. Autonomic responses to exercise: deconditioning/inactivity. Auton Neurosci. 2015;188:32–5.
15. Levine BD, Pawelczyk JA, Ertl AC, Cox JF, Zuckerman JH, Diedrich A, Biaggioni I, Ray CA, Smith ML, Iwase S, Saito M, Sugiyama Y, Mano T, Zhang R, Iwasaki K, Lane LD, Buckey JC, Jr, Cooke WH, Baisch FJ, Eckberg DL, Blomqvist CG. Human muscle sympathetic neural and haemodynamic responses to tilt following spaceflight. J Physiol. 2002;538:331–40.
16. Levine BD, Zuckerman JH, Pawelczyk JA. Cardiac atrophy after bed-rest deconditioning: a nonneural mechanism for orthostatic intolerance. Circulation. 1997;96:517–25.
17. Brilla LR, Stephens AB, Knutzen KM, Caine D. Effect of strength training on orthostatic hypotension in older adults. J Cardiopulm Rehabil. 1998;18:295–300.
18. Dorfman TA, Levine BD, Tillery T, Peshock RM, Hastings JL, Schneider SM, Macias BR, Biolo G,

Hargens AR. Cardiac atrophy in women following bed rest. J Appl Physiol. 2007;1985(103):8–16.
19. Mtinangi BL, Hainsworth R. Increased orthostatic tolerance following moderate exercise training in patients with unexplained syncope. Heart. 1998;80:596–600.
20. George SA, Bivens TB, Howden EJ, Saleem Y, Galbreath MM, Hendrickson D, Fu Q, Levine BD. The international PoTS registry: evaluating the efficacy of an exercise training intervention in a community setting. Heart Rhythm. 2016;13:943–50.
21. Mundel T, Perry BG, Ainslie PN, Thomas KN, Sikken EL, Cotter JD, Lucas SJ. Postexercise orthostatic intolerance: influence of exercise intensity. Exp Physiol. 2015;100:915–25.
22. Macdonald JR, Macdougall JD, Hogben CD. The effects of exercising muscle mass on post exercise hypotension. J Hum Hypertens. 2000;14:317–20.
23. Halliwill JR, Buck TM, Lacewell AN, Romero SA. Postexercise hypotension and sustained postexercise vasodilatation: what happens after we exercise? Exp Physiol. 2013;98:7–18.
24. Ogoh S, Ainslie PN. Cerebral blood flow during exercise: mechanisms of regulation. J Appl Physiol. 2009;1985(107):1370–80.
25. Gotshall RW, Gootman J, Byrnes WC, Fleck SJ, Valocivch TC. Noninvasive characterization of the blood pressure response to the double-leg press exercise. J Exer Physiol. 1999;2.
26. Macdonald JR. Potential causes, mechanisms, and implications of post exercise hypotension. J Hum Hypertens. 2002;16:225–36.
27. Pstras L, Thomaseth K, Waniewski J, Balzani I, Bellavere F. The Valsalva manoeuvre: physiology and clinical examples. Acta Physiol (Oxf). 2016;217:103–19.
28. Arimoto M, Kijima A, Muramatsu S. Cardiorespiratory response to dynamic and static leg press exercise in humans. J Physiol Anthropol Appl Human Sci. 2005;24:277–83.
29. Singh SJ, Morgan MD, Hardman AE, Rowe C, Bardsley PA. Comparison of oxygen uptake during a conventional treadmill test and the shuttle walking test in chronic airflow limitation. Eur Respir J. 1994;7:2016–20.
30. Friden C, Jansson E, Osterlund T, Grooten WJ, Opava CH, Rickenlund A. Criterion validity of the submaximal astrand bicycle test to estimate aerobic capacity in people with rheumatoid arthritis. Ann Rheum Dis. 2014;73:1200.
31. American Heart Association. Target heart rates. American Heart Association. 2015. Available at https://www.heart.org/HEARTORG/HealthyLiving/PhysicalActivity/FitnessBasics/Target-Heart-Rates_UCM_434341_Article.jsp#.V43z2pOLQxF. Accessed 16 July 2016.
32. Engelbert RHH, Juul-Kristensen B, Pacey V, De Wandele I, Smeenk S, Woinarosky N, Sabo S, Russek L, Scheper MC, Simmonds J. International physical therapy management guidelines for children, adolescents and adults diagnosed with Joint Hypermobility Syndrome/Ehlers-Danlos Syndrome—hypermobility type. 2017.
33. Loiola Souto A, Moreira Lima L, Aparecida Castro E, Peixoto Veras R, Segheto W, Camargos Zanatta T, Aparecida Doimo L. Blood pressure in hypertensive women after aerobics and hydrogymnastics sessions. Nutr Hosp. 2015;32:823–8.
34. May M, Jordan J. The osmopressor response to water drinking. Am J Physiol Regul Integr Comp Physiol. 2011;300:R40–6.
35. Halliwill JR, Sieck DC, Romero SA, Buck TM, Ely MR. Blood pressure regulation X: what happens when the muscle pump is lost? Post-exercise hypotension and syncope. Eur J Appl Physiol. 2014;114:561–78.
36. Figueroa JJ, Basford JR, Low PA. Preventing and treating orthostatic hypotension: as easy as A, B, C. Cleve Clin J Med. 2010;77:298–306.
37. NHS CHOICES. Physical activity for adults 18–64 years. https://www.nhs.uk/Livewell/fitness/Pages/physical-activity-guidelines-for-adults.aspx. Accessed July 2016.

Medication in PoTS: An Overview

Nicholas Gall

The next section of this book will deal with the use of medications in PoTS. As is clear from many of the other chapters and indeed the review articles in the literature, while the diagnosis of PoTS is very much focused on a heart rate increase, there do seem to be more widespread abnormalities in cardiovascular and respiratory control but also symptoms in other territories. Any therapeutic approach, therefore, will rely on excluding other underlying conditions, treating individual systemic symptoms and should be particularly focused on the non-pharmacological therapies of increased fluid and salt intake, compression clothing and exercise. In many cases, however, the non-pharmacological approach may be insufficient to provide benefit and indeed in some cases, symptoms may be so significant that medications are required to allow patients to function, at least to some extent and may even be required to allow them to feel that they can exercise. While there are guidelines in the literature [1] and indeed there is now guidance from the Canadian Cardiac Society [2], there is no clear consensus about which medications to use and when. In addition, as is detailed in the individual drug chapters to come, while there is some evidence of potential benefit in individual patients and while there are small studies using a number of the medications, there are no major trials undertaken to prove benefit in the longer term. In general, the medications we use are not licensed in the UK nor abroad in the US amongst others and therefore it is important to emphasise to the patient that medications are used off-label although that is an acceptable approach in certain circumstances, as detailed by the GMC [3].

In general, patients are young and more often female and there will be less concern that renal excretion or liver metabolism will significantly affect the doses provided however, an assessment of biochemistry is clearly always appropriate. We recommend a blood test undertaken on a yearly basis for that purpose although that is purely arbitrary. As the pathophysiology of PoTS is uncertain and is potentially different in different individuals, it is therefore not unsurprising that different patients react to different medications in different ways. In addition, allergic responses may make some medications poorly tolerated and indeed in a small number of cases lactose in the medication may not be tolerated.

As many of the patients are female and of reproductive age, it is also important to bear in mind the potential for pregnancy and as detailed in chapter 'Pregnancy and Postural Tachycardia Syndrome'

N. Gall (✉)
Department of Cardiology, King's College Hospital, London SE5 9RS, UK
e-mail: nickgall@doctors.org.uk

N. Gall et al. (eds.), *Postural Tachycardia Syndrome*, https://doi.org/10.1007/978-3-030-54165-1_27

of this textbook, while some of the medications are known to be safe, others are not known and therefore should be avoided in that circumstance.

The abnormalities in physiology appear to relate to a combination of an inappropriately fast heart rate, sometimes low and particularly variable BP and abnormalities in blood volume control, the medications used often have actions to affect those individual pathophysiologies. There is no clear guidance as to which medications to use in what order, but a logical approach would be to prescribe medications to affect one of those abnormalities, slowly and gradually increasing the dose to provide efficacy. Alternative drugs providing the same benefit, for instance ivabradine and beta-blockers could be either added together to provide additional benefit or used alternatively if one is not tolerated. Doses should be slowly and gradually increased according to patient's symptoms with some regard to haemodynamic variables such as heart rate or blood pressure but in general the smallest dose of medication should be used to provide therapeutic benefit in each case. If benefit is found with one particular medication but more benefit is required, it may be worth considering prescribing an additional medication, taking note of drug-drug interactions, with effects on a different aspect of the pathophysiology. Polypharmacy is always a particular danger in complex areas of medicine and while there are some interactions, many of the commonly used are prescribed altogether. It is always important to ensure that, not only are medications started to improve symptoms but medications which provide no benefit should be stopped. Patient's symptoms often wax and wane according to other associated illnesses, with the menstrual cycle and with the weather, particularly in the summer and therefore whether a particular medication provides benefit may need to be assessed in the longer term; however all of the medications used do tend to produce rapid changes in physiology and therefore prolonged treatment awaiting benefit is not required. It is clearly important to emphasise that the non-pharmacological approaches remain paramount and it may well be that without that bedrock, medications may provide little support.

Many of the review articles in the field provide lists of medications which can be used [4–6] and, as will be defined in individual chapters, much of the evidence may be relatively limited. Not every physician will have experience with every medication and at times, particularly with the injectable medications, there may be significant risks and it may be that if such an approach is considered enlisting the assistance of a centre where there is experience or with colleagues in an alternative specialty where there may be greater experience, for example in renal medicine for EPO, may be needed. From personal experience, much can be gained with the use of the more commonly prescribed medications but often as more and more medications are prescribed, the incremental benefit may be smaller.

As is clear from the other chapters, there are no long-term, randomised controlled trials in the area and therefore there is no guidance as to which medications to use in which circumstance. With alternative physiologies perhaps predominating in different patients, it may well be clear that one medication which has provided benefit in one patient may provide absolutely no benefit in another, emphasising differences in physiology rather than necessarily indicating a diagnostic error.

Boris (2018) [7] details their experience of managing PoTS in children. They describe their standard approach to management and assessed this using a clinical database as to which medications were being taken, noting which provided symptomatic improvement assessing efficacy based on both patient-reported symptom improvement and maintenance of the medication dose to indicate that the medications were being taken with five or more repeat prescriptions at a consistent dose. 708 patients were involved in their assessment, 77.5% being female, ranging from 6 to 18 years with a significant majority of the patients in their teenage years. They note that lightheadedness was a particularly common symptom for which medications were prescribed and noted that overall more than half of the patients found benefit from those medications. They note that other medications used for other symptoms, such as headache, nausea, dysmotility, pain and insomnia were limited by side-effects but still had the potential to provide benefit in a small number of patients. None of the medications assessed provided benefit to more than 50% of patients and they note that lightheadedness and pain were often more effectively treated than other symptoms, such as gastrointestinal dysmotility. Their assessment highlights multiple individual medications being prescribed for symptom improvement: the median number of therapies per patient included two for lightheadedness, two for headache, one for nausea, one for dysmotility, one for pain and two for insomnia. This represents a retrospective analysis of their practice and therefore will be limited to some extent in that regard and as a specialist centre, patients may be more unwell than others seen in more general settings.

A number of medications may be prescribed for other purposes which can worsen orthostatic intolerance such as many commonly prescribed medications for hypertension. While hypertension may coexist, it is a rare finding because of the demographic who suffer PoTS in general. There may be some symptoms where vasoactive medications are prescribed to improve one symptom which may worsen another and therefore the prescription will become a balance of which are the most important symptoms to treat. For example, it is recognised that the serotonin norepinephrine reuptake inhibitor anti-depressants can worsen PoTS however as they can provide benefit treating pain or depression, which may lead to improved activity, in some cases the benefit outweighs the worsening of symptoms. Therefore, it is important that the physician managing the case overall can take an overview of all of the medications prescribed to ensure interactions are not missed but also to guide the best therapeutic approach for individual symptoms.

It is important to recognise that any therapy can be associated with a placebo effect. There is a growing understanding of this both in a positive sense, as shown in the syncope trials [8], patients are well-recognised to note benefit from both medications and from interventions. In addition, if there is a perceived suggestion that a particular medication may produce adverse effects, for instance when prescribing statins for hypercholesterolaemia, side effects may occur [9]. How much of the therapeutic benefit that is noted with any individual medication may well therefore be affected by a super-added placebo effect however as the basis of the therapeutic approach to PoTS is symptom improvement with the aim in the longer term to wean and stop medications, the placebo effect may be of benefit. Patients do however react to different medications in different ways and therefore the placebo effect is not an explanation for the entire therapeutic approach. It will only be with true double-blind, randomised controlled trials that an understanding of this area will be understood however [10].

While there is no accepted standard approach to prescribing medications in PoTS, a recent review from experts in the field [11] does provide a suggested therapeutic approach, emphasising the use of different medications to affect different parts of the symptomatology.

Those individual medications will be detailed in chapters 'Midodrine', 'Ivabradine', 'β-blockers', 'Fludrocortisone', 'Octreotide', 'Clonidine', 'Other Medications: Desmopressin, Pyridostigmine Erythropoietin and SSRIs'.

References

1. Sheldon RS, Grubb BP, Olshansky B, et al. 2015 heart rhythm society expert consensus statement on the diagnosis and treatment of postural tachycardia syndrome, inappropriate sinus tachycardia, and vasovagal syncope. Heart Rhythm. 2015;12:e41–e63.
2. Raj SR, Guzman JC, Harvey P, et al. Canadian Cardiovascular Society Position Statement on Postural Orthostatic Tachycardia Syndrome (POTS) and Related Disorders of Chronic Orthostatic Intolerance. Can J Cardiol. 2020; 36(3):357–72. https://doi.org/10.1016/j.cjca.2019.12.024.
3. GMC prescribing guidance. Available at: https://www.gmc-uk.org/ethical-guidance/ethical-guidance-for-doctors/prescribing-and-managing-medicines-and-devices/prescribing-unlicensed-medicines.
4. Zadourian A, Doherty TA, Swiatkiewicz I, Taub PR. Postural orthostatic tachycardia syndrome:

prevelance, pathophysiology and management. Drugs. 2018;78:983–94.
5. Ruzieh M, Grubb BP. Orthostatic intolerance and postural tachycardia syndrome: new insights into pathophysiology and treatment. Herzschr Elektrophys. 2018;29:183–186.
6. Bryarly M, Fu PLTQ, Vernino S, Levine BD. Postural torthostatic tachycardia syndrome. JACC. 2018;73:1207–28.
7. Boris JR, Bernadzikowski T. Utilisation of medications to reduce symptoms in children with postural orthostatic tachycardia syndrome. Cardiol Young. 2018;28:1386–92.
8. Pournazari P, Sahota I, Sheldon R. High remission rates in vasovagal syncope. JACC Clin Electrophysiol. 2017;3:384–92.
9. Gupta A, Thompson D, Whitehouse A, et al. Adverse events associated with unblinded, but not with blinded, statin therapy in the Anglo-Scandinavian Cardiac Outcomes Trial—Lipid-Lowering Arm (ASCOT-LLA): a randomised double-blind placebo-controlled trial and its non-randomised non-blind extension pharse. Lancet. 2017;389:2473–81.
10. Nwazue VC, Arnold AC, Raj V, et al. Understanding the placebo effect in clinical trials for postural tachycardia syndrome. Clin Exp Pharmacol Physiol. 2014;41:325–30.
11. Miller AJ, Raj SR. Pharmacotherapy for postural tachycardia syndrome. Autonom Neurosci Basic Clin. 2018;215:28–36.

Midodrine

Nicholas Gall

The detailed pathophysiology of PoTS remains uncertain but, as detailed elsewhere, one of the likely mechanisms relates to impaired peripheral vasoconstriction leading to cardiac under-filling, reduced preload and lower BP, thus affecting the adequacy of forward perfusion. Interventions such as compression clothing have been suggested to affect this aspect and vasoconstricting medications have been proposed as a therapeutic approach. One of the most commonly used medications in this area is midodrine which has also been studied for the prevention of vasovagal syncope. Raj and colleagues [1] have proposed the use of midodrine to reduce the risk of vasovagal syncope as part of the POST 4 trial which has now completed recruitment and is awaiting publication.

Midodrine [2] is a pro-drug which undergoes hydrolysis in both the intestines and in the plasma to produce desglymidodrine, which is an agonist of peripheral alpha-1 adrenergic receptors, producing both veno- and arteriolar constriction, therefore increasing cardiac output and peripheral resistance. It does not cross the blood–brain barrier and therefore does not produce more central effects. It is rapidly converted into its active metabolite and therefore has a short half-life. The half-life of its metabolic product is around 2.5 hours and therefore its clinical effects usually will last for around four hours.

It can affect adrenoreceptors elsewhere, for instance in the bladder and ureter, leading to some of the potential side effects. It is felt to be contraindicated in those with significant heart and other vascular diseases, hypertension, significant renal failure, those with problematic urinary retention, proliferative diabetic retinopathy, phaeochromocytoma, hyperthyroidism and narrow-angle glaucoma. Other than the hypertensive side effects, many patients note tingling in the scalp which is usually insufficient to prevent its use but some use that as a guide as to when the medication is working. Some patients may note headache, nausea, flushing, rash and particularly urinary retention and a small number may not be able to continue using the medication because of these side-effects. Perhaps a larger number, through personal experience, may not find clinical benefit from the medication and will stop for that reason.

It is not known to be safe in pregnancy and therefore it is generally recommended that it is avoided although there are case reports of patients going through pregnancy successfully without problem [3]. It should be avoided in severe renal failure but is not affected by liver function impairment.

There are interactions, however these are generally few and it is worth consulting a

N. Gall (✉)
Department of Cardiology, King's College Hospital, London SE5 9RS, UK
e-mail: nickgall@doctors.org.uk

N. Gall et al. (eds.), *Postural Tachycardia Syndrome*, https://doi.org/10.1007/978-3-030-54165-1_28

formulary for an up-to-date list, for instance the British National Formulary app.

As it produces vasoconstriction, there is some concern that it can lead to hypertension and therefore it is important to monitor blood pressure with its use. There is concern particularly that high blood pressure may occur while the patient is supine and therefore it is generally suggested that patients avoid lying flat having taken midodrine for four hours after the last dose. If patients do need to lie flat, then being somewhat propped up and assessing their BP would be appropriate. The medication often begins to produce its effect within 30–45 minutes and therefore many patients will take their first dose as they get out of bed in the morning but can also take it half an hour before rising. They will often note the effects wearing off and therefore can have further doses every four hours, ensuring that they do not take a dose within four or five hours of going to bed. While it is not mandatary, it is clearly important to ensure that BP does not rise excessively while taking this medication and purely arbitrarily, in our practice, we give patients the first dose and monitor their blood pressure over several hours to ensure that no significant events occur. In general, because of the demographic of PoTS patients, we tend not to see significantly high blood pressure. While on the medication subsequently, we advise patients to assess their BP on occasion at home, perhaps every few weeks.

In terms of dosing, we start with 2.5 mg three times a day and assess for clinical benefit. As it does seem to produce rapid effects, patients will often be aware of its efficacy within a few days. If patients tolerate the starting dose, we allow them to increase their dose every few weeks by 2.5 mg at each dose point, as long as their BP is well-controlled. The maximum licenced dose in the UK is 10 mg three times a day although the Canadian guidance suggests that doses up to 15 mg can be used [4]. We have found that patients often note the effects of the medication and can predict what is required at each dose point. We therefore allow patients to take different amounts at different times on different days according to their symptoms, as long as they do not exceed the maximum daily amount. At times, patients may take an extra dose into the evening if they are staying out late.

As detailed elsewhere, there are no long-term assessments of the use of midodrine in PoTS patients but it has been studied in a number of small studies.

Gordon et al. [5] studied 21 subjects who fulfilled criteria for PoTS, the majority being female. They were given midodrine in addition to other medication interventions and assessed their symptoms after the dose; in addition, heart rates were monitored while tilted. Midodrine reduced both the tilt-related heart rate increase but also improved patient's symptoms.

In a retrospective, questionnaire-based assessment of PoTS patients studied at the Mayo Clinic [6], patients reported an improvement in symptoms with midodrine and also with beta-blockers. In a study examining the effects of midodrine and octreotide [7] on postural heart rate, nine patients with PoTS and six with orthostatic intolerance were studied while standing for one hour. Neither medication alone led to an increase in standing time but the combination increased their standing time significantly. Both medications separately and in combination reduced standing heart rate.

It remains unclear as to whether it is possible to predict which patients may respond to midodrine however a number of small studies have been undertaken looking at various biomarkers including plasma copeptin [8], erythrocytic hydrogen sulphide [9], mid-regional pro-adrenomedullin [10] and flow-mediated vasodilatation [11]. While these are clearly areas of interest, the data originate from small studies in children and therefore will require a significant degree of validation. The same group [12] have also assessed the use of midodrine over 3–6 months and showed improvements in postural heart rate and in symptom score although again this was a small study in children.

It could be postulated that midodrine would be more likely to produce therapeutic benefit in patients where there is a failure of peripheral vasoconstriction rather than in patients with other potential PoTS mechanisms. Ross and colleagues [13] investigated patients who were defined as neuropathic versus hyperadrenergic and assessed the effects of midodrine versus placebo and examined the effects of tilt testing, measuring calf vascular resistance and calf venous capacitance in addition. They noted improvements in heart rate in the neuropathic cohort from midodrine when compared to placebo which was associated with an increase in calf vascular resistance. A similar effect was not seen in the hyperadrenergic patients although there seemed to be some benefit from a placebo effect.

In conclusion, midodrine is a commonly used medication in PoTS because of its peripheral vasoconstrictive effects which potentially leads to symptomatic improvement by improving pre-load. Small studies have been undertaken and certainly there is some experimental data to suggest the potential for benefit although different subtypes of PoTS may benefit preferentially. It is therefore recognised in the international guidelines [14] as a potential therapy.

References

1. Raj SR, Faris PD, McRae M, Sheldon RS. Rationale for the prevention of syncope trial IV: Assessment of midodrine. Clin Auton Res. 2012;22(6):275–80.
2. Midodrine, for severe orthostatic hypotension. Drug Ther Bull. 2016;54(5):54–6.
3. Glatter KA, Tuteja D, Chiamvimonvat N, Hamdan M, Park JK. Pregnancy in postural orthostatic tachycardia syndrome. PACE Pacing Clin Electrophysiol. 2005;28(6):591–3.
4. Raj SR, Guzman JC, Harvey P, et al. Canadian Cardiovascular Society Position Statement on Postural Orthostatic Tachycardia Syndrome (POTS) and Related Disorders of Chronic Orthostatic Intolerance. Can J Cardiol. 2020; 36(3):357–72. https://doi.org/10.1016/j.cjca.2019.12.024.
5. Gordon VM, Opfer-Gehrking TL, Novak V, Low PA. Hemodynamic and symptomatic effects of acute interventions on tilt in patients with postural tachycardia syndrome. Clin Auton Res. 2000;10(1):29–33.
6. Lai CC, Fischer PR, Brands CK, Fisher JL, Porter C-BJ, Driscoll SW, et al. Outcomes in adolescents with postural orthostatic tachycardia syndrome treated with midodrine and beta-blockers. Pacing Clin Electrophysiol [Internet]. 2009 [cited 2019 Nov 27];32(2):234–8. https://www.ncbi.nlm.nih.gov/pubmed/19170913.
7. Hoeldtke RD, Bryner KD, Hoeldtke ME, Hobbs G. Treatment of postural tachycardia syndrome: A comparison of octreotide and midodrine. Clin Auton Res. 2006;16(6):390–5.
8. Zhao J, Tang C, Jin H, Du J. Plasma copeptin and therapeutic effectiveness of midodrine hydrochloride on postural tachycardia syndrome in children. J Pediatr [Internet]. 2014 [cited 2019 Nov 27];165(2):290–294.e1. https://www.ncbi.nlm.nih.gov/pubmed/24857518.
9. Yang J, Zhao J, Du S, Liu D, Fu C, Li X, et al. Postural orthostatic tachycardia syndrome with increased erythrocytic hydrogen sulfide and response to midodrine hydrochloride. J Pediatr. 2013;163(4).
10. Zhang F, Li X, Ochs T, Chen L, Liao Y, Tang C, et al. Midregional pro-adrenomedullin as a predictor for therapeutic response to midodrine hydrochloride in children with postural orthostatic tachycardia syndrome. J Am Coll Cardiol [Internet]. 2012 [cited 2019 Nov 27];60(4):315–20. https://www.ncbi.nlm.nih.gov/pubmed/22813609.
11. Liao Y, Yang J, Zhang F, Chen S, Liu X, Zhang Q, et al. Flow-mediated vasodilation as a predictor of therapeutic response to midodrine hydrochloride in children with postural orthostatic tachycardia syndrome. Am J Cardiol [Internet]. 2013 [cited 2019 Nov 27];112(6):816–20. https://www.ncbi.nlm.nih.gov/pubmed/23735645.
12. Chen L, Wang L, Sun J, Qin J, Tang C, Jin H, et al. Midodrine hydrochloride is effective in the treatment of children with postural orthostatic tachycardia syndrome. Circ J [Internet]. 2011 [cited 2019 Nov 27];75(4):927–31. https://www.ncbi.nlm.nih.gov/pubmed/21301135.
13. Ross AJ, Ocon AJ, Medow MS, Stewart JM. A double-blind placebo-controlled cross-over study of the vascular effects of midodrine in neuropathic compared with hyperadrenergic postural tachycardia syndrome. Clin Sci. 2014;126(4):289–96.
14. 2015 Heart Rhythm Society Expert Consensus Statement on the Diagnosis and Treatment of Postural Tachycardia Syndrome, Inappropriate Sinus Tachycardia, and Vasovagal Syncope | Heart Rhythm Society [Internet]. [cited 2019 Nov 27]. https://www.hrsonline.org/clinical-resources/2015-heart-rhythm-society-expert-consensus-statement-diagnosis-and-treatment-postural-tachycardia.

Ivabradine

Tushar V. Salukhe

Sinus tachycardia in response to postural stress is the fundamental to diagnosis and the source of many symptoms in PoTS patients. This typically occurs in the absence of sustained or precipitous hypotension. It is plausible that the postural tachycardia is a reflex to venous pooling and subsequent sluggish venous return. If tachycardia is necessary to maintain blood pressure and cerebral perfusion, attempting to mitigate symptoms by blunting sinus tachycardia may appear counterproductive, yet sequential publications have documented symptom reduction after therapies specifically targeting sinus tachycardia [1–3]. These observations underscore the importance of tachycardia in symptom production.

The rationale for selective sinus node modulation in PoTS patients was borne from two fundamental observations. Symptoms reduction with beta-blockers is often offset by side effects of peripheral drug action, in particular hypotension [1, 2]. Secondly, the contribution of abnormal sympathetic tone in PoTS patients was negligible compared to that of patients with inappropriate sinus tachycardia and is comparable to healthy controls [3]. Sympathetic attenuation with beta blockade, though effective in many, is a blunt approach.

T. V. Salukhe (✉)
Royal Brompton Hospital and Imperial College London, Sydney Street, London SW36NP, UK
e-mail: t.salukhe@rbht.nhs.uk; T.salukhe@imperial.ac.uk

Ivabradine inhibits *If*, mixed Na^+-K^+ channels expressed with high density in sino-atrial node myocytes, thereby selectively reducing sinoatrial rate without affecting myocardial contractility or hypotension. This selective action received attention to prompt investigation into its utility in PoTS and to date is evidenced by two non-randomised, single-centre, observational case studies in PoTS patients [4, 5].

Both studies demonstrated a reduction in fatigue and palpitations in ~60–70% of patients with the introduction of Ivabradine. These series started Ivabradine at 2.5 mg BD or 5 mg BD achieving a mean dose of 10.7 mg/24 h over 15 months. A significant proportion of patients in both series were also taking volume expanders (fludrocortisone) or peripheral vasoconstrictors (midodrine), although co-therapy was not predictive of positive symptomatic response.

Side effects were reported in 10–25% of patients, which seldom led to drug cessation. The most common reason for stopping treatment was lack of efficacy. Side effects were mainly in the form of temporary visual disturbances, described as light spots (phosphenes) or increased fatigue.

The results of these small studies, limited by their design, is encouraging and would justify further evaluation in more robust prospective randomized study, but no further conclusions can be drawn.

Ivabradine for the treatment of PoTS remains unlicensed in the United Kingdom. Its use by

N. Gall et al. (eds.), *Postural Tachycardia Syndrome*, https://doi.org/10.1007/978-3-030-54165-1_29

specialist centers has largely been justified by specialists on the grounds of lack of alternative treatments and the excellent safety profile of ivabradine in patients with heart failure and angina. The ongoing frustration for patients with PoTS and PoTS specialists is that identification of responders is difficult and like other treatment options, such as midodrine, beta-blockers or fludrocortisone, trial and error of individual and combination therapy is still common practice. Tilt testing can be valuable for documentation of a significant postural tachycardia with concomitant symptoms before considering Ivabradine treatment, but is not clearly predictive of a positive response to treatment. There is no role for tilt testing in monitoring Ivabradine treatment and success should be assessed by symptom improvement.

Lifestyle changes, education and cognitive support remain the foundation of managing patients with PoTS. Pharmacological support can provide an invaluable respite from symptoms, but treatment will need to be tailored to the individual, often through trial and error, while also remaining mindful that the needs of the individual will also change with time.

References

1. Raj SR, Black BK, Biaggioni I, Paranjape SY, Ramirez M, Dupont WD, Robertson D. Propranolol decreases tachycardia and improves symptoms in the postural tachycardia syndrome: Less is more. Circulation. 2009;120(9):725–34.
2. Lai CC, Fischer PR, Brands CK, Fisher JL, Porter CB, Driscoll SW, Graner KK. Outcomes in adolescents with postural orthostatic tachycardia syndrome treated with midodrine and beta-blockers. Pacing Clin Electrophysiol. 2009;32(2):234–8.
3. Nwazue VC, Paranjape SY, Black BK, Biaggioni I, Diedrich A, Dupont WD, Robertson D, Raj SR. Postural tachycardia syndrome and inappropriate sinus tachycardia: role of autonomic modulation and sinus node automaticity. J Am Heart Assoc. 2014;3(2).
4. Sutton R, Salukhe TV, Franzen-McManus AC, Collins A, Lim PB, Francis DP. Ivabradine in treatment of sinus tachycardia mediated vasovagal syncope. Europace. 2014;16(2):284–8.
5. McDonald C, Frith J, Newton JL. Single centre experience of ivabradine in postural orthostatic tachycardia syndrome. Europace. 2011;13(3):427–30.

β-blockers

P. Boon Lim

One major pathophysiological manifestation of PoTS includes palpitations due to sinus tachycardia during orthostatic challenge. In a majority of patients, this is an appropriate reflex tachycardia due to activation of baroreceptors during an orthostatic challenge, with the prevailing view of pooling in the lower limbs reducing venous return therefore resulting in the activation of the medullary centres in the brainstem to promote ventricular inotropy and chronotropy mediated by the sympathetic nervous system.

Rationale for Us of β-blockers

The rationale for β-blockers (β adrenergic receptor antagonists) is to target tachycardia symptoms, which may drive symptoms such as light-headedness, palpitations and shortness of breath. However, the tachycardia is often secondary to low stroke volume due to other mechanisms, including neurohumoral dysregulation, peripheral venous pooling and relative hypovolaemia.

Large doses of β-blockers may decrease heart rate excessively or lower blood pressure, which may lead to worsening symptoms. Lower doses of β-blockers are therefore usually used for PoTS. The β-blocker which is recommended is propranolol, a non-selective lipophilic drug which crosses the blood brain barrier, and blocks both the β1 and β2 adrenergic receptors. In particular β2 blockade can lead to peripheral vasoconstriction, which could then promote a secondary reflex lowering of heart rate.

Clinical Trials Evidence

Although the evidence is sparse, propranolol is currently a Class IIb recommendation in the Heart Rhythm Society consensus document [1], as it may be effective in controlling symptoms and reducing tachycardia [1, 2]. A small study showed exercise training is superior to long-acting propranolol in restoring upright haemodynamics, renal-adrenal responsiveness and improving quality of life [3].

A Meta-analysis of 8 studies looking into the efficacy of β-blockers in children demonstrated that small doses led to an improvement in heart-rate increment during standing, with improved symptoms scores [4].

If beta-blockers are to be prescribed, this should be given (at low doses initially) to patients in whom palpitations are a dominant symptom profile, and patients should be told about the possibility of worsening dizziness due

P. B. Lim (✉)
Imperial Syncope Unit, Imperial College Healthcare NHS Trust, Hammersmith Hospital, Du Cane Road, W12 0HS London, UK
e-mail: pblim@imperial.ac.uk

N. Gall et al. (eds.), *Postural Tachycardia Syndrome*, https://doi.org/10.1007/978-3-030-54165-1_30

to hypotension or relative bradycardia whilst not upright.

Recommendations for Use of Beta Blockers

Propranolol 10–20 mg bd may be tried in PoTS, higher doses are not advised due to potential intolerance [5]. There is no evidence on the use of other beta blockers in adults [1].

Prior to commencing any form of drug therapy in patients with PoTS, physicians should ensure that all patients are adhering to all conservative strategies, with particular focus on maximising fluid intake.

References

1. Sheldon RS, Grubb BP 2nd, Olshansky B, Shen W-K, Calkins H, Brignole M, Raj SR, Krahn AD, Morillo CA, Stewart JM, Sutton R, Sandroni P, Friday KJ, Hachul DT, Cohen MI, Lau DH, Mayuga KA, Moak JP, Sandhu RK, Kanjwal K. 2015 heart rhythm society expert consensus statement on the diagnosis and treatment of postural tachycardia syndrome, inappropriate sinus tachycardia, and vasovagal syncope. Heart Rhythm. 2015;12:e41-63.
2. Miller A, Raj SR. Pharmacotherapy for postural tachycardia syndrome. Auton Neurosci. 2018;215:28–36.
3. Fu Q, VanGundy TB, Shibata S, Auchus RJ, Williams GH, Levine BD. Exercise training versus propranolol in the treatment of the postural orthostatic tachycardia syndrome. Hypertension. 2011;58:167–75.
4. Deng-X, Zhang Y, Liao Y, and Du J. Efficacy of β-blockers on postural tachycardia syndrome in children and adolescents: A systematic review and meta-analysis. Front Pediatr. 2019;7:460.
5. Raj SR, Black BK, Biaggioni I, Paranjape SY, Ramirez M, Dupont WD, Robertson D. Propranolol decreases tachycardia and improves symptoms in the postural tachycardia syndrome: Less is more. Circulation. 2009;120:725–34.

Fludrocortisone

Melvin D. Lobo

Introduction

Many PoTS patients are hypovolemic and respond well to increased fluid and blood volume [1, 2]. In addition it has been demonstrated that some PoTS patients also have low levels of aldosterone [3]. Fludrocortisone is a synthetic mineralocorticoid used in the treatment of patients with adrenal insufficiency [4]. Functionally it is similar to aldosterone, the body's primary endogenous mineralocorticoid, and is structurally analogous to cortisol, but has been modified to enhance its mineralocorticoid potency.

Fludrocortisone: Mechanism of Action

In a similar fashion to aldosterone, fludrocortisone acts on mineralocorticoid receptors in the kidney to promote sodium reabsorption and potassium excretion by increasing the density of sodium channels on the apical border of renal tubular cells and also increasing the density of Na^{+}-K^{+}-ATPase on the basolateral membrane [5]. The end result is to increase plasma sodium concentration and thereby blood pressure as well as decreasing plasma potassium levels. Thus electrolytes and renal function need monitoring during fludrocortisone therapy. In the longer term, it is believed that fludrocortisone also acts to sensitise vascular smooth muscle cells to circulating catecholamines [6, 7].

There is a much milder effect of fludrocortisone on glucocorticoid receptors—the glucocorticoid potency of fludrocortisone is up to 10 times that of endogenous cortisol whilst its mineralocorticoid affinity is 200–400 times greater [8].

Pharmacology

Fludrocortisone is rapidly and well absorbed following oral administration and is 80% protein bound in plasma [9]. Metabolism of fludrocortisone is not well understood although the CYP3A family is likely to be involved and thus strong inhibitors/inducers of CYP3A should not be concomitantly prescribed during therapy with fludrocortisone [10].

M. D. Lobo (✉)
Barts BP Centre of Excellence, Barts Heart Centre, St Bartholomew's Hospital, West Smithfield, London EC17BE, UK
e-mail: m.d.lobo@qmul.ac.uk

M. D. Lobo
Barts NIHR Cardiovascular Biomedical Research Centre, Charterhouse Square, William Harvey Research Institute, Queen Mary University London, London EC1M6BQ, UK

N. Gall et al. (eds.), *Postural Tachycardia Syndrome*, https://doi.org/10.1007/978-3-030-54165-1_31

Adverse Effects

Common adverse reactions of fludrocortisone arise as a direct consequence of its potent mineralocorticoid activity and include retention of sodium and water, hypertension, congestive heart failure and hypokalaemia. Less commonly stomach upset, abdominal pain and bloating and nausea have been described as well as headache, insomnia and mood changes.

Indication in POTS

The use of fludrocortisone in patients with PoTS has not been evaluated in randomised controlled clinical trials although there is limited literature to support its efficacy in the setting of neurogenic orthostatic hypotension [11]. Beneficial effects of fludrocortisone on chronic nausea and abdominal pain were demonstrated in a small uncontrolled study in children with PoTS although cardiovascular effects were not assessed [12].

By convention a dose of 0.1–0.2 mg is used daily either as a single dose or in split doses although there is no real need for the latter. Use of fludrocortisone mandates monitoring of electrolytes and renal function as mentioned above, initially 1 week following a dose change and thereafter at 4-6monthly intervals when at a steady dose. In the Heart Rhythm Society Expert Consensus Statement 2015, fludrocortisone was given a Class 2B recommendation for use in PoTS [13].

References

1. Fouad FM, Tadena-Thome L, Bravo EL, Tarazi RC. Idiopathic hypovolemia. Ann Intern Med. 1986;104(3):298–303.
2. Jacob G, Shannon JR, Black B, Biaggioni I, Mosqueda-Garcia R, Robertson RM, et al. Effects of volume loading and pressor agents in idiopathic orthostatic tachycardia. Circulation. 1997;96(2):575–80.
3. Raj SR, Biaggioni I, Yamhure PC, Black BK, Paranjape SY, Byrne DW, et al. Renin-aldosterone paradox and perturbed blood volume regulation underlying postural tachycardia syndrome. Circulation. 2005;111(13):1574–82.
4. Charmandari E, Nicolaides NC, Chrousos GP. Adrenal insufficiency. Lancet. 2014;383(9935):2152–67.
5. Bastl CP, Hayslett JP. The cellular action of aldosterone in target epithelia. Kidney Int. 1992;42(2):250–64.
6. Chobanian AV, Volicer L, Tifft CP, Gavras H, Liang CS, Faxon D. Mineralocorticoid-induced hypertension in patients with orthostatic hypotension. New Engl J Med. 1979;301(2):68–73.
7. Davies B, Bannester R, Sever P, Wilcox C. The pressor actions of noradrenaline, angiotensin II and saralasin in chronic autonomic failure treated with fludrocortisone. Br J Clin Pharmacol. 1979;8(3):253–60.
8. Oelkers W, Buchen S, Diederich S, Krain J, Muhme S, Schoneshofer M. Impaired renal 11 beta-oxidation of 9 alpha-fluorocortisol: an explanation for its mineralocorticoid potency. J Clin Endocrinol Metablsm. 1994;78(4):928–32.
9. Banda J, Lakshmanan R, Vvs SP, Gudla SP, Prudhivi R. A highly sensitive method for the quantification of fludrocortisone in human plasma using ultra-high-performance liquid chromatography tandem mass spectrometry and its pharmacokinetic application. Biomed Chromatogr. 2015;29(8):1213–9.
10. Rendic S. Summary of information on human CYP enzymes: human P450 metabolism data. Drug Metab Rev. 2002;34(1–2):83–448.
11. Schreglmann SR, Buchele F, Sommerauer M, Epprecht L, Kagi G, Hagele-Link S, et al. Pyridostigmine bromide versus fludrocortisone in the treatment of orthostatic hypotension in Parkinson's disease—A randomized controlled trial. Eur J Neurol. 2017;24(4):545–51.
12. Fortunato JE, Wagoner AL, Harbinson RL, D'Agostino RB Jr, Shaltout HA, Diz DI. Effect of fludrocortisone acetate on chronic unexplained nausea and abdominal pain in children with orthostatic intolerance. J Pediatr Gastroenterol Nutr. 2014;59(1):39–43.
13. Sheldon RS, Grubb BP 2nd, Olshansky B, Shen WK, Calkins H, Brignole M, et al. 2015 heart rhythm society expert consensus statement on the diagnosis and treatment of postural tachycardia syndrome, inappropriate sinus tachycardia, and vasovagal syncope. Heart Rhythm. 2015;12(6):e41-63.

Octreotide

Melvin D. Lobo

Introduction

Octreotide is a synthetic octapeptide analogue of the natural hormone somatostatin [1]. Its main indication for use is in the treatment of acromegaly and also to minimise side effects during cancer chemotherapy [2]. It is likely to improve orthostatic symptoms in patients with PoTS through splanchnic vasoconstriction.

Octreotide: Mechanism of Action

Octreotide binds to somatostatin receptors and acts as a potent inhibitor or growth hormone, glucagon and insulin [3]. In addition it suppresses luteinising hormone, decreases splanchnic blood flow and inhibits the release of numerous gastrointestinal peptides include serotonin, gastrin, vasoactive intestinal peptide and pancreatic polypeptide.

Pharmacology

Octreotide has a much longer half life than somatostatin and binds with high affinity to the specific somatostatin receptor sub-type 2 (SST2).

Adverse Effects

Common side effects of therapy with Octreotide (which are dose dependent in severity) include nausea, abdominal cramps and diarrhoea, flatulence and fat malabsorption. During treatment of acromegaly with octreotide, a third of patients were noted to develop gallstones although symptomatic gallbladder disease was uncommon [3, 4].

Indication in POTS

Octreotide can be administered by intravenous, intramuscular or subcutaneous injection and longer acting versions now exist which are given via the intramuscular route. There is limited data to support the use of Octreotide in PoTS and its use has not been recommended in any guidelines/expert consensus statements to date. In two small, uncontrolled trials, it was demonstrated that Octreotide by either subcutaneous or intramuscular injection improved symptoms

M. D. Lobo (✉)
Barts BP Centre of Excellence, Barts Heart Centre, St Bartholomew's Hospital, West Smithfield, London EC17BE, UK
e-mail: m.d.lobo@qmul.ac.uk

M. D. Lobo
Barts NIHR Cardiovascular Biomedical Research Centre, Charterhouse Square, William Harvey Research Institute, Queen Mary University London, London EC1M6BQ, UK

N. Gall et al. (eds.), *Postural Tachycardia Syndrome*, https://doi.org/10.1007/978-3-030-54165-1_32

of orthostatic intolerance as well as fatigue in patients with PoTS [5, 6]. The use of Octreotide to attenuate post-prandial hypotension has shown some promise albeit in patients who did not have PoTS and this is an area worthy of further research in PoTS patients who often report severe post-prandial lassitude due to splanchnic pooling [7–9].

References

1. Bauer W, Briner U, Doepfner W, Haller R, Huguenin R, Marbach P, et al. SMS 201–995: A very potent and selective octapeptide analogue of somatostatin with prolonged action. Life Sci. 1982;31(11):1133–40.
2. Lamberts SWJ, Hofland LJ. Anniversary review: Octreotide, 40 years later. Eur J Endocrino l. 2019;181(5):R173–83.
3. Lamberts SW, van der Lely AJ, de Herder WW, Hofland LJ. Octreotide. New Engl J Med. 1996;334(4):246–54.
4. Moschetta A, Stolk MF, Rehfeld JF, Portincasa P, Slee PH, Koppeschaar HP, et al. Severe impairment of postprandial cholecystokinin release and gall-bladder emptying and high risk of gallstone formation in acromegalic patients during Sandostatin LAR. Aliment Pharmacol Ther. 2001;15(2):181–5.
5. Hoeldtke RD, Bryner KD, Hoeldtke ME, Hobbs G. Treatment of postural tachycardia syndrome: A comparison of octreotide and midodrine. Clin Auton Res. 2006;16(6):390–5.
6. Hoeldtke RD, Bryner KD, Hoeldtke ME, Hobbs G. Treatment of autonomic neuropathy, postural tachycardia and orthostatic syncope with octreotide LAR. Clin Auton Res. 2007;17(6):334–40.
7. Alam M, Smith G, Bleasdale-Barr K, Pavitt DV, Mathias CJ. Effects of the peptide release inhibitor, octreotide, on daytime hypotension and on nocturnal hypertension in primary autonomic failure. J Hypertens. 1995;13(12 Pt 2):1664–9.
8. Jansen RW, Lenders JW, Peeters TL, van Lier HJ, Hoefnagels WH. SMS 201–995 prevents postprandial blood pressure reduction in normotensive and hypertensive elderly subjects. J Hypertens Suppl. 1988;6(4):S669–72.
9. Jansen RW, Peeters TL, Lenders JW, van Lier HJ, v't Laar A, Hoefnagels WH. Somatostatin analog octreotide (SMS 201–995) prevents the decrease in blood pressure after oral glucose loading in the elderly. J Clin Endocrinol Metabol. 1989;68(4):752–6.

Clonidine

Carmela Maniero and Melvin D. Lobo

Abbreviations

α	alpha
β	beta
BP	blood pressure
MSA	multiple system atrophy
OH	orthostatic hypotension
PAF	pure autonomic failure
PoTS	Postural Tachycardia Syndrome

Introduction

The conventional classification of PoTS in subtypes (hyperadrenergic, neuropathic and volume dysregulation) is based on clinical evaluation and review of symptoms but, as they are the final common pathway resulting from a number of different pathophysiologic mechanisms [1], they can overlap in the same patient, making pharmacological treatment complex.

C. Maniero (✉) · M. D. Lobo
Barts BP Centre of Excellence, Barts Heart Centre, St Bartholomew's Hospital, West Smithfield, London EC17BE, UK
e-mail: carmen.maniero@nhs.net; m.d.lobo@qmul.ac.uk

C. Maniero · M. D. Lobo
Barts NIHR Cardiovascular Biomedical Research Centre, Charterhouse Square, William Harvey Research Institute, Queen Mary University London, London EC1M6BQ, UK

This chapter will focus on the use of Clonidine, a central sympatholytic, to improve BP control and alleviate symptoms in particular in 3 groups of patients:

- hyperadrenergic PoTS with increased BP
- patients with supine hypertension
- patients with severe neurogenic orthostatic hypotension (OH).

Clonidine: Mechanism of Action and Pharmacokinetics

Clonidine (2-((2,6-dichlorophenyl) amino)-2-imidazoline hydrochloride) is an Imidazoline derivative that acts as a central α-2 adrenergic agonist.

Anatomically, its site of action is the rostral ventrolateral medulla in the brainstem, whose afferents regulate vasomotor and chronotropic targets. Clonidine terminates the presynaptic release of norepinephrine and inhibits the sympathetic outflow. It can also reduce serum catecholamine levels [2]. Moreover, it increases the parasympathetic outflow from the medulla by preventing the action of cardio-inhibitory vagal neurons in the nucleus ambiguus.

Besides its central action it can act directly on peripheral pre-synaptic α-2 adrenergic receptors in the heart and vessels, thus preventing release of norepinephrine and local smooth vessel β-adrenergic activation.

N. Gall et al. (eds.), *Postural Tachycardia Syndrome*, https://doi.org/10.1007/978-3-030-54165-1_33

Altogether, treatment with Clonidine mediates increased vasodilation, reduced cardiac output and heart rate and reduced blood pressure.

As a centrally acting agent, Clonidine does not cause tolerance or reflex tachycardia. It is especially useful as fourth or fifth line antihypertensive drug, in patients with labile hypertension, significant BP variability and with a relevant component of anxiety. Oral Clonidine, at small doses, may be used in patients with symptomatic BP surges thanks to its short-lasting action. Other therapeutic indications include pain management, attention-deficit/hyperactivity disorder, and symptomatic treatment of opioid withdrawal, as adjuvant to induce sedation or for epidural analgesia.

Pharmacokinetics

Clonidine's pharmacokinetics differs according to the formulation prescribed.

For oral tablets the bioavailability varies between 75 and 100%. Peak plasma concentration is achieved in about 2 hours, with the maximal blood pressure reduction achieved between 3 and 8 hours. Clonidine is 20–40% protein bound in plasma. More than half of Clonidine is excreted unmodified in the urine and its half-life is between 6 and 24 hours.

The Clonidine transdermal adhesive system is a 0.2 mm thick patch composed of a drug reservoir, a membrane that controls delivery rate, and a pliable backing. Clonidine is released at a constant rate, with "zero-order" kinetics similar to continuous infusion. Clonidine patch formulations come in doses of 2.5, 5, and 7.5 mg contained in a timed matrix delivery system and deliver 0.1, 0.2, or 0.3 mg/day of Clonidine for 7 days, respectively. The elimination half-life while the patch is adherent varies from 26 to 55 hours.

Clonidine patches should be applied preferably on the chest or upper arms as these sites correspond to the higher average Clonidine concentration [3]. The amount released depends mainly on the contact surface area of the patch, especially in the early phases of treatment as the drug is sequestered in the stratum corneum.

Adverse Effects

As a central acting sympatholytic Clonidine also acts as a central nervous system depressant, causing or worsening fatigue, brain fog and drowsiness. It can also cause postural hypotension, sodium and water retention, and dry mouth. The spectrum of side effects makes the use of Clonidine in PoTS patients particularly challenging as they can overlap with symptoms associated to the syndrome including brain fog, fatigue, worsening of postural BP drop and of orthostatic intolerance. It is however possible to minimise this by starting with small doses and using a long-acting transdermal formulation.

Clonidine can act as a depressor of sinus and atrioventricular nodes and cause significant bradycardia, especially in patients with chronic kidney disease and sick sinus syndrome.

Sudden discontinuation of Clonidine, particularly when used at high doses and in association with β-blockers, can cause sympathetic surge with rebound hypertension. This is less common for the transdermal formulation, likely due to residual drug accumulation in the skin.

Besides these side effects secondary to its mechanism of action, it is important to recognise that transdermal Clonidine can cause additional skin reactions such as erythema, changes in skin color with hyperpigmentation or depigmentation, vesicular rash, excoriation, which may require treatment with corticosteroid creams.

Indication in PoTS/Dysautonomia

There are no randomized clinical trials on the use of Clonidine in PoTS, therefore most of the literature and also guidelines including the Heart Rhythm association Consensus on PoTS, Inappropriate Sinus Tachycardia and Vasovagal Syncope, mention the use of sympatholytic agents as supported by a class IIb Recommendation (level of Evidence E) [4].

We describe potential uses of Clonidine in the following settings.

Hyperadrenergic PoTS

The spectrum of symptoms of hyperadrenergic PoTS (palpitations, tachycardia, anxiety, orthostatic hypertension with BP raise $\geq$10 mmHg) and the finding of plasma norepinephrine levels $\geq$600 pmol/L after standing are suggestive of marked sympathetic activation, therefore the reduction in sympathetic outflow by Clonidine may be beneficial.

A study on a small group of patients with hyperadrenergic postural intolerance found that Clonidine improved symptoms and haemodynamic. As expected, it lowered blood pressure, heart rate, cardiac input but also raised peripheral vascular resistance and plasma norepinephrine levels on standing and improved plasma volume [5].

In our practice we would recommend to start with a small oral dose, and increase it up to 0.1–0.2 mg two to three times daily, or switch to a transdermal formulation if tolerated and when prolonged action is required or when patients are unable to tolerate oral administration.

Neuropathic PoTS—Peripheral Adrenergic Failure: Control of Supine Hypertension

Patients with neuropathic PoTS or with autonomic failure may present with supine hypertension, increased sympathetic activity being the shared pathophysiologic mechanism in these two types of orthostatic intolerances.

Nocturnal hypertension is associated with increased cardiovascular risk and target organ damage and requires treatment, which represents a challenge as these patients present with postural intolerance and, in case of autonomic failure, postural hypotension.

Shibao et al. tested Clonidine as an overnight medication in 23 patients with autonomic failure (either with MSA or with PAF) and observed significant reduction of supine BP and reduction in nocturnal natriuresis compared to placebo [6]. The BP effect was observed in both subgroups although the mechanism underlying supine hypertension is believed to be different-residual sympathetic tone unrestrained by the lack of baroreflex buffering in MSA and damage to postganglionic sympathetic neurons in PAF.

Treatment of Severe Hypotension in PoTS: Use as a Pressor Agent

While Clonidine lowers blood pressure in patients with essential hypertension, it can "paradoxically" raise blood pressure in patients with autonomic failure or PoTS, by acting as an agonist of peripheral post-junctional α_2- and α_1-adrenergic receptors in the venous bed. This novel use for clonidine was described by Robertson et al. who analyzed the pressor response of patients with idiopathic orthostatic hypotension to oral Clonidine and found that BP was significantly raised for several hours with durable improvement of symptoms [7].

References

1. Raj SR. The Postural Tachycardia Syndrome (POTS): Pathophysiology, diagnosis & management. Indian Pacing Electrophysiol J. 2006;6(2):84–99.
2. Kanagy NL. Alpha(2)-adrenergic receptor signalling in hypertension. Clin Sci (Lond). 2005;109(5):431–7.
3. Hopkins K, Aarons L, Rowland M. Absorption of clonidine from a transdermal therapeutic system when applied to different body sites. In: Webers M and Mathias CJ, editors. Mild hypertension. Current controversies and newapproaches. 1984.
4. Sheldon RS, Grubb BP, Olshansky B, Shen WK, Calkins H, Brignole M, et al. 2015 heart rhythm society expert consensus statement on the diagnosis and treatment of postural tachycardia syndrome, inappropriate sinus tachycardia, and vasovagal syncope. Heart Rhythm. 2015;12(6):e41-63.
5. Gaffney FA, Lane LB, Pettinger W, Blomqvist CG. Effects of long-term clonidine administration on the

hemodynamic and neuroendocrine postural responses of patients with dysautonomia. Chest. 1983;83(2 Suppl):436–8.

6. Shibao C, Gamboa A, Abraham R, Raj SR, Diedrich A, Black B, et al. Clonidine for the treatment of supine hypertension and pressure natriuresis in autonomic failure. Hypertension. 2006;47(3):522–6.
7. Robertson D, Goldberg MR, Hollister AS, Wade D, Robertson RM. Clonidine raises blood pressure in severe idiopathic orthostatic hypotension. Am J Med. 1983;74(2):193–200.

Other Medications: Desmopressin, Pyridostigmine, Erythropoietin and SSRIs

Mehran Asgari and Melvin D. Lobo

A review of the literature identifies differences in the definition for POTS and wide variations in treatment and outcomes. This syndrome appears to describe a group of conditions with differing pathophysiology, which requires treatment tailored to the true underlying disorder. Most of these treatments are covered in other chapters on pharmacological approaches in this text book; however patients with PoTS may continue to be symptomatic despite being treated with a combination of volume expander (fludrocortisone) and vasoconstrictor (midodrine). Here consideration is limited to four additional classes of therapy which may be of benefit when conventional approaches have failed:

- anti-diuretic treatment (Desmopressin)
- acetylcholinesterase inhibition (pryidostigmine)
- Colony stimulating factors (erythropoietin)
- Selective serotonin reuptake inhibitors (SSRI).

Desmopressin

Desmopressin acetate (DDAVP) is a synthetic version of arginine vasopressin, a natural anti-diuretic hormone (ADH), which binds to V2 receptors in the collecting duct of the kidney and results in translocation of aquaporin channels to the distal nephron and increased reasbsorption of free water from the urine [1]. Desmopressin has specific attributes that make it theoretically attractive as a volume expander as it displays enhanced antidiuretic potency and a prolonged half-life and duration of action compared to endogenous ADH. However due to selective targeting of the V2 receptor, it is not thought to have much in the way of pressor activity.

Desmopressin might promote acute blood volume expansion and reduce upright tachycardia and therefore be of benefit in patients with PoTS. Whilst there is limited data to support use of desmopressin in patients with orthostatic hypotension, few studies have addressed its potential utility in PoTS [2]. In a 'proof of concept' crossover study of 30 adults with PoTS, a single dose of oral DDAVP (0.2 mg) significantly attenuated tachycardia and improved symptoms compared to placebo [3].

M. Asgari (✉)
Department of Cardiology, Wirral University Teaching Hospital NHS Foundation Trust, Merseyside C49 5PE, UK
e-mail: Mehran.asgari@nhs.net

M. D. Lobo
Barts BP Centre of Excellence, Barts Heart Centre, St Bartholomew's Hospital, West Smithfield, London EC17BE, UK

M. D. Lobo
Barts NIHR Cardiovascular Biomedical Research Unit, Charterhouse Square, William Harvey Research Institute, Queen Mary University London, London EC1M 6BQ, UK

N. Gall et al. (eds.), *Postural Tachycardia Syndrome*, https://doi.org/10.1007/978-3-030-54165-1_34

Potential side effects include hyponatraemia, oedema and headache. Desmopressin acetate can be given at a dose of 0.1–0.2 mg at night on a daily basis and serum electrolyte levels (especially sodium) must be monitored routinely during therapy. This is all the more important for patients with PoTS who are already encouraged to maintain high fluid intake which might increase the risk of developing hyponatremia [4].

Pyridostigmine Bromide

Pyridostigmine bromide is a small molecule reversible acetylcholinesterase inhibitor that enhances the effect of acetylcholine by inhibiting its breakdown in the synaptic cleft and thereby increasing bioavailability of acetylcholine for interaction with both nicotinic and muscarinic receptors [5]. This would theoretically improve sympathetic nervous system signaling and peripheral vascular resistance (nicotinic effects) as well as suppressing heart rate (muscarinic effects) which could be beneficial in PoTS as well as other conditions causing orthostatic hypotension. Pyridostigmine is a quaternary amine, poorly absorbed from the gastrointestinal tract and does not cross the blood–brain barrier. A starting dose of 30 mg twice daily can be up-titrated to a maximum of 90 mg three times daily (or 180 mg daily of the long acting formulation) depending on efficacy/tolerability. Commonly reported side effects include increased colonic motility (diarrhoea), abdominal cramps, nausea, muscle twitching and headaches. Pryidostigmine can also cause shortness of breath necessitating caution when prescribing in patients who have coexistent asthma.

Limited data from four single dose trials have demonstrated modest haemodynamic improvements with pyridostigmine when used for neurogenic orthostatic hypotension [5]. Using a randomized crossover design, Raj et al. have demonstrated that a single dose of 30 mg pyridostimine significantly attenuated tachycardia in patients with PoTS along with a concomitant decrease in symptom burden [6]. A retrospective analysis of a large single centre experience with pyridostigmine in PoTS reported that most patients tolerated the drug with careful dose titration and this was accompanied by improvement in symptoms of fatigue, palpitations, presyncope and syncope in about 50% of the patients [7]. Moreover symptom reduction correlated with clinically significant reduction in orthostatic heart rate and increase in diastolic BP compared to baseline. Longer term prospective studies evaluating the effects of pyridostigmine in PoTS with continued daily adminstration are lacking.

Erythropoietin (EPO)

Erythropoietin (EPO) is a growth factor produced by the kidneys that stimulates the production of red blood cells by promoting the division and differentiation of committed erythroid progenitors in the bone marrow [8]. It is usually reserved for the treatment of anaemia associated with conditions such as chronic kidney disease, or drug therapy such as chemotherapy/antiretroviral therapy. Synthetic forms of EPO contain the identical amino acid sequence of isolated natural erythropoietin and have the same biological activity as endogenous erythropoietin and are high cost clinical therapies. EPO therapy requires the subcutaneous route of administration: one of the most common complaints is pain at the site of injection. EPO therapy increases the risk of myocardial infarction, stroke and venous thromboembolism and has been associated with increased mortality in certain populations [9]. Safety monitoring requires haemoglobin and haematocrit levels to be closely monitored every 3–4 weeks with the haematocrit level kept below 50%.

Limited data indicate there is a role for use of EPO in treatment of orthostatic hypotension [10]. However only two studies to date have assessed the use of EPO in PoTS, one of which demonstrated improvement in orthostatic symptoms in 3 out of 8 patients [11]. In a retrospective single centre analysis, Kanjwal et al.demonstrated improvement in orthostatic symptoms in 27 out of 39 patients with PoTS refractory to all other therapies. Of note EPO improved seated diastolic BP without any effect on other haemodynamic parameters [12].

Based upon current data which is insufficient and its high cost, use of EPO should be restricted to only the most severe and refractory cases of PoTS. It is recommended to obtain full blood count, total iron binding capacity, serum iron and ferritin levels before EPO therapy. Hematocrit (HCT) levels must be monitored monthly and should remain less than 50%.

Selective Serotonin Reuptake Inhibitors (SSRI)

SSRI therapy has been found to be helpful in the prevention of neurocardiogenic syncope [13]. Some experts continue to recommend the use of these drugs to improve cardiovascular symptoms in PoTS despite scanty supporting evidence [15]. In a study of 39 patients with PoTS, sertraline was found to have only modest pressor effects which were not associated with heart rate reduction or improvement in symptoms [16]. Similarly use of serotonin-norepineprhine reuptake inhibitors (SNRI) should be viewed with caution in this population as no published data supports their use and a single centre study of the norepineprhine reuptake transporter inhibitor atomexitine in 27 patients with PoTS demonstrated an acute increase in standing heart rate and symptom burden with no reported benefits [17].

On the basis of the data to date, it may be reasonable to attempt a trial of SSRI therapy for psychological manifestations of PoTS rather than as an approach to managing neurocardiogenic symptoms [18].

References

1. Richardson DW, Robinson AG. Desmopressin. Ann Intern Med. 1985;103(2):228–39.
2. Ahmad RA, Watson RD. Treatment of postural hypotension. Rev Drugs. 1990;39(1):74–85.
3. Coffin ST, Black BK, Biaggioni I, Paranjape SY, Orozco C, Black PW, et al. Desmopressin acutely decreases tachycardia and improves symptoms in the postural tachycardia syndrome. Heart Rhythm. 2012;9(9):1484–90.
4. Raj SR. Postural tachycardia syndrome (POTS). Circulation. 2013;127(23):2336–42.
5. Gales BJ, Gales MA. Pyridostigmine in the treatment of orthostatic intolerance. Annals Pharmacoth. 2007;41(2):314–8.
6. Raj SR, Black BK, Biaggioni I, Harris PA, Robertson D. Acetylcholinesterase inhibition improves tachycardia in postural tachycardia syndrome. Circulation. 2005;111(21):2734–40.
7. Kanjwal K, Karabin B, Sheikh M, Elmer L, Kanjwal Y, Saeed B, et al. Pyridostigmine in the treatment of postural orthostatic tachycardia: a single-center experience. Pacing Clin Electrophy. 2011;34(6):750–5.
8. Elliott S, Pham E, Macdougall IC. Erythropoietins: a common mechanism of action. Exp Hematol. 2008;36(12):1573–84.
9. Fishbane S, Besarab A. Mechanism of increased mortality risk with erythropoietin treatment to higher hemoglobin targets. Clin J Am Soc Nephrol. 2007;2(6):1274–82.
10. Gupta V, Lipsitz LA. Orthostatic hypotension in the elderly: diagnosis and treatment. Am J Med. 2007;120(10):841–7.
11. Hoeldtke RD, Horvath GG, Bryner KD. Treatment of orthostatic tachycardia with erythropoietin. Am J Med. 1995;99(5):525–9.
12. Kanjwal K, Saeed B, Karabin B, Kanjwal Y, Sheikh M, Grubb BP. Erythropoietin in the treatment of postural orthostatic tachycardia syndrome. Am J Ther. 2012;19(2):92–5.
13. Guzman JC, Armaganijan LV, Morillo CA. Treatment of neurally mediated reflex syncope. Cardiol Clin. 2013;31(1):123–9.
14. Sharma T, Guski LS, Freund N, Gotzsche PC. Suicidality and aggression during antidepressant treatment: systematic review and meta-analyses based on clinical study reports. BMJ. 2016;352:i65.
15. Grubb BP. Postural tachycardia syndrome. Circulation. 2008;117(21):2814–7.
16. Mar PL, Raj V, Black BK, Biaggioni I, Shibao CA, Paranjape SY, et al. Acute haemodynamic effects of a selective serotonin reuptake inhinitor in postural tachycardia syndrome: a radnomized crossover trial. J Psychopharmacol. 2014;28(2):155–61.
17. Green EA, Raj V, Shibao CA, Biaggioni I, Black BK, Dupont WD, et al. Effects of norepinephrine reuptake inhibition on postural tachycardia syndrome. J Am Heart Assoc. 2013;2(5):e000395.
18. Bryarly M, Phillips LT, Fu Q, Vernino S, Levine BD. Postural Orthostatic Tachycardia Syndrome: JACC Focus Seminar. J Am Coll Cardiol. 2019;73(10):1207–28.

Assessing Benefit in PoTS

Nicholas Gall

As has been detailed in a number of the other chapters in this text, we remain uncertain as to the detailed pathophysiology that produces PoTS and indeed it is likely that multiple pathophysiologies will contribute to the symptoms in each individual patient, not only in the cardiovascular autonomic system but also in other areas. The effects of any therapeutic approach in other territories will be assessed by the individual treating physician and may involve validated assessments, for instance headache questionnaires. We recognise PoTS on the basis of a significant heart rate rise on standing although, as is detailed elsewhere, this was an arbitrary definition based on a limited understanding of the pathophysiology and certainly there is no single haemodynamic measure which can provide an entire understanding of whether a particular therapy has provided benefit. While we do recognise that an inappropriate tachycardia is present in most patients and indeed it may be present much of the time to varying degrees, there are patients who have a normal heart rate at rest and it increases significantly on activity. Therefore, while it is entirely acceptable to assess the effects of interventions to slow heart rate on the basis of a standing heart rate or a daytime or average heart rate on Holter monitoring, there is no doubt that patient's symptoms might not improve concurrent with this heart rate fall. If this were a pure heart rate issue, then medications such as beta blockade and ivabradine would provide a perfect therapeutic approach which experience suggests that they do not. In addition, more interventional therapies such as sinus node ablation would also provide such benefit and in general that approach is not felt to be indicated in many patients [1]. In general, therefore, we rely on patient-reported symptomatic improvement to define whether the patient improves, over and above changes in haemodynamic measures. It may well be that assessing the haemodynamic effects on a stand/tilt test, looking for the magnitude of heart rate increase and the variability in blood pressure oscillation may provide some assessment however that is not a validated approach and as patient's symptoms are often complex and multi-systemic, aiming for improvement in one particular haemodynamic variable is unlikely to provide an improvement in patient's overall functioning.

As has been detailed elsewhere [2], the placebo effect can be very important in any therapy and indeed many therapies may rely on the placebo effect to a significant degree and that will clearly affect PoTS patients. As there are no randomised controlled trials of medication use in the long-term, defining how important the

N. Gall (✉)
Department of Cardiology, King's College Hospital, London SE5 9RS, UKe-mail: nickgall@doctors.org.uk

N. Gall et al. (eds.), *Postural Tachycardia Syndrome*, https://doi.org/10.1007/978-3-030-54165-1_35

placebo effect is remains difficult. Providing a caring and understanding approach to patients may well enhance this. It is important to recognise that patient symptoms do wax and wane, varying during the day with many patients describing symptoms to be worse in the mornings and better in the evenings which has been validated in haemodynamic terms [3]. Nwazue and colleagues investigated the placebo effect in PoTS patients by performing a prospective, randomised crossover trial where PoTS patients either received open-label no treatment, that is a medication which they knew would provide no benefit and a blinded placebo. They assessed subsequently the standing heart rate after each intervention at two hours and four hours and noted that there was no difference between either intervention although there was a decrease over time. This reiterated the impression that the heart rate increase is often more significant in the earlier part of the day but also suggests that PoTS patients are no more susceptible to a placebo effect than others. They note that up to 35% of patients may respond to placebo in clinical trials.

It is also recognised by clinicians in the field that patients often will describe worsening of their symptoms with the menstrual cycle, patients will often note a significant deterioration with intercurrent illness and certainly in hot weather, symptoms can at times significantly deteriorate. Many patients will also note deterioration if they push themselves too hard in some way. In that regard therefore an assessment of symptoms while important, does need to take into account this natural variability prior to taking the decision to change or escalate therapy.

There are no validated symptom questionnaires in PoTS however the Compass 31 questionnaire, which is used to assess autonomic symptoms in those with more significant autonomic dysfunction, has been used [4]. Rea and colleagues used the Compass 31 autonomic symptoms assessment in PoTS patients and compared the results to other validated questionnaires assessing fatigue and affective symptoms. They assessed 32 patients with PoTS, 32 healthy controls and compared its use in its originally intended patient cohort, in patients with autonomic failure and neuropathy. They detail that the compass 31 questionnaire assesses autonomic symptoms in a number of different territories including effects on pupils, bladder, gastrointestinal symptoms, sweating, orthostatic intolerance and blood vessel control. They noted more autonomic symptoms in PoTS patients than in controls. They also assessed autonomic physiology with standard autonomic function tests. After thorough statistical assessment, fatigue, orthostatic and pupillomotor symptoms specifically differentiated PoTS patients from controls. They note that much of the pupilomotor domain relates to light sensitivity and therefore may reflect the migraine associations of PoTS. They note that the vasomotor symptoms did not differentiate which was perhaps surprising and also note that a number of PoTS symptoms, for instance flushing which is frequently described by PoTS patients were not assessed.

It is well recognised that PoTS patients have reduced quality of life and that has been assessed using the SF-36 questionnaire correlated with autonomic symptoms [5]. 94 patients were assessed and were clearly shown to have significant impairments in a number of territories including pain, general health, social functioning, vitality, role functioning and physical functioning. Symptom severity and disability status correlated with impaired quality of life although this was by no means the entire effect. It is recognised that quality-of-life measures in PoTS patients are often significantly impaired and equivalent to other chronic and significant conditions [6]. It is certainly possible that the use of this questionnaire may allow an understanding of benefit although it has not been used in such a manner to date.

Another study [7] undertaken in 624 PoTS patients with a smaller control group used various validated questionnaires to assess quality of life, pain, sleep quality, fatigue and an assessment of suicidal behaviour, noting significant impairments in quality-of-life, pain, sleep/fatigue and increases in suicide risk. The use of such validated questionnaires therefore may provide insight into patient symptoms although again they have not been used prospectively to assess therapeutic benefit. They may however be used in individual practices on a serial basis to provide a more objective assessment.

While a reliance on symptomatic improvement can define whether a patient is improving and whether a particular therapeutic approach has provided benefit, there are other methods which can be used to assess how effective an individual therapy has been. As detailed elsewhere, increased fluid and salt intake is usually of great benefit in PoTS patients and at times it is worthwhile trying to validate how well a patient may be hydrated. Guidelines suggest increasing salt intake to 10 to 12 g of salt on a daily basis [1] however in many cases it can be difficult to define whether a patient is achieving the required amount. An earlier study in vasovagal patients [8] suggested that aiming to increase salt intake, as reflected by a 24 h urinary sodium excretion of more than 170 mmol, seems to provide benefit and that has been further assessed in PoTS patients [9] and could therefore be used to define that the sodium intake is sufficient. Aiming to see perhaps 2.5 to 3 L of urinary excretion in that 24 h period is arbitrary but clearly smaller volumes will reflect inadequate hydration.

Zhang and colleagues [9] used the 170 mmol per 24 h cut off to assess PoTS patients, focusing on 30 children, 20 female, with a mean age of 11 who fulfilled criteria for PoTS although their criteria were somewhat different to that in the guidelines. They assessed 24 h urinary sodium excretion and found that PoTS patients had lower excretion than a matched control group and after salt supplementation there was a significant improvement in salt excretion which predicted symptom improvement. They noted that baseline sodium excretion predicted the likelihood of benefit with those with an excretion above 124 mmol per 24 h less likely to benefit.

Exercise has clearly been shown to provide therapeutic benefit in PoTS [10]; the degree of conditioning can be assessed using the cardiopulmonary exercise test through the VO_{2max} assessment. This can therefore define how much benefit may be expected, to some extent, by further exercise.

A number of biomarkers have been proposed as assessments in PoTS [11] including flow mediated vasodilatation, plasma pro-adrenomedullin and erythrocytic hydrogen sulphide although these have often been assessed in very small trials. Other small studies have suggested that limited increase in systolic or diastolic pressure or increases in heart rate on standing may predict benefit from midodrine or metoprolol respectively. Although there are theoretical reasons why they may provide an assessment, they are usually experimental, not commonly available and certainly not validated in large populations.

In conclusion, therefore, while there are methods to assess certain aspects of the therapeutic approach, for instance the degree of hydration or the level of fitness and other symptomatic questionnaire-based assessments or biomarkers have been studied, there are no formalised assessments currently available, although these are clearly urgently needed.

References

1. Sheldon RS, Grubb BP, Olshansky B et. Al. 2015 Heart Rhythm Society Expert Consensus Statement on the diagnosis and treatment of postural tachycardia syndrome, inappropriate sinus tachycardia, and vasovagal syncope. Heart Rhythm. 2015; 12:e41–e63.
2. Pournazari P, Sahota I, Sheldon R. High remission rates in vasovagal syncope. JACC: Clin Electrophysiol. 2017; 3:384–392.
3. Nwazue VC, Arnold AC, Raj V et al. Understanding the placebo effect in clinical trials for postural tachycardia syndrome. Clin Exp Pharmacol Physiol. 2014; 41:325–330.
4. Rea NA, Campbell CL, Cortez MM. Quantitative assessment of autonomic symptom burden in postural tachycardia syndrome (PoTS). J Neurol Sci. 2017;377:35–41.
5. Benrud-Larson LM, Dewar MS, Sandroni P, Rummans TA, Haythonthwaite JA, Low PA. Quality of life in patients with postural tachycardia syndrome. Mayo Clin Proc. 2002;77:531–7.

6. KYKD. Grubb BP. The postural tachycardia syndrome: a concise guide to diagnosis and management. J Cardiovasc Electrophysiol. 2006; 17:108–12.
7. Pederson CL, Brook JB. Health-related quality of life and suicide risk in postural tachycardia syndrome. Clin Auton Res. 2017;27:75–81.
8. El-Sayed H, Hainsworth R. Salt supplement increases plasma volume and orthostatic tolerance in patients with unexplained syncope. Heart. 1996;75:134–40.
9. Zhang Q, Liao Y, Tang C, Du J, Jin H. Twenty-four-hour urinary sodium excreation and postural orthostatic tachycardia syndrome. J Paediat. 2012;161:281–4.
10. Bryarly M, Phillips LT, Fu Q, Vernino S, Levine BD. Postural orthostatic tachycardia syndrome. JACC. 2019;73:1207–28.
11. Lin J, Jin H, Du J. Assessment of therapeutic biomarkers in the treatment of children with postural tachycardia syndrome and vasovagal syncope. Cardiol Young. 2014;24:792–6.

Additional Therapeutic Considerations

Clinical Aspects of Paediatric PoTS

Philip R. Fischer, Lesley Kavi and William Whitehouse

Postural Tachycardia Syndrome or Postural Orthostatic Tachycardia Syndrome (PoTS) is similar physiologically in adolescents and adults. Nonetheless, the clinical presentations, diagnostic criteria [1], and, potentially, the treatment and prognosis vary by age.

Clinical Presentation of PoTS in Adolescents

The incidence of adolescent PoTS is unknown. There are data, however, about the incidence of chronic fatigue, and chronic fatigue is linked to autonomic dysfunction[2]. Approximately 31% of US early adolescent girls struggle with morning fatigue at least twice weekly [3]. In Holland, 21% of adolescent girls and 7% of adolescent boys have had significant fatigue for at least three months [4]. A community study in the UK suggested that 1.1% of adolescents have chronic disabling fatigue [5]. Thus, it could well be that at least 1% of adolescents have autonomic dysfunction, including postural orthostatic tachycardia syndrome. Clearly, there are more than the number of PoTS patients who have orthostatic intolerance to some degree since more than 25% of adolescents sometimes feel dizzy when they assume an upright posture [6].

Typically, PoTS presents during early adolescence, around the start of a growth spurt and, for girls, within a year of menarche [7–9] It is extremely rare for PoTS to present much before the onset of pubertal changes. Some older adolescents and young adults, however, report PoTS symptoms beginning separate from the time of pubertal hormone changes. About two-thirds of adolescents with PoTS are females.

It seems likely that anyone can develop PoTS, but there are clear predisposing factors in addition to potential influences of pubertal hormone changes [7]. PoTS is less common in blacks than in whites and Asians and is found in about 15% of first degree relatives of PoTS patients, indicating a probable genetic predisposition. Over half of people affected with PoTS have a significant degree of hypermobility, again suggesting either a genetic or, perhaps, a structural physical predisposing factor. Anecdotally, many patients are high achievers, hinting at a possible biochemical predisposition, however, the observation could just be due to ascertainment bias: high achievers in high achieving families getting access to the medical teams who can make the diagnosis. The actual onset of symptoms often follows a period of physical illness, such as mononucleosis or an injury, such as a concussion. Some people have suggested that immunisation, such as for human papilloma

P. R. Fischer (✉) · L. Kavi · W. Whitehouse
Institution Mayo Clinic, 200 First Street SW, Rochester, MN 55905, USAe-mail: fischer.phil@mayo.edu

N. Gall et al. (eds.), *Postural Tachycardia Syndrome*, https://doi.org/10.1007/978-3-030-54165-1_36

virus, can trigger PoTS, but that impression lacks support of controlled epidemiological studies and could be due to recall bias [10].

Symptoms of PoTS are similar in adolescents and adults. Fatigue and postural dizziness are nearly uniform. Pain is also common, usually headache and or abdominal discomfort but also sometimes extremity or back pain. Cloudy thinking and a sense of forgetfulness are common. Heat and cold intolerance are also common.

Diagnostic Criteria

The key physical finding of PoTS is postural tachycardia. Other associated findings can include abnormally large pupils and, when upright, facial pallor and mottled dusky distal extremities.

The diagnosis of adolescent PoTS is based on typical symptoms (chronic fatigue and orthostatic intolerance) along with an excessive postural tachycardia in the absence of another obvious cause of those findings (such as severe anxiety with a panic attack during postural challenge) [9]. Based on data from active standing tests (ASTs) and head-up tilt tests (HUTTs), a postural tachycardia rise of more than 40 beats per minute is considered "excessive" in adolescents [6, 11]. Standardised HUTTs may be more reliable than ASTs (due to muscle use facilitating blood flow during standing), but there is a loose correlation between results [$p = 0.04$ in one study [12]]. In the UK, there is currently no agreed consensus on whether ASTs or HUTTs are more sensitive in adolescents. In a recent unpublished survey of 61 patients under the age of 18 by the national charity, PoTS UK, 62% of patients reported receiving their diagnosis following a HUTT. There are a variety of protocols for ASTs and HUTTs in current practice (Box 1, Box 2). ASTs and HUTTs require neither medication nor venous access, however, beat-to-beat Blood Pressure (BP) and Heart Rate (HR) are essential for HUTTs.

Box 1 Example of an Active Standing Test (AST)

Resting supine 5 minutes	BP	HR
Stand up (≤ 1 min)	BP	HR
Standing up for 3 minutes	BP	HR
Standing up for 10 minutes	BP	HR

Use a common place automated sphygmomanometer that can simultaneously record BP and HR non-invasively from the brachial artery. Use largest cuff that comfortably fits around the upper arm. If BP or HR are high at baseline after 5 min supine, ask them to relax and repeat baseline in a few minutes.

In adolescents with orthostatic intolerance a rise in HR of ≥ 40 bpm without OH at the time, and with typical symptoms (chronic fatigue, orthostatic intolerance etc.), confirms the diagnosis of PoTS.

Orthostatic Hypotension (OH) is a drop in BP systolic ≥ 20 mmHg, or BP diastolic ≥ 10 mmHg, or BP systolic < 90 mmHg.

Box 2 Example of a Head-Up Tilt Test (HUTT) for PoTS

Resting supine 5 minutes	BP	HR
Resting supine 10 minutes	BP	HR
60° Head-Up Tilt (≤ 1 min)	BP	HR
60° Head-Up Tilt 3 minutes	BP	HR
60° Head-Up Tilt 10 minutes	BP	HR

Use an automated tilt table.

Use continuous beat-to-beat finger BP and HR recording, in addition to a common place automated sphygmomanometer on the opposite arm to record brachial BP and HR at these specific times.

Can be combined with continuous video-EEG, respiratory bands, and end-tidal CO_2 recording.

In adolescents with orthostatic intolerance a rise in HR of ≥ 40 bpm without OH at the time, and with typical symptoms (chronic fatigue, orthostatic intolerance etc.), confirms the diagnosis of PoTS.

A longer HUTT (up to 50 min) may be required if investigating Transient Loss of Consciousness, e.g. syncope.

Orthostatic Hypotension (OH) is a drop in BP systolic ≥ 20 mmHg, or BP diastolic ≥ 10 mmHg, or BP systolic < 90 mmHg.

Orthostatic hypotension (OH) and PoTS are both on the spectrum of autonomic dysfunction and sometimes overlap, e.g. in the same person on different occasions. Vasovagal syncope, with orthostatic hypotension (a systolic blood pressure drop of more than 20 mm Hg or a drop in diastolic pressure of more than 10 mmHg with postural challenge), is a common cause of fainting in adolescents. Patients who have hypotension prior to manifesting tachycardia during tilt likely have orthostatic hypotension rather than PoTS. Typically, PoTS patients are chronically tired and only rarely faint while patients with vasovagal syncope are not bothered by daily fatigue and "just" faint.

Treatment of PoTS in Adolescents

The treatment of adolescents with PoTS has been incompletely studied. In fact, there are very few comparative studies of various treatments in either adults or adolescents with PoTS [13, 14]. For now, management decisions are often based on personal experience of the treating physician and extrapolated adult data and expert reviews [15]. It is hoped that this current publication can serve as a sort of "expert consensus" to guide management.

1. Non-Pharmacological Measures (see also Sect. 5, Chapters 27 & 28)

   Non-pharmacologic measures are essential in managing adolescents with PoTS [7, 9] First, steps should be taken to increase the circulating blood volume. Fluid intake should be very generous; it is often suggested that adolescents should drink so much water that their urine appears clear like water, apart from an early morning urine which can be pale yellow. Salt intake should be increased since intravascular salt helps "hold on" to the fluid; if affirmation of adequate salt intake is needed, the daily output of sodium (in a 24 h urine collection) should be more than 170 mmol. In the UK, Slow sodium is available and is an easy way to add salt without disrupting the family's healthy low salt diet. For a teenager or young adult, a reasonable starting dose is 50 mmol of sodium (3 g of salt) twice a day increasing to 100 mmol of sodium (6 g salt) twice a day. For small or younger patients start at a lower dose of 2 mmol sodium/kg/day (0.12 g/kg/day salt) in 2 divided doses.

   Manoeuvers to temporarily increase BP can help with acute orthostatic symptoms, e.g. drinking a large glass of water before trying to get out of bed in the morning [16] Compression stockings can also help return otherwise pooled vascular volume to the circulation.

   Second, exercise is vitally important. Gentle morning exercises involving the contraction of large muscle groups can get blood flowing. Aerobic exercise is important to improve vascular tone and to correct any concurrent deconditioning. Patients should exercise daily, starting with a duration of aerobic exercise that does not lead to excessive post-exertional fatigue and then building the duration by a few minutes every week until reaching the target of 30 min of daily aerobic exercise. However, some patients will not be able to maintain their previous levels of activity even though they should still get daily aerobic exercise.

Third, cognitive behavioral therapy is effective in reducing symptoms of PoTS and in facilitating functional restoration. Intensive programs can lead to quick improvement in tolerance of normal daily activities in PoTS patients who had been debilitated [17].

Regular school attendance should be facilitated wherever possible to maintain academic activity, peer interaction, and to prevent social isolation.

2. Drug therapy of PoTS in adolescents (see also Chapters 27–35)

Medications do not cure PoTS, but they can help improve blood flow and functional ability while non-pharmacologic measures are being instituted [7, 8] Beta blockers (such as metoprolol tartrate, 25 mg orally first thing in the morning and then again mid-day) are commonly used with good effect. While low-dose propranolol has proven effective in adults [18], there is anecdotal evidence that some adolescents feel more fatigued on propranolol. Various beta blockers have different receptor specificity and varying ability to cross the blood–brain barrier; thus, when one beta blocker is incompletely effective, another may be tried.

Fludrocortisone, a selective mineralocorticoid, starting with 50 mcg daily and increasing to 0.1 mg twice daily according to response, is sometimes used for its ability to foster fluid and salt retention. However, there are no clear data demonstrating that this is more effective than generous oral fluid and salt intake, which should accompany its use.

Midodrine, an alpha-adrenergic receptor agonist, can improve peripheral vascular tone and increase peripheral vascular resistance, venous return and cardiac output. It may be used three times daily with the final dose at least three to four hours before lying down at night (to prevent supine headaches due to increased blood flow, and supine hypertension); starting at a low dose (2.5 mg) and increasing incrementally to as much as 10 mg can help avoid some of the bothersome side effects such as a tingling sensation in the scalp.

Selective serotonin reuptake inhibitors (SSRIs) can have a helpful adjunctive effect, presumably by increasing serotonin-mediated vascular and intestinal flow.

Ivabradine is a selective channel inhibitor which slows the sinoatrial (SA) node, the natural cardiac pacemaker. It shows some promise in adults [19] and in a UK review of 13 PoTS patients under the age of 18 treated with ivabradine, 63% reported improvement of symptoms. In these patients, mean Ivabradine dose after up titration was 0.1 mg/kg per dose [20].

Other medications have been used in small numbers of patients without proven efficacy. These include stimulants such as methylphenidate and amphetamines to decrease mental clouding, modafanil to facilitate wakefulness, and even erythropoietin to build blood volume.

Of course, concurrent comorbidities [21] should be managed while treating patients with PoTS. Nearly half of adolescents with PoTS are iron deficient with a low ferritin level (<20 ng/mL), even without anemia; iron supplementation is helpful [22, 23]. In some areas, many PoTS patients are vitamin D deficient [22]. Vitamin D deficiency has also been associated with chronic pain [24].

Anxiety and depression occur in a third or more of PoTS patients; SSRI treatment can often help these comorbidities while also helping the symptoms of PoTS. Gastrointestinal dysmotility is often part of PoTS but could be treated with motility agents such as erythromycin, metoclopramide, or, rarely, octreotide. Chronic pain in PoTS patients should not be treated with opiates but can respond to gabapentin (gradually escalating doses, as needed, up to 1200 mg three times daily), pregabalin, and amitriptyline. Hypermobility spectrum disorder and hypermobile Ehlers Danlos syndrome (hEDS) are fairly common in patients with PoTS, and require recognition and advice. The diagnostic criteria for EDS and hypermobility have recently been revised. (see https://ehlers-danlos.

com/wp-content/uploads/hEDS-Dx-Criteria-checklist-1.pdf, [25]).

Mast cell activation disorders can co-occur with PoTS: and beta blockers can worsen symptoms of mast cell activation [26].

PoTS can be debilitating for adolescents. With appropriate management, however, functional restoration is expected, even before the PoTS resolves. In complex cases fatigue and other debilitating symptoms sometimes persist when the postural tachycardia improves, and as with those with complex additional symptoms, a multidisciplinary rehabilitation approach is best, as with young people with CFS/ME. Prognosis in adolescent PoTS is unclear; In one study, over time, the vast majority of patients reported improvement of symptoms, and approximately one fifth reported full recovery [27].

References

1. Sheldon RS, Grubb BP II, Olshansky B, Shen WK, Calkins H, Brignole M, et al. 2015 Heart Rhythm Society Expert Consensus Statement on the Diagnosis and Treatment of Postural Tachycardia Syndrome, Inappropriate Sinus Tachycardia, and Vasovagal Syncope. Heart Rhythm. 2015;12(6):e41–63.
2. Wyller VB, Godang K, Mørkrid L, Saul JP, Thaulow E, Walløe L. Abnormal thermoregulatory responses in adolescents with chronic fatigue syndrome: relation to clinical symptoms. Pediatrics. 2007;120:e129–37.
3. Ghandour RM, Overpeck MD, Huang ZJ, Kogan MD, Scheidt PC. Headache, stomachache, backache, and morning fatigue among adolescent girls in the United States: associations with behavioral, sociodemographic, and environmental factors. Arch Pediatr Adolesc Med. 2004;158:797–803.
4. ter Wolbeek M, van Doornen LJ, Kavelaars A, Heijnen CJ. Severe fatigue in adolescents: a common phenomenon? Pediatrics. 2006;117:e1078–86.
5. Rimes KA, Goodman R, Hotopf M, Wessely S, Meltzer H, Chalder T. Incidence, prognosis, and risk factors for fatigue and chronic fatigue syndrome in adolescents: a prospective community study. Pediatrics. 2007;119:e603–9.
6. Skinner JE, Driscoll SW, Porter CB, Brands CK, Pianosi PT, Kuntz NL, et al. Orthostatic heart rate and blood pressure in adolescents: reference ranges. J Child Neurol. 2010;25:1210–5.
7. Johnson JN, Mack KJ, Kuntz NL, Brands CK, Porter CJ, Fischer PR. Postural orthostatic tachycardia syndrome: a clinical review. Pediatr Neurol. 2010;42:77–85.
8. Kizilbash SJ, Ahrens SP, Bruce BK, Chelimsky G, Driscoll SW, Harbeck-Weber C, et al. Adolescent fatigue, PoTS, and recovery: a guide for clinicians. Curr Probl Pediatr Adolesc Health Care. 2014;44(5):108–33.
9. Stewart JM, Boris JR, Chelimsky G, Fischer PR, Fortunato JE, Grubb BP, et al. Pediatric Writing Group of the American Autonomic Society. Pediatric disorders of orthostatic intolerance. Pediatrics 2018;141:e20171673.
10. Butts BN, Fischer PR, Mack KJ. Human papillomavirus vaccine and postural orthostatic tachycardia syndrome: a review of current literature. J Child Neurol. 2017;32:956–65.
11. Singer W, Sletten D, Opfer T, Brands CK, Fischer PR, Low PA. Postural tachycardia in children and adolescents: what is normal? J Pediatr. 2012;160:222–6.
12. Fischer PR, Brands CK, Porter CJ, Kuntz NL, Mack KJ, Risma JM, et al. High prevalence of orthostatic intolerance in adolescents in a general pediatric referral clinic. (abstract) Clin Autonom Res. 2005;15:340.
13. Wells R, Elliott AD, Mahajan R, Page A, Iodice V, Sanders P, et al. Efficacy of therapies for postural tachycardia syndrome: a systematic review and meta-analysis. Mayo Clin Proc. 2018;93:1043–53.
14. Hasan B, Almasri J, Marwa B, Klaas KM, Fischer PR. treatment of postural orthostatic tachycardia syndrome with medication: a systematic review. J Child Neurol. 2020 (in press)
15. Miller AJ, Raj SR. Pharmacotherapy for postural tachycardia syndrome. Autonom Neurosci: Basic Clin. 2018;215:28–36.
16. Ma J, Hu W, Wu D. Drinking cold water increases blood pressure in healthy young students. Blood Press Monit. 2014;19:118–9.
17. Bruce BK, Weiss KE, Ale CM, Harrison TE, Fischer PR. Development of an interdisciplinary pediatric pain rehabilitation program: the first 1000 consecutive patients. Mayo Clin Proc Inn Qual Out. 2017;1:141–9.
18. Raj SR, Black BK, Biaggioni I, Paranjape SY, Ramirez M, Dupont WD, et al. Propranolol decreases tachycardia and improves symptoms in the postural tachycardia syndrome: less is more. Circulation. 2009;120:725–34.
19. Barzilai M, Jacob G. The effect of ivabradine on the heart rate and sympathovagal balance in postural tachycardia syndrome patients. Rambam Maimonides Med J.2015 Jul 30;6(3).
20. Donne GD, Roses-Noguer F, Til J, Salukhe T, Prasad S, Daubeney P. Ivabradine in the pediatric population: preliminary findings. J Am Coll Cardiol. 2016;67(13):774.

21. Ojha A, Chelimsky TC, Chelimsky G. Comorbidities in pediatric patients with postural orthostatic tachycardia syndrome. J Pediatr. 2011;158:20–3.
22. Antiel RM, Caudill JS, Burkhardt BE, Brands CK, Fischer PR. Iron insufficiency and hypovitaminosis D in adolescents with chronic fatigue and orthostatic intolerance. South Med J. 2011;104:609–11.
23. Jarjour IT, Jarjour LK. Low iron storage and mild anemia in postural tachycardia syndrome in adolescents. Clin Auton Res. 2013;23:175–9.
24. Turner MK, Hooten WM, Schmidt JE, Kerkvliet JL, Townsend CO, Bruce BK. Prevalence and clinical correlates of vitamin D inadequacy among patients with chronic pain. Pain Med. 2008;9:979–84.
25. Tinkle B, Castori M, Berglund B, Cohen H, Grahame R, Kazkaz H, et al. Hypermobile Ehkers-danlos syndrome: clinical description and natural history. Am J Med Genet (Seminars in Medical Genetics). 2017;175C:48–69.
26. Seneviratre SL, Maitland A, Afrin L. Mast cell diseases in Ehlers-danlos syndrome. Am J Med Genet (Seminars in Medical Genetics). 2017;175C:226–36.
27. Bhatia R, Kizilbash SJ, Ahrens SP, Killian JM, Kimmes SA, Knoebel EE, et al. Outcomes of adolescent-onset postural orthostatic tachycardia syndrome. J Pediatr. 2016;173:149–53.

Pregnancy and Postural Tachycardia Syndrome

Daniel Borlase and Cathy Nelson-Piercy

The exact incidence and prevalence of Postural Tachycardia Syndrome (PoTS) is unclear, probably owing to the nature of the disease's heterogeneous manifestations and underdiagnosis. It affects women five times more than men and usually affects women of childbearing age [1]. There are an ever increasing number of diagnoses being made as patients and clinicians alike become more informed about this neuro-cardiovascular condition. It is therefore encountered with increasing frequency in pregnancy and those with an established diagnosis will often seek information specifically about their condition and pregnancy. While it is important not to underestimate the impact PoTS may have on the quality of life of its sufferers, it is important to reassure women that there is no evidence that PoTS is associated with life threatening sequelae for either the mother or her baby [2].

D. Borlase (✉)
MRCOG MRCP, Consultant Obstetrician and Gynaecologist, University Maternity Hospital, Limerick, Republic of Ireland
e-mail: daniel.borlase@hse.ie

C. Nelson-Piercy
FRCOG FRCP, Professor of Obstetric Medicine, Consultant Obstetric Physician, Guy's & St. Thomas' Foundation Trust, London, UK

Cardiovascular Changes in Normal Pregnancy

Pregnancy is associated with significant changes in cardiovascular physiology. By eight weeks gestation cardiac output has already increased by approximately 20%. This rises further to a maximum of 40% to 50% above baseline by the beginning of the third trimester. The increase in cardiac output is a compensatory mechanism for the significant reduction in systemic vascular resistance caused by the developing vascular placental bed and peripheral vasodilatation mediated by a combination of nitric oxide, oestrogens and prostaglandins [3]. The increase in cardiac output is largely due to an increase in stroke volume, although heart rate does contribute to a lesser degree. Resting heart rate in pregnancy is increased by an average of 10 to 15 beats per minute above the baseline and this should not change significantly with position [3]. Blood pressure normally falls during the first and second trimesters owing to the changes in systemic vascular resistance and rises slowly back to baseline, or just exceeding baseline by the end of the third trimester. Blood pressure is more likely to be influenced by position and even women without PoTS often complain of orthostatic symptoms, particularly in the second to third trimesters owing to caval compression from the gravid uterus [4].

N. Gall et al. (eds.), *Postural Tachycardia Syndrome*, https://doi.org/10.1007/978-3-030-54165-1_37

Labour is associated with further significant physiological changes to cardiac function. Cardiac output increases by 15% in the first stage of labour and more than trebles up to 50% by the time full cervical dilatation is reached at the end of the first stage of labour [3]. Uterine contractions cause autotransfusion of up to 500 ml of blood from the uterus back into the central circulation. Along with the relief of pressure on the inferior vena cava following delivery, autotransfusion increases a further 500 ml to 1000 ml immediately after delivery. The vast volumes of blood re-entering the circulation further increases cardiac output by up to 80%, which then rapidly declines to near normal ranges within an hour postpartum [3].

Postural Tachycardia Syndrome in Pregnancy: The Effects on Mother and Her Baby

PoTS is five times more likely to affect women of childbearing age [4, 5]. Most newly diagnosed women are between the ages of 15 and 40 years and it may present for the first time in pregnancy [2]. The condition may not be considered as a potential diagnosis in pregnancy as many of the presenting symptoms mimic those of pregnancy itself. Diagnosis may also be difficult as the objective parameters used for the diagnosis of the condition can be affected by the associated haemodynamic changes. Furthermore, tilt table testing is generally contraindicated in pregnancy although there are no definitive data to support its risks in pregnancy.

There is an increasing body of evidence supporting the overall safety of PoTS in pregnancy for both the mother and her baby; however the changes in symptom severity throughout pregnancy are varied and somewhat unpredictable. A recent systematic review of the literature suggests that 60% to 70% of women experience either an improvement or report stable symptoms throughout pregnancy [4]. Physiologically, pregnancy is associated with a 50% increase in plasma volume and this may in part be responsible for the observed improvement [4]. Approximately 40% can expect an exacerbation of their symptoms which appears to be most evident in the first trimester and has been associated with a concurrent diagnosis of hyperemesis gravidarum. A small case series of 22 patients with PoTS had a 59% risk of developing severe nausea and emesis during the first trimester which is significantly greater than the background risk of 2% [6]. What is not clear is whether the reported exacerbations of PoTS in these cases are as a cause or consequence of this nausea and vomiting in the early stages of pregnancy. Powless et al. identified that women who did not require treatment for PoTS prior to pregnancy were the least likely to report exacerbations during pregnancy. Patients already on treatment were more likely to develop exacerbations and require an increase in pre-existing medications. The introduction of second or third agents to treat exacerbations was seldom required [7]. There has been no reported effect of parity on the frequency and severity of exacerbations of PoTS in pregnancy.

There is no evidence that pregnancy outcomes are worse for mothers or their offspring as a direct consequence of PoTS. The rates of miscarriage and stillbirth are not increased above background risk and the same applies for the rates of spontaneous preterm birth and perinatal morbidity and mortality [2].

PoTS is not a contraindication for vaginal delivery and caesarean section should be reserved for the usual obstetric indications [2]. There are a small number of published reports of elective caesarean sections being performed in patients with very severe symptoms to mitigate the risks of haemodynamic instability on cardiovascular physiology and placental blood flow in labour [1].

Contraception

There have been no studies that investigate the effect of different methods of contraception on PoTS. Therefore, methods can be recommended using the usual FSRH (Faculty of Sexual and Reproductive Healthcare) guidelines [8].

However, migraine is common in PoTS and may limit the use of the combined contraceptive pill.

There is some evidence that women with PoTS experience exacerbations in their symptoms during menstruation [9]. It is possible that methods of contraception that induce amenorrhoea may improve symptoms. These include the progesterone only subdermal implant, levenogestrol releasing intrauterine systems and progesterone only depot injection. The combined pill may be taken continuously every 63 days with a 7 day break between (tricycling) resulting in 4 periods per year and there is emerging evidence that it can be taken continuously throughout the year with no breaks (and therefore no menstruation), although this is an unlicensed use [8].

Pre-Pregnancy Management of PoTS

As with all chronic medical conditions, women contemplating a pregnancy should be encouraged to discuss their PoTS with the medical practitioners managing their condition to address any concerns that the disease may have on the outcomes of a pregnancy or vice versa. Women with PoTS should be reassured that the risk of adverse outcomes during pregnancy and at delivery is no greater than the general population.

A pre-pregnancy counselling appointment with a general practitioner, cardiologist or obstetric physician should identify the phenotype and severity of a patient's symptoms, how they are managed and whether they are controlled. A baseline recording of the heart rate and blood pressure should be taken in the supine and standing positions so that any symptom changes in pregnancy can be identified. It is prudent to also identify any associated or concurrent medical problems, particularly those which often co-exist with PoTS and how these affect her quality of life. In the absence of other cardiac risk factors, and providing the patient has been formally diagnosed, an echocardiogram and Holter monitoring is unlikely to yield any further information and would not be indicated at this stage.

Many women with PoTS require medication to achieve symptom relief and will naturally be concerned about the effect this may also have on her developing fetus. Owing to a paucity of data on the effects of some medications in pregnancy, the fewest number of medications, at the lowest effective doses should be used to manage symptoms. The wide varieties of medications used in PoTS have very different mechanisms of action and therefore all have potentially different ways of affecting a pregnancy and the developing fetus. As with all women planning a pregnancy, folic acid at a dose of at least 400 μg should be recommended for at least 12 weeks prior to conception and for the first 12 weeks of pregnancy to reduce the risks of neural tube (spina bifida, anencephaly) embryopathy.

Early Pregnancy Management of PoTS

Owing to the early changes in cardiac physiology it is important that women with a diagnosis of PoTS are referred to an obstetrician on discovery of their pregnancy, especially if they have not been seen in the preconception period. A detailed assessment should follow that is described in the above pre-pregnancy section and a record made of any symptom deterioration. Patients with PoTS should be referred to an anaesthetist during the pregnancy to discuss plans for analgesia in labour and how regional anaesthesia may impact on symptoms should they arise in labour [10]. There is no indication for serial growth scans for the fetus in this condition unless the patient is taking high dose beta-blockers. The severity of a patient's symptoms will guide the amount of support the woman needs and the number of medical reviews required during the pregnancy; however, pregnancy itself need not be managed any differently to routine antenatal care. Continuity of midwifery care is very important in women with PoTS.

Conservative Management of PoTS in Pregnancy

Pregnancy should not affect the conservative measures used in the management of PoTS. For the majority of patients, these conservative measures alone are enough to improve symptoms. Women not requiring medication are less likely to experience exacerbations of symptoms in pregnancy [1, 5]. An increase in salt intake from 6 to 10 g per day and a total fluid intake of approximately 3 L per day increases circulating plasma volume and is associated with symptom improvement [5]. Care should be taken if hypertensive diseases such as pregnancy induced hypertension or pre-eclampsia develop, when fluid restriction is often required post partum. Improvement in physical fitness particularly with aerobic exercise, has been shown to improve symptoms of PoTS, and this should continue to be encouraged in pregnancy. Elasticated compression tights can also be used to improve the return of fluid from the peripheral to central circulation [4]. Caffeine intake should be limited as it causes diuresis which may deplete fluid volume and cause tachycardia [9]. As with all pregnant women the increasing size of the gravid uterus causes compression of the inferior vena cava in the supine position. Women should be encouraged to lie in the left lateral position whilst lying down if at all possible and avoid lying flat on their backs to minimise the risk of aorta-caval compression.

Pharmacological Management of PoTS in Pregnancy

There are many ways in which drugs can improve the symptoms of orthostatic intolerance associated with PoTS. Medication may aim to increase plasma volume, while others target vasoconstriction. Beta-blockers exhibit a negative chronotropic effect to control heart rate directly. Not all pharmacological options are efficacious and some are associated with intolerable side effects. Furthermore, the decisions on treatment options will likely be affected by patient choice and on the relative safety profiles of these medications in pregnancy. Table 1 summaries the common medications used for the management of PoTS and their relative safety profiles in pregnancy. Pregnancy is associated with increases in drug volume of distribution owing to increases in both intravascular (plasma volume) and extravascular fluid content. Drug elimination is also augmented owing to increases in both hepatic and renal excretion. Dosages of some medication may therefore require upward titration to provide the same desired effects as in the non-pregnant patient.

Medications for PoTS in Pregnancy: The Rate Controllers

There have been no studies directly comparing the use of cardioselective and non-cardioselective β-blockers for the treatment of PoTS in pregnancy. Studies outside of pregnancy suggest that as well as reducing heart rate, non-selective blockade has the additional benefit of reducing peripheral vasodilatation and therefore propranolol is usually the β-blocker of choice [5]. Propranolol has been shown to reduce standing tachycardia without causing orthostatic hypotension and is particularly advantageous for patients with the primary hyperadrenergic subtype of PoTS [5]. Propranolol has also been used in the prevention of migraine in pregnancy, a condition which often coexists with PoTS and thus may have dual benefit in these cases. The majority of safety data surrounding β-blockade in pregnancy comes from studies investigating gestational hypertension. Labetalol is a non-selective β-blocker with coexistent α–adrenoceptor blocking properties and is considered first line for treating hypertension in pregnancy. Its use in PoTS however, is limited. There is no convincing evidence that β-blockers have any teratogenic effects; however there is evidence to suggest that they may cause a reduction in average birth weight by 200 to 230 g, which is not clinically significant [12]. Beta blockers have also been associated with

Table 1 The common medications used in the management of PoTS, their pharmacology, side effects and potential concerns on their use in pregnancy

Medication	Mechanism of action	FDA class	Safety in pregnancy	Safety in breastfeeding	Common side effects
Propranolol	Beta-adrenoreceptor antagonist to Beta-1 and Beta-2 adrenoreceptors causing: Direct reduction in heart rate Reduction in peripheral vasodilatation	C	SAFE	SAFE	– Presyncope/Syncope – Bronchospasm/dyspnoea (Avoid in asthma) – Diarrhoea – Fatigue
Midodrine	Alpha-1-adrenoreceptor agonist causing: – Arterial and venous vasoconstriction – Reduction in peripheral venous pooling – Increases blood pressure in the upright position	C	INSUFFICIENT DATA	INSUFFICIENT DATA	– Headache – Urinary retention – Supine hypertension – Chills – Piloerection
Fludrocortisone	Aldosterone mimetic causing: – Increased salt and water retention – Increasing total plasma volume	C	SAFE	SAFE	– Hypokalaemia – Headache – Hirsuitism – oedema
Desmopressin (DDAVP)	Synthetic analogue of Antidiuretic Hormone (ADH) causing: – Increased fluid reabsorption at the collecting ducts – Increasing total plasma volume	B	SAFE	SAFE	– Hyponatraemia – Nausea – Headaches – Fluid retention
Pyridostigmine	Acetylcholinesterase inhibitor causing: – Increased concentration of acetylcholine at muscarinic receptors – Augments parasympathetic tone – Reduction in heart rate	C	SAFE	SAFE	– Significant GI upset – Hypersalivation – Nausea and Vomiting
Ivabradine	Reduction of conduction speed at the Sinoatrial node	X	AVOID	AVOID	– Arrhythmias – AV nodal block – Presyncope/Syncope – Headache
Somatostatin analogues (E.g. Octreotide)	Inhibitors of Growth Hormone and Vasoactive Intestinal Peptide causing: – Systemic vasoconstriction – Reduction in heart rate	B	PROBABLY SAFE	PROBABLY SAFE	– GI upset – Presyncope – Impaired glucose tolerance/diabetes mellitus – Alopecia

Table 1 undefined

Medication	Mechanism of action	FDA class	Safety in pregnancy	Safety in breastfeeding	Common side effects
Clonidine	Alpha-2-receptor agonist causing: Reduction in Heart rate	C	SAFE	PROBABLY SAFE	– Presyncope/postural hypotension – Dry mouth – Headache – Sexual dysfunction

neonatal hypotension, bradycardia and hypoglycaemia when used in higher dosages [11]. The doses used in managing PoTS are safe and can therefore be used [13].

Ivabradine controls heart rate by specifically reducing conduction speed at the sinoatrial node. It has no effect on other cardiac ionic currents and therefore does not impact on stroke volume or other cardiovascular parameters. Ivabradine was initially developed for the management of angina pectoris and like many other pharmacological options for PoTS it is not licensed for this indication either in or outside of pregnancy. Some animal studies have suggested teratogenicity and it therefore relatively contraindicated in pregnancy [2].

Medication for PoTS in Pregnancy: The Volume Expanders

Fludrocortisone mimics aldosterone, which aims to increase salt and water retention thereby increasing total plasma volume. This may be more effective in patients with the hypovolaemic subtype of PoTS. Fludrocortisone is a mainstay treatment in patients with Addison's disease and is safe in pregnancy [13]. Patients may require upward titration in the third trimester owing to the anti-mineralcorticoid effects of progesterone. Care should be taken to monitor electrolytes, specifically potassium as it can cause hypokalaemia. In some instances fludrocortisone may need to be reduced or even stopped in cases of gestational hypertensive disease such as pre-eclampsia.

Desmopressin, or DDAVP, is a synthetic analogue of anti-diuretic hormone (ADH). Desmopressin also acts as a volume expander by increasing fluid reabsorption at the level of the collecting ducts [5]. Hyponatraemia is a potential complication and patients should be monitored for this. Desmopressin has been used safely in pregnancy for the management of Von Willebrand's disease and diabetes insipidus [3].

Medications for PoTS in Pregnancy: The Vasoconstrictors

Midodrine is an alpha-1-adrenoreceptor agonist, which causes both arterial and venous vasoconstriction thus reducing peripheral venous pooling and increasing blood pressure in the upright position. It has been shown to be effective in the management of PoTS, particularly the neurogenic subclass [5]. In the few case studies published no teratogenic effects are reported, but there are no rigorous data confirming its safety in pregnancy or breastfeeding and it should only to be used when treatments with better safety profiles such as beta-blockers and fludrocortisone are unable to control symptoms effectively [2, 13]. Side effects include piloerection, supine hypertension, headaches and urinary retention which along with the regular dosing regimens, can dissuade patients from this treatment option [5].

Somatostatin analogues such as octreotide are inhibitors of a wide variety of hormones, particularly growth hormone (GH) and vasoactive intestinal peptide (VIP) and are usually used in the management of acromegaly, carcinoid syndrome and neuroendocrine tumours. Given intramuscularly or subcutaneously, octreotide has been used in the treatment of refractory PoTS particularly in combination with midodrine. Since acromegaly is commonly associated with subfertility there are very limited data on the use of octreotide in pregnancy. It should be avoided in pregnancy unless there is a clear benefit. This is relevant, as patients presenting with PoTS on octreotide are most likely to have severe symptoms and may be on a multitude of medications concurrently.

Medications for PoTS in Pregnancy and Breastfeeding: Pyridostigmine

Pyridostigmine is an acetylcholinesterase inhibitor, which increases the concentration of acetylcholine in the autonomic ganglia and muscarinic receptors [5]. It is most often used in the management of myasthenia gravis and has been successfully used in the management of PoTS. It reduces tachycardia and symptoms of the disease by up to 50% [5]. The World Health Organisation classifies this as safe in pregnancy and breastfeeding [2]. Side effects are common. Up to 20% of patients report significant gastrointestinal side effects owing to its effect of increasing gastric motility and therefore compliance may be affected [2, 5].

Medications for PoTS in Pregnancy and Breastfeeding: Clonidine

The centrally acting alpha-2 receptor agonist, clonidine, has been used in the treatment of PoTS with good outcomes in patients with high sympathetic nervous system activity such as those with the hyperadrenergic subtype of the disease [5]. Patients with the neurogenic subgroup are less likely to tolerate its side effects as it can paradoxically cause symptoms of orthostatic hypotension. It appears to be safe in pregnancy and has similar properties to methyldopa, which has been widely used for hypertension in pregnancy.

Medications for PoTS in Pregnancy and Breastfeeding: Selective Serotonin Reuptake Inhibitors

Patients with PoTS do not have higher levels of depression or anxiety than the population in general. However, SSRIs have a mildly vasoconstrictive effect and have been used to treat symptoms of PoTS, although there have been no studies to investigate their efficacy [14].

SSRIs may also be prescribed for anxiety or depression independent of or related to chronic illness. The safety of these medications in pregnancy is continually subject to controversy. Many of the studies highlighting the risks are fraught with inconsistent methodology. The most robust studies show very little evidence of teratogenicity or adverse outcomes. The National Institute for Health and Clinical Excellence (NICE) states that the association between major congenital malformations and all SSRIs is not statistically significant [15]. Patients requiring SSRIs prior to pregnancy are encouraged to remain on these medications as the risks to the mother's mental wellbeing of withdrawal of these drugs is likely to be far greater than the risk to the fetus.

Intrapartum Considerations in Patients with PoTS

The physiological fluid shifts during labour and in the immediate puerperal period have the potential to exacerbate the symptoms of PoTS. The more severe a patient's symptoms, both prior to and during pregnancy, the worse these exacerbations could potentially be in labour. A birth plan should be discussed during pregnancy with both obstetric and midwifery teams to identify the most appropriate place for the woman to deliver, which is usually on or close to an obstetric-led unit. Analgesia options should also be discussed prior to labour and an anaesthetist would normally have seen the woman during pregnancy. Severe stress responses to labour pain may contribute to an extreme tachycardic response and so regional anaesthesia could be considered early in active labour to manage this [10]. Haemodynamic parameters should be monitored closely, particularly during the second stage when Valsalva may be associated with significant cardiac changes [10]. If these do not stabilise between contractions and the mother is symptomatic then operative delivery should be considered. Patients with PoTS should avoid prolonged periods of dehydration and fluid-volume status should be closely monitored both during and after labour. There is no evidence suggesting the use of electronic fetal monitoring in women with PoTS influences neonatal outcome. Theoretically however, women with severe symptoms during pregnancy or those who are identified as having significant changes in blood pressure and heart rate during labour should have continuous fetal monitoring. Intramuscular oxytocin alone or in combination with ergot alkaloids is often used for the management of the third stage of labour and its use is not contraindicated in patients with PoTS. Intravenous use of oxytocin in the management of both labour dystocia and postpartum haemorrhage is not contraindicated, although its delivery should be slow owing to the potential side effects of hypotension and reflex tachycardia. Prostaglandins often used for induction of labour and to treat post partum haemorrhage, are all safe in patients with PoTS.

Postural Tachycardia Syndrome and the Puerperium

Immediately after delivery there is a significant fluid volume shift with autotransfusion of up to a litre of blood from the uterus back into the maternal circulation. These haemodynamic changes reach equilibrium within an hour after delivery by which time women usually report stable symptoms [4]. Excessive postpartum diuresis may contribute to a reduced plasma volume, which may delay this recovery. A minority of patients experience deterioration in their symptoms, although most will resolve to baseline by six months [2]. Patients with PoTS who remain symptomatic should only be discharged from hospital when their symptoms have stabilised. Women should be supported by a partner or carers at home, and consideration should be given to the mother with autonomic disturbance when nursing a newborn baby. Both beta-blockers and fludrocortisone are safe to continue postpartum when breastfeeding. There are no data for midodrine and ivabradine and these are usually avoided (See Table 1).

References

1. Morgan K, Chojenta C, Taverner M, Smith A, Loxton D. Postural orthostatic tachycardia syndrome during pregnancy: a systematic review of the literature. Auto Neurosci Basic Clin. 2018;215:106–18.
2. Bhatia M, Kavi L, Nelson-Piercy C. Postural tachycardia syndrome and pregnancy. Obstetric Gynaecol. 2018;20:119–23.
3. Nelson-Piercy C. Handbook of Obstetric Medicine. 5th Edition. Baton Rouge. 2015.
4. Ruzieh M, Grub BP. Overview of the management of postural tachycardia syndrome in pregnant patients. Auto Neurosci Basic Clin. 2018;215:102–5.
5. Zadourian A, Doherty TA, Swiatkiewicz I, Taud PR. Postural orthostatic tachycardia syndrome: prevalence, pathophysiology and management. Drugs. 2018; 78:983–994.
6. Blitshteyn S, Poya H, Bett GCL. Pregnancy in postural tachycardia syndrome: clinical course and maternal and fetal outcomes. J Mater Fetal Neonat Med. 2012;25:1631–4.
7. Powless CA, Harms RW, Watson WJ. Postural tachycardia syndrome complicating pregnancy. J Mater Fetal Neonatal Med. 2010;23:850–3.
8. Faculty of Sexual and Reproductive Healthcare Clinical Guidelines.
9. https://www.fsrh.org/standards-and-guidance/ (Accessed 22nd February 2020).
10. Peggs KJ, Nguyen H, Enayat D, Keller NR, Al-Hendy A, Raj SR. Gynecologic disorders and menstrual cycle lightheadedness in postural tachycardia syndrome. Int J Gynaecol Obstet. 2012;118(3):242–6.
11. McEvoy MD, Low PA, Hebbar L. Postural orthostatic tachycardia syndrome: anesthetic implications in the obstetric patient. Obstetr Anesthesia. 2007;104:166–7.
12. Lide B, Haeri S. A care report and review of postural orthostatic tachycardia syndrome in pregnancy. Am J Perinatol. 2015;5:33–6.

13. Cauldwell M, et al. Birth weight in pregnancies complicated by maternal heart disease. Heart. 2019;105:391–8.
14. Potsuk.org (2017) Postural Tachycardia Syndrome (PoTS and Pregnancy) https://www.potsuk.org/pregnancy (Accessed 20th February 2019).
15. Miller AJ, Raj SR. Pharmacotherapy for postural tachycardia syndrome. Auton Neurosci. 2018;215:28–36.
16. National Institute for Health and Care Excellence. Antenatal and Postnatal Mental Health. National Clinical Guideline Number 192. London. NICE. 2016.

Anaesthetic Considerations

Peter William Vaughan Wicks and Roger Cordery

Literature relating to the perioperative care of the patient with PoTS is limited to a small case series and a number of individual case reports. Although there is very little evidence base for decision making during the perioperative period, knowledge of the underlying pathophysiological mechanisms can allow an understanding of the possible response to anaesthetic techniques and can guide the delivery of safe perioperative care.

Pathophysiological Mechanisms

PoTS is the manifestation of a number of pathophysiological processes which may occur either on their own or co-exist in the individual. The Heart Rhythm Society consensus document describes five underlying pathophysiological mechanisms [1].

- **Peripheral autonomic denervation**: Reduced sympathetic tone resulting from autonomic neuropathy leads to venous pooling in the lower limbs and splanchnic beds. The requirement for a compensatory increase in cardiac output to maintain perfusion pressure on standing results in the clinical features of PoTS [1].

  Anaesthetic Consequences: There is a potential for an increased hypotensive response to general/neuraxial anaesthesia and positional changes during anaesthesia.

- **Hypovolaemia**: 70% of patients with PoTS have reduced blood volume. A small study identified a total blood volume deficit of 689mls ± 270mls compared with predicted ideal blood volume. There is a failure of renin and aldosterone levels to rise in response to this reduced volume state [2].

  Anaesthetic Consequences: There is potential for an exaggerated response to blood loss, positive pressure ventilation or pneumoperitoneum.

- **Hyperadrenergic PoTS**: Standing upright for 10 min results in an increase in systolic blood pressure of > 10 mmHg associated with a rise in plasma norepinephrine levels of > 600 pg/mL. Sympathetic activation symptoms (palpitations, anxiety, and tremor) predominate in these patients [3].

  Anaesthetic Consequences: There is a heightened response to isoprenaline in these patients and beta agonists should be titrated carefully. Patients have the potential for an exaggerated response to laryngoscopy, surgical stimulation and agents which

P. W. V. Wicks
Department of Anaesthesia, University Hospital Southampton, Tremona Rd, Southampton SO16 6YD, UK

R. Cordery (✉)
Department of Perioperative Medicine, Barts Heart Centre, St Bartholomew's Hospital, West Smithfield, London EC17BE, UK
e-mail: rogercordery@nhs.net

N. Gall et al. (eds.), *Postural Tachycardia Syndrome*, https://doi.org/10.1007/978-3-030-54165-1_38

result in catecholamine release (ketamine, desflurane) [4].

- **Deconditioning**: Poor exercise tolerance and deconditioning seen in patients with PoTS leads to a reduced left ventricular mass, stroke volume and blood volume. Reduced stroke volume requires a tachycardic response to impaired cardiac filling on standing. Exercise training can improve the cardiovascular manifestations of deconditioning.

  Anaesthetic Consequences: There is the potential for poor compliance with post operative rehabilitation programmes which may affect recovery. Decreased ability for early post operative mobilisation may increase chance of postoperative venous thromboembolic and respiratory complications [5, 6].

- **Anxiety and Hypervigilance**: Patients with PoTS have higher levels of anxiety and somatic hypervigilance. Although it has been shown this is not the primary cause of the exaggerated heart rate response to standing there may be a psychological contribution to the symptoms felt by the patient [6].

  Anaesthetic Consequences: Somatic hypervigilance may predispose to increased postoperative pain. Anxiety has been associated with increased postoperative chronic pain [7].

Anaesthetic Management

Preoperative

In addition to a routine anaesthetic history and examination, preoperative assessment of patients with PoTS should involve the following:

1. Focused questioning of symptoms to allow identification of possible underlying pathophysiological mechanisms and establishing factors which can trigger symptoms in the patient.
2. Identification of any conditions associated with PoTS with relevance to anaesthetic management. (Table 1)
3. Review of the patient's usual medical therapy. Medications used for the treatment of PoTS and their potential implications to anaesthesia are described in Table 2. Where possible medications should be continued throughout the perioperative period to prevent worsening of symptoms which may affect engagement with rehabilitation and recovery.
4. Providing reassurance and consideration of preoperative anxiolysis.

Intraoperative

The lack of academic literature means that the optimal anaesthetic technique for the patient with PoTS is unknown. The main intraoperative considerations relate to the potential for haemodynamic instability and the possibility of an exaggerated response to hypovolaemia (Table 2) [10].

In a case series of thirteen patients with PoTS undergoing elective general anaesthesia, three patients developed prolonged intraoperative hypotension despite relative stability during induction. In two of these patients, the changes were associated with positional changes. All were treated effectively with ephedrine or phenylephrine boluses with no postoperative effects [10]. Given this potential for haemodynamic instability, invasive monitoring should be considered for surgery where blood loss or major fluid shifts are likely. Vigilance is required during positional changes with an anticipation for the need for vasopressor therapy. Intravenous boluses of crystalloid solutions have been used as an effective treatment of tachycardia associated with postural changes [11] and the correction of relative hypovolaemia may reduce haemodynamic instability.

Table 1 Conditions Associated with PoTS [8, 9]

Chronic Fatigue Syndrome
Ehlers-Danlos Syndrome
Mitral Valve Prolapse
Inflammatory Bowel Disease

Table 2 Pharmacological treatment and consequences to anaesthetics [1, 4]

Midodrine	• Prodrug acting on peripheral Alpha-1 adreno-receptors	• Potential for supine hypertension
Fludrocortisone	• Sodium retention and increased sensitivity to circulating catecholamines	• 50% have hypokalaemia and 10% hypomagnesemia • Risk of adrenal insufficiency with long term doses greater than 0.3 mg/d
Propranolol	• Non-selective beta-antagonist used for symptomatic improvement	• Enhances effect of muscle relaxants and antagonises neostigmine • Enhances antihypertensive effect and relative resistance to beta agonist therapy
Pyridostigmine	• Enhances sympathetic ganglionic neurotransmission blunting orthostatic tachycardia	• Unpredictable response of non-depolarising neuromuscular blockers
Clonidine	• Alpha-2 agonist useful in hyperadrenergic PoTS	• Enhanced sedative and hypotensive effect with anaesthetics • Rebound hypertension with abrupt withdrawal
Methyldopa	• Central sympatholytic agent useful in hyperadrenergic PoTS	• Enhanced hypotensive effect with anaesthetics

Agents which produce a tachycardia should be avoided where possible. Patients with hyperadrenergic PoTS may produce an exaggerated response to stimulation of the sympathetic system [12] and care should be taken with the administration of beta-agonists and agents which result in catecholamine release such as ketamine.

Neuraxial anaesthesia has been safely used in obstetric patients with PoTS, although consideration needs to be taken for the possibility of pronounced hypotension and its potential consequences for the foetus and mother. In hyperadrenergic PoTS an early epidural to inhibit an exaggerated sympathetic response to labour may be of benefit. Caesarean section under regional anaesthesia and general anaesthesia have been described [9, 13, 14]. There are no descriptions in the literature of the use of neuraxial anaesthesia in the non-parturient.

The presence of anxiety and somatic hypervigilance in PoTS patients may place them at increased risk of severe postoperative pain. A pre-emptive multimodal analgesic approach should be used with consideration of the use of regional anaesthetic techniques.

Postoperative

Postoperative care and rehabilitation may present a challenge as a result of deconditioning, chronic fatigue and orthostatic symptoms. A planned multidisciplinary approach should be used with engagement of the patient's primary PoTS physician where required. Effective symptom control will allow early mobilisation and engagement with rehabilitation. This should involve continuation of the patient's regular medications in addition to avoiding drugs that may stimulate a tachycardia. Increased postoperative pain should be anticipated and effective rescue analgesia should be prescribed.

References

1. Sheldon RS, Grubb BP, Olshansky B, et al. 2015 Heart rhythm society expert consensus statement on the diagnosis and treatment of postural tachycardia syndrome, inappropriate sinus tachycardia, and vasovagal syncope. Heart Rhythm. 2015;12(6):e41–63.
2. Raj SR, Biaggioni I, Yamhure PC, Black BK, Paranjape SY, Byrne DW, Robertson D. Renin-aldosterone paradox and perturbed blood volume regulation underlying postural tachycardia syndrome. Circulation. 2005;111:1574–82.

3. Garland EM, Raj SR, Black BK, Harris PA, Robertson D. The hemodynamic and neurohumoral phenotype of postural tachycardia syndrome. Neurology. 2007;69:790–8.
4. Mustafa HI, Fessel JP, Barwise J, et al. Dysautonomia: Perioperative Implications. Anesthesiology. 2012;116(1):205–15.
5. Fu Q, Vangundy TB, Galbreath MM, Shibata S, Jain M, Hastings JL, Bhella PS, Levine BD. Cardiac origins of the postural orthostatic tachycardia syndrome. J Am Coll Cardiol. 2010;55:2858–68.
6. Masuki S, Eisenach JH, Johnson CP, Dietz NM, Benrud-Larson LM, Schrage WG, Curry TB, Sandroni P, Low PA, Joyner MJ. Excessive heart rate response to orthostatic stress in postural tachycardia syndrome is not caused by anxiety. J Appl Physiol. 2007;102:896–903.
7. Stamenkovic DM, Rancic NK, Latas MB, Neskovic V, Rondovic GM, Wu JD, et al. Preoperative anxiety and implications on postoperative recovery: what can we do to change our history. Minerva Anestesiol. 2018;84:1307–17.
8. Benarroch EE. Postural tachycardia syndrome: a heterogeneous and multifactorial disorder. Mayo Clin Proc. 2012;87(12):1214–25.
9. Corbett W, Reiter C, JSchultz J , Kanter R, Habib R. Anaesthetic management of a parturient with the postural orthostatic tachycardia syndrome: a case report. British J Anaesthes. 2006; 97(2):196–9.
10. Rabbitts JA, Groenewald CB, Jacob AK, Low PA, Curry TB. Postural orthostatic tachycardia syndrome and general anesthesia: a series of 13 cases. J Clin Anesth. 2011;23(5):384–92.
11. Jacob G, Shannon JR, Black B, Biaggioni I, Mosqueda-Garcia R, Robertson RM, Robertson D. Effects of volume loading and pressor agents in idiopathic orthostatic tachycardia. Circulation. 1997;96:575–80.
12. Abe H, Nagatomo T, Kohshi K, Numata T, Kikuchi K, Sonoda S, Mizuki T, Kuroiwa A, Nakashima Y. Heart rate and plasma cyclic AMP responses to isoproterenol infusion and effect of beta-adrenergic blockade in patients with postural orthostatic tachycardia syndrome. J Cardiovasc Pharmacol. 2000;36(Suppl 2):S79–82.
13. McEvoy M, Low P, Hebbar L. Postural orthostatic tachycardia syndrome: anesthetic implications in the obstetric patient. Anesth Analg. 2007;104(1):166–7.
14. Lide B, Haer S. A Case Report and Review of Postural Orthostatic Tachycardia Syndrome in Pregnancy. Am J Perinatol Rep. 2015;5:e33–6.

Respiratory Specific Diagnostic Tests and Physiotherapy Intervention for Patients with PoTS Presenting with Breathlessness

Charles C. Reilly, Sarah V. Floyd and Kai K. Lee

Breathlessness in Patients with PoTS

Breathlessness is a highly prevalent symptom in patients with PoTS [1, 2]. Cohort studies suggest that $\geq 65\%$ of patients experience significant breathlessness [2]. However, little is known about the aetiology of breathlessness in this patient group, but it is most likely to be multifactorial. Recent data from Reilly CC et al. suggests that dysfunctional breathing is common in patients with PoTS resulting in inappropriate breathlessness [1].

In the context of PoTS, patients often attribute their breathlessness to changes in their breathing pattern, frequency or quality alongside cardiac symptoms such as tachycardia and/or palpitations. For many patients with PoTS, their breathlessness can be episodic, triggered by physical activity or stressful thoughts and events [1].

C. C. Reilly (✉)
Consultant Physiotherapist in Chronic Respiratory Disease / NIHR Clinical Lecturer, King's College Hospital NHS Foundation Trust, London, UK
e-mail: charles.reilly@nhs.net; charles.c.reilly@kcl.ac.uk

S. V. Floyd
Respiratory Specialist Physiotherapist, King's College Hospital NHS Foundation Trust, London, UK

K. K. Lee
Consultant in Respiratory Medicine, King's College Hospital NHS Foundation Trust, London, UK

Respiratory Specific Clinical Investigations to Assess Breathlessness in Patients with PoTS

The assessment of breathlessness in PoTS should be performed in a similar fashion to the usual investigation pathways for other patients.

Based on clinical experience, we recommend that the following investigations be considered in the assessment of a patient with PoTS presenting with chronic and/or disproportionate breathlessness. The appropriateness of each investigation should be guided by the degree of suspicion from the clinician as determined by the clinical history and examination findings.

Lung function testing: Spirometry is a simple non-invasive test that can provide a valuable insight into likely underlying lung pathophysiology. The forced expiratory volume in one second (FEV_1) and forced vital capacity (FVC) parameters can highlight obstructive lung defects due to diseases such as chronic obstructive pulmonary disease (COPD) and asthma, or restrictive lung defects due to obesity, interstitial lung diseases or chest wall disease. In patients with obstructive spirometry, measurement of fraction of exhaled nitric oxide (FeNO) is

N. Gall et al. (eds.), *Postural Tachycardia Syndrome*, https://doi.org/10.1007/978-3-030-54165-1_39

recommended to assess for airway inflammation where asthma is suspected. Since bronchodilator reversibility testing with the use of beta-agonists may not be preferred in patients with PoTS, a bronchial challenge test e.g. methacholine may be considered instead to screen for airway hypersensitivity. Measurement of static lung volumes may be considered if a restrictive lung pattern is found on spirometry [3].

Chest radiograph: a chest radiograph should be considered in patients with chronic symptoms to exclude underlying major structural lung pathology but especially in those with acute breathlessness. For example, pneumothorax should be considered in patients with co-existent Ehlers-Danlos Syndrome who complain of acute breathlessness and chest pain. Other possible abnormal radiographic findings include hyperinflation due to chronic obstructive airways diseases, a raised hemi-diaphragm suggestive of respiratory muscle weakness, increased interstitial markings due to parenchymal lung diseases or signs of pulmonary oedema due to heart failure.

Hyperventilation provocation test: this test will help to determine if a patient may have hyperventilation syndrome (HVS), the most common dysfunctional breathing pattern. A positive hyperventilation provocation test is defined as: end-tidal carbon dioxide ($etCO_2$) at rest or 10 min post-voluntary hyperventilation < 4.3 kPa. Capillary blood gas with a significant reduction in $PaCO_2$ and a Nijmegen score $> 23/60$ will additionally support this diagnosis [1, 4].

Cardiopulmonary exercise text (CPET): if available, CPET can be useful in identifying the significant factors underlying a patient's breathlessness and can be particularly useful in patients with disproportionate symptoms. CPET can also identify dysfunctional breathing patterns (DB) [1, 5] and therefore may supersede the need for some of the tests listed above.

Respiratory muscle testing: although not considered routine, investigations for respiratory muscle weakness should be prompted by the presence of symptoms such as significant/intolerable breathlessness when lying flat, bending forwards i.e. to tie shoes laces or to pick something up off the floor, sitting in a bath or standing in a swimming pool and/or where the patient reports significant sleep disturbance specifically due to breathlessness or gasping for breath. Respiratory muscle function testing should include multiple tests [6] which include: sitting and lying vital capacity (VC) (drop in VC $\geq 30\%$ suggestive of diaphragm weakness), a sniff nasal inspiratory pressure (SNIP) and/or maximum inspiratory pressure measured at the mouth (MIP). Both the SNIP and MIP provide measures of inspiratory muscle strength; reference ranges are available for the clinical diagnosis of inspiratory muscle strength [6]. If respiratory muscle weakness is suggested or there is significant breathlessness related to sleep disturbance then overnight pulse oximetry is recommended.

Dysfunctional Breathing Patterns in Patients with PoTS

Dysfunctional breathing (DB) is an umbrella term describing breathing disorders where chronic changes in breathing pattern result in inappropriate breathlessness and other symptoms in the absence or disproportinate to the magnitude of physiological respiratory or cardiac disease [7]. There is no consensus definition of dysfunctional breathing or gold standard diagnostic criteria. The most widely recognised form of dysfunctional breathing is hyperventilation syndrome (HVS); this term is often also used synonymously with dysfunctional breathing, whereas in fact it is just one type of breathing pattern disorder.

To appropriately describe dysfunctional breathing, *Boulding R and colleagues* [7] suggest the following classification: **(1) Hyperventilation syndrome**: associated with symptoms both related to respiratory alkalosis and independent of hypocapnia; **(2) Periodic deep sighing**: frequent sighing with an irregular breathing pattern; **(3) Thoracic dominant breathing**: can often manifest in somatic disease, if occurring without disease it may be considered dysfunctional and results in dyspnoea; **(4) Forced abdominal expiration**: these patients utilise inappropriate and excessive abdominal muscle contraction to aid expiration; **(5) Thoraco-abdominal asynchrony**: where there is a delay between rib cage and abdominal contraction resulting in ineffective breathing mechanics. DB is not a continuously symptomatic state but a syndrome of episodic symptoms that occur with or without recognizable provocation [7–9].

It is estimated that DB/HVS affects 10% of the general population and is more prevalent in women than in men [10]. Recent data by Reilly CC et al. demonstrated that patients with PoTS who reported significant breathlessness at rest or disproportionate breathlessness on exertion, and/or symptoms of air hunger, excessive yawing or sighing, had DB/HVS [1].

DB/HVS may coexist with chronic respiratory diseases such as asthma [10] and chronic obstructive pulmonary disease [11] although whether the relationship is causal or coincidental remains unclear. More frequently DB occurs in the absence of respiratory disease.

Unexplained breathlessness and '*air hunger*' are the predominant symptoms of DB/HVS [12, 13]. DB/HVS can result in significant patient morbidity and an array of non-respiratory symptoms including: chest tightness, dizziness, palpitations, pins and needles most noted in the feet, hands or around the mouth [12, 13]. The presence of these symptoms can themselves result in anxiety and panic, which can provoke further breathing irregularity.

While orthostatic tachycardia is the hallmark of PoTS, orthostasis also initiates increased minute ventilation and decreased end – tidal CO_2 in many patients. Hyperpnea in PoTS is related to sympathetic baroreflex stimulation and almost complete cardiovagal baroreflex withdrawal [24] resulting in hypocapnia. PoTS patients have decreased central chemosensitivity to CO_2 but conversely peripheral chemosensitivity to hypoxia is enhanced [14]. It is hypothesised that the enhanced hypoxic sensitivity may contribute to the long-term facilitation of sympathoexcitation in patients with PoTS, resulting in chronic hyperventilation/ dysfunctional breathing patterns. The hypocapnia resulting from chronic/intermittent hyperventilation reduces cerebral blood flow and contributes to light-headedness and to cognitive impairment during daily life. It also lowers the excitatory threshold for nerve fibres resulting in paraesthesiae and reduces the Bohr effect so that haemoglobin releases oxygen less easily. Acute on chronic hyperventilation results in a reduction in peripheral vascular resistance and reduced mean arterial blood pressure (MAP). The reduced MAP exacerbates or triggers PoTS symptoms of light headiness and fainting, as well as increasing heart rate to compensate for the reduced venous return and lowered cardiac output, and maintain blood pressure [1, 14, 15]. It must be acknowledged that psychological influences such as stress, anxiety and depression, which are prevalent in patients with PoTS [16, 17], may also predispose patients to DB/HVS.

Physiotherapy as a Potential Treatment for DB/HVS in Patients with PoTS

Reilly CC, et al. reported that a physiotherapy intervention, which focussed on breathing retraining for patients with PoTS and dysfunctional breathing, improved patients breathing pattern and symptom burden [1].

When to Refer to Respiratory Physiotherapy

- All patients with a formal diagnosis of PoTS that report symptoms of breathlessness at rest, on exertion or with disproportionate breathlessness on activity and/or breath-holding, sighing and excessive yawning should be referred to respiratory physiotherapy for a breathing pattern assessment. If a patient has a physiotherapist diagnosed dysfunctional breathing pattern, they should be provided with advice and breathing exercises to help treat/manage their dysfunctional breathing pattern and associated breathlessness [1].

- Ideally patients should be established/optimised with regards to their cardiac symptoms. However, this should not be a pre-requisite given the complexity of PoTS[1].
- Early access to physiotherapy is recommended, as early physiotherapy intervention for DB/HVS may result in better outcomes.

What Physiotherapy Interventions can be helpful in the management of DFB/HVS in PoTS?

- Patient education: focusing on the patient's understanding of: (1) respiratory physiology, specifically respiratory control and normal breathing pattern (2) the mind—body link and how external factors such as anxiety, stress and lifestyle influences breathing patterns resulting in breathlessness [1].
- Breathing re-training should include the following techniques: (1) breathing control at rest and during activity, (2) controlled pause technique [1].
- In addition, the following physiotherapy treatments should be considered: sinus management, airway clearance techniques, postural exercises and exercise advice.

Physiotherapy Good Practice Points

- Patients should be provided with information regarding stress and lifestyle management e.g. pacing and relaxation techniques
- Each patient should be provided with an individualised self-management plan.
- In addition, the link between anxiety and hyperventilation should not be overlooked, and where appropriate, patients should be referred for psychological support or counselling.

References

1. Reilly CC, et al. Breathlessness and dysfunctional breathing in patients with postural orthostatic tachycardia syndrome (PoTS): The impact of a physiotherapy intervention. Auton Neurosci. 2020;223:102601.
2. Boris JR, Bernadzikowski T. Demographics of a large paediatric postural orthostatic tachycardia syndrome program. Cardiol Young. 2018;28(5):668–74.
3. Nicholson PJ. The updated ATS/ERS spirometry technical standards. Occupational Medicine (Oxford, England). 2020:kqaa030.
4. van Dixhoorn J, Duivenvoorden HJ. Efficacy of Nijmegen Questionnaire in recognition of the hyperventilation syndrome. J Psychosom Res. 1985;29(2):199–206.
5. Ross RM. ATS/ACCP statement on cardiopulmonary exercise testing. Am J Respir Crit Care Med. 2003;167(10):1451–1451.
6. Steier J, et al. The value of multiple tests of respiratory muscle strength. Thorax. 2007;62(11):975–80.
7. Boulding R, et al. Dysfunctional breathing: a review of the literature and proposal for classification. Eur Respir Rev. 2016;25(141):287–94.
8. Depiazzi J, Everard ML. Dysfunctional breathing and reaching one's physiological limit as causes of exercise-induced dyspnoea. Breathe (Sheff). 2016;12(2):120–9.
9. Vidotto LS, et al. Dysfunctional breathing: what do we know? J Bras Pneumol. 2019;45(1):e20170347.
10. Thomas M, et al. The prevalence of dysfunctional breathing in adults in the community with and without asthma. Primary Care Respirat J J Gener Pract Airways Group. 2005;14(2):78–82.
11. Law N, et al. Dysfunctional breathing is more frequent in chronic obstructive pulmonary disease than in asthma and in health. Respir Phy Neurobiol. 2018;247:20–3.
12. Bott J, et al. Guidelines for the physiotherapy management of the adult, medical, spontaneously breathing patient. Thorax. 2009;64(Suppl 1):i1–51.
13. Gardner WN. The pathophysiology of hyperventilation disorders. Chest. 1996;109(2):516–34.
14. Taneja I, et al. Baroreceptor unloading in postural tachycardia syndrome augments peripheral chemoreceptor sensitivity and decreases central chemoreceptor sensitivity. Am J Physiol Heart Circulat Physiol . 2011;301(1):H173–9.
15. Fortune JB et al. Cerebral blood flow and blood volume in response to O2 and CO2 changes in normal humans. J Trauma. 1995; **39**(3):463–71; discussion 471–2.
16. Pederson CL, Brook JB. Health-related quality of life and suicide risk in postural tachycardia syndrome. Clin Auton Res. 2017;27(2):75–81.
17. McDonald C, et al. Postural tachycardia syndrome is associated with significant symptoms and functional impairment predominantly affecting young women: a UK perspective. BMJ Open. 2014;4(6):e004127.

Psychological and Psychiatric Support; When, Why and What to Do

Morwenna Opie, Vidya Raj and Amy C. Arnold

Introduction

This chapter offers a clinically-focused review of the limited available research pertaining to psychological and cognitive influences in PoTS patients. We will discuss common psychological co-morbidities in patients with PoTS, and the indications and goals for referral to psychiatric and affiliated services.

We examine treatment interventions with empirical support in other long term conditions (LTCs) including Cognitive Behavioural Therapy (CBT), Mindfulness-Based Cognitive Therapy (MBCT), and Acceptance and Commitment Therapy (ACT); considering some of the key relevant therapeutic aspects of these approaches. Of necessity, as this section is sparse on condition-specific research data, it relies heavily on the authors' collective clinical experience. Pharmacological interventions will also be reviewed, including contraindications for some commonly prescribed medications in this patient group. It is our clinical experience that PoTS patients can be either highly sensitive to medications or occasionally appear unresponsive to them.

Understanding the complex interaction of psychological and physiological processes in PoTS and other LTCs (long term conditions) is challenging. The conceptual separation of body and mind seems especially ill-fitting to disorders like PoTS, which involve the autonomic nervous system and can impact aspects of attention and cognitive functioning. Attempting to tease out these dynamically-interrelated influences makes it clear that trying to understand symptoms as either exclusively physical or psychological is unhelpful for either effective formulation or treatment. PoTS patients can present to clinicians as anxious, and may have received diagnoses of anxiety disorders previously. Having been told their symptoms are "all in their head" can be confusing, distressing and lead to resistance to engaging with mental health services, which can be a beneficial adjunct to standard medical care if sensitively and appropriately delivered.

M. Opie (✉)
Department Clinical Health Psychology, Royal Cornwall Hospital Treliske, Cornwall, Truro TR1 3LJ, UK
e-mail: morwenna.opie-moran@nhs.net

V. Raj
Departments of Psychiatry, Cardiac Sciences and Family Medicine, University of Calgary, Calgary, AB, Canada
e-mail: vidya.raj@ahs.ca

A. C. Arnold
Department of Neural and Behavioral Sciences, Penn State College of Medicine, Hershey, PA, US
e-mail: aca17@psu.edu

A. C. Arnold
Division of Clinical Pharmacology, Vanderbilt University Medical Center, Nashville, TN, US

N. Gall et al. (eds.), *Postural Tachycardia Syndrome*, https://doi.org/10.1007/978-3-030-54165-1_40

We emphasise that in patient interactions, every health professional influences the psychology of their patients. As yet, there are few psychological magic bullets for PoTS patients; however, patient experience speaks to the transformative power of diagnosis, acceptance, and being taken seriously. Hope and understanding are arguably some of the most powerful therapeutic interventions for LTCs. Isolation and taking on the patient identity can become factors in a patient's mental decline. Patients who feel able to take the lead in actively managing their condition appear to do best. Recognising that, as well as attending to physiological considerations as medical and allied-health practitioners, we have the potential to influence patients' psychological well-being, simply acknowledging and validating their difficulties opens up powerful therapeutic opportunities in consultations. Helping PoTS patients access psychological and psychiatric support when appropriate, destigmatising these approaches, and breaking down the division between mind and body, can be enormously helpful.

Key Considerations in PoTS

- PoTS is not a mental health condition. It is distinct from anxiety and associated reactive depressions, which are common in many LTCs and can affect QoL and involve "invisible" scary and unpredictable symptoms.
- There is contradictory evidence on whether there are increased rates of mental health problems such as anxiety and depressive disorders in patients with PoTS. This is, in part, a function of methodology (such as use of somatically focused measures to assess mood and anxiety symptoms) and relates to an outdated separation of mind and body (which is particularly inappropriate in considering disorders of the autonomic nervous system).
- Impaired attention appears to be highly prevalent and troublesome in PoTS. Cognitive dysfunction or "brain fog" is often cited by patients as the most troubling of their many symptoms, and is often present even in the supine and seated positions when classical orthostatic symptoms are minimized.
- A patient's attention to unpleasant physiological sensations is a fine balance between avoiding under-attention to physical cues (and preventing syncope/over-exertion) and over-attention (can lead to hyper-vigilance and exaggerated fight/flight responses and behavioural avoidance).
- PoTs can negatively impact on many areas which compromise mental health (e.g. sleep, mobility, appetite, relationships, activities), thus making usual coping strategies less accessible.
- In the absence of a single disease pathway or 'cure', psychological support can be an important consideration in supporting the many changes required to help patients achieve optimal functioning. Psychological support, however, may not be necessary in all PoTS patients.
- In combination with research from other chronic health conditions, there is reasonable rationale for why therapeutic interventions such as CBT and MBCT/ACT can play a useful part in the multidisciplinary treatment of PoTS.
- There are some emerging data indicating elevated suicidality within this patient group. Safety screening and asking about thoughts around self-harm should be a routine part of clinical contact with any healthcare provider.
- Referral to psychiatric and psychological services should be done sensitively. This is required to avoid stigmatization and, given that many patients have previously been told their condition is "all in their head", creating resistance to engaging. Inter-disciplinary collaboration can assist with this.
- Pharmacological approaches need to be considered with awareness of some of the documented relative contraindications in PoTS patients.

Quality of Life

There is clear evidence for reduced QoL in PoTS patients, even those with relatively mild orthostatic intolerance symptoms on tilt [1–3]. The finding that physical health related QoL reduction is similar in PoTS to CHF and COPD is tragic [1], particularly given that PoTS patients are typically pre-menopausal women previously in an active and productive period of their lives. This is of course also a critical time when coping strategies, relationships, and life-goals are still developing, and education still ongoing. Data on functional impacts have largely come from self-report questionnaires with resulting questions about validity; however, these results capture powerful statistics about the breath of disability. One study reported that 76% of PoTS patients need help with routine activities such as shopping, and 30% need help with personal care [4]. In a separate study, 23% of PoTS respondents were wheelchair users, 50% of school aged patients were unable to continue to attend education, and 41% of patients reported financial loss associated with health-related changes [5]. Such profound and rapid changes are likely to be important factors in impaired QoL and mental distress. Recent work looking at suicidal ideation in PoTS patients found elevated suicidal ideation well above the general population and equivalent to psychiatric in-patient groups [4]. Clearly, this is of great concern and requires further investigation. Research suggests that part of this increased suicidal ideation is associated with sleep disturbance [6]. Indeed, there is evidence that sleep is also implicated in compromised QoL in PoTS, as well as in cognitive impairment, pain, and fatigue [7].

Mood Disorders

There is some debate about whether patients with PoTS are more prone to mental health difficulties. Of course, patients with PoTS are not immune to mood disorders which are prevalent among the general population. The Office of National Statistics cited a prevalence as high as one-fifth of adults who experienced anxiety or depression in their 2015 data collection, with rates being even higher in women [8]. Rates of depressive disorders are more than twice as common as the national average in other LTCs with similar impacts on QoL as PoTS, such as COPD [9, 10]. Overall, despite limited research in this area, it is reasonable to assume that patients with PoTS are equally (but not more) likely to have compromised mood as patients with other chronic health issues.

McGrady et al. documented increased rates of depression associated with positive tilt table tests for autonomic dysfunction [11]. The psychiatric profiles of patients with PoTS were examined in more detail in a study by Raj et al. [12]. This study found that patients did not have an increased prevalence of major depression compared to the general population. Subjects typically had mild depression, and interestingly depression scores were inversely related to time since diagnosis, suggesting some process of adjustment and acceptance tends to operate over time [12]. Moon et al. similarly observed a mean self-rated depression score that fell in the mild range in adolescent and adult PoTS patients compared with normative population scores [3]. The orthostatic intolerance symptoms most strongly associated with depression in this study were impaired concentration, chest discomfort, palpitations, lightheadedness, and nausea.

In summary, there is consistent evidence of mild-moderate depression in PoTS. Several studies found a positive correlation between depression scores and self-rated orthostatic symptom burden, but not with HR variability [3], which may be a red-herring for assessing the severity of the syndrome as a whole. One study reported less mood disturbance with increasing time from diagnosis, which is consistent with a reactive/adjustment mood disorder hypothesis [12]. Of great concern, however, is increased suicidality in this patient group, which is associated with impaired sleep, and likely reflects how distressing living with PoTS can be [4, 6]. It is consequently important to screen for suicidal ideation and we recommend this should be a routine part of any clinical contact.

Anxiety and PoTS

In clinical anxiety, mind (worry, fearful cognitions, perceptions of threat and ability to cope) and body (somatic symptoms such as a racing heart, sweating, altered breathing, attention changes) are dynamically interrelated, both feeding into a vicious cycle. Patients with PoTS are typically perceived as anxious, but it is important to recongise that there is significant overlap between somatic aspects of anxiety and PoTS symptomology. In the case of patients with PoTS, in order to understand what is driving and maintaining distress and tailor treatment appropriately, separating the two conceptually can be important.

A series of elegant studies have addressed whether PoTS patients mistakenly appear anxious due to overlap of their orthostatic symptoms with the physiological symptoms of anxiety (e.g. elevated heart rate, palpitations, sweating, difficulty concentrating), or truly experience anxiety (consisting of both physiological and psychological symptom components) [7, 12–14]. These studies consistently conclude that the former is true. For example, Khurana et al. demonstrated by provoking somatic anxiety using both orthostatic and pharmacological stimuli, that panic-like symptoms in PoTs are phenomenally distinct from anxiety disorders [13]. Patients with PoTS, however, do show mildly elevated levels of anxious thinking compared with the general population, and this anxiety focuses on worries about somatic symptoms (particularly cardiovascular) [7].

Adding to this complexity, patients can naturally become anxious about managing independently despite their symptoms. They can fear staying safe, experiencing a faint (hemodynamic or non-hemodynamic), as well as have anxious thoughts about the future and the impact that their illness could have on it. Such thoughts, while understandable and rational, can feed into the clinical picture if untreated, amplifying symptoms and distress. Thus it is still clinically important to consider a comorbid anxiety disorder in patients with PoTS.

Our clinical experience accords with the research finding that the critical drivers in panic disorder and generalized anxiety, such as thoughts about threat, inability to cope, and responses associated with avoidance, are not the drivers or the primary maintaining factors in PoTS. Patients do, however, describe a sense in which they feel their body responding 'excessively anxiously' to situations, and in excess of how they cognitively perceive a threat. They report a sense in which the subtlety of the system is absent, that anxiety can rocket from 0 straight to 100, and some describe a subsequent stalling of cognitive processing, and a feeling of the brain stalling in its flexibility and speed.

All of this speaks to the complex processes at work that we are just beginning to understand more fully. Currently, details are of academic interest, with active research ongoing about what attentional and functional aspects may be involved. In the meantime, the finding that patients experience heightened and extreme sympathetic arousal, and unsubtle physiological changes, is not in dispute. Optimising our capacity to navigate stressors is an essential part of optimising our well-being, especially when our health is compromised and affected by stress. There is therefore a role in PoTS for various types of psychological input typically used to improve anxiety management.

Cognitive Issues

Difficulties with "brain-fog," mental clarity, and feeling 'not entirely present' have been cited as the most troubling symptoms of PoTS [5]. In fact, a survey-based study by Ross et al. found that over 95% of PoTS patients report brain fog, with most experiencing symptoms on a daily basis [15]. These cognitive issues can greatly impair the ability of these patients to participate in occupational and educational activities, thus resulting in reduced QoL and in some cases disability. PoTS patients can often tolerate palpitations when reassured that they are not harmful, and dizziness if reassured that they will not faint, but cognitive difficulties can be refractory even in those well-adjusted to other symptoms.

Despite this high prevalence and clinical impact, only a handful of studies to date have examined the profile of cognitive impairment in PoTS. Raj et al. highlighted that PoTS patients experience significant problems with attention, to a level comparable to patients with attention deficit hyperactivity disorder (ADHD) [12]. Unlike the latter neurodevelopmental condition which emerges in childhood, the presence of inattention symptoms was not reported in PoTS patients prior to orthostatic symptom onset. Compromised attention was noted as an important source of disability.

Recent work by Arnold et al. detected impaired selective attention, cognitive processing speed, and executive function in adult PoTS patients when in the semi-recumbent position [16]. These deficits were selective, with patients having similar reaction time, sustained attention and verbal fluency compared with healthy control subjects. This study, however, did not examine the impact of orthostatic stress on cognitive measures and noted that future studies examining performance on tilt might deliver more prominent findings since patients often report that their cognitive symptoms are worse when upright. Stewart et al. have demonstrated that adolescent PoTS patients with comorbid chronic fatigue syndrome have impaired working memory during graded orthostatic stress, with normal functioning in this domain in the supine position [17]. They further hypothesized from their work that there may be an uncoupling of the neurovascular unit during orthostatic stress in these PoTS patients that contributes to their cognitive dysfunction [18, 19]. As recently reviewed, other hypothesized theories for reported cognitive difficulties include central norepinephrine dysregulation and structural and functional brain abnormalities, which may also contribute to increased vulnerability to autonomic and psychiatric symptoms in PoTS [20].

It has also been hypothesized that significant mood and anxiety difficulties could be causal factors in cognitive dysfunction in patients with PoTS. One study by Anderson et al. examined for changes in cognition during tilt table testing and concluded that impaired attention and short-term memory in PoTS patients versus healthy controls were largely explained by psychological factors including higher levels of anxiety and mood disorders [7]. Although rates of clinically significant depression were higher in this smaller sample, it is worth noting that the mood assessment tool used here, the Hamilton Depression scale, is heavily comprised of somatic factors that overlap with PoTS symptoms (sleep disturbance, motor activity, fatigue and gastrointestinal changes). In contrast, Arnold et al. found no correlation between measures of cognitive impairment and self-reported depression or anxiety symptoms in adult PoTS patients [16]. Thus, the contribution of mood difficulties to cognitive dysfunction in PoTS remains unclear and requires further investigation.

To date, it remains unclear whether cognitive dysfunction in PoTS is a result of orthostatic stress, fatigue, sleep issues, or part of syndrome-specific processes such as central norepinephrine dysregulation. Similarly, we have yet to establish whether the mismatch between subjective patient perceptions and results of objective neuropsychological testing is a consequence of lack of testing specificity or because compromised interception is part of the syndrome itself. In addition, PoTS patients often have comorbidities known to negatively influence cognitive function, and associated with psychiatric difficulties, including autoimmune disorders, chronic pain, irritable bowel syndrome, fibromyalgia, and hypermobile Ehlers-Danlos Syndrome [21–24]. Poor sleep can of course also affect cognitive function, and PoTS patients often report sleep disruption and symptoms of unrefreshing sleep, which may in part be linked with symptoms of hyperarousal [25–27]. It seems likely that an integrated treatment approach targeting these interacting factors will be needed to optimise cognitive outcomes; however, there are no studies examining potential treatment approaches for cognitive difficulties in PoTS.

In summary, studies have shown selective impairment of measures of cognitive function in PoTS including attention, cognitive processing speed, memory function, and executive function. The precise profile of cognitive dysfunction in PoTS patients varies among studies perhaps due to the neuropsychological tests used, postural position, comorbidities and length of illness, inclusion of adolescent versus adult patients, and sites of recruitment. It remains unclear whether cognitive issues are posturally related, or represent different symptom pathways or disease processes. The subtle changes detected on neuropsychological testing often do not match the global and incapacitating deficits reported by patients, leaving more work to be done in this area.

Eating Disorders

Many patients with PoTS have weight change associated with the timing of onset of their symptoms. This may be due to direct changes in hunger-signaling pathways, or changes in eating habits made by patients to manage symptoms established by trial and error (many patients anecdotally report a little-and-often eating strategy works best for them). Those who report early satiety and anorexia as a salient symptom are more likely to end up in treatment for an eating disorder (ED). It would seem important to educate mental health professionals about PoTS, as there are likely to be many missed PoTS diagnoses amongst referrals, particularly in the case of eating disorders services.

A clear defining characteristic of anorexia nervosa (AN) is distortion of body image. A patient with PoTS is more likely to report wishing to eat more but finding themselves unable to do so, and experiencing nausea or symptom escalation when they do. A referral to a gastroenterologist with an interest in autonomic dysfunction, who would work in tandem with a dietician, would be most pertinent to assess for the presence of an ED. Patients with PoTS are not immune to developing AN, which is relatively common in the general population (1 in 250 women, NHS Choices, 2015), and indeed many find restriction easier if appetite is suppressed by their altered physiology. Patients with AN commonly report feeling 'physically out of control' as a trigger for the over-control manifested in their eating behaviours, and in this context PoTS, where feeling physically out of control is commonly reported, could be a risk factor for AN.

In essence, this is another reminder of the importance of widespread physician and healthcare provider education, and also the importance of protective psychological support for patients made vulnerable by their PoTS symptoms.

Psychological Misdiagnosis

To appropriately support anyone with compromised mental health is critical, and there is good reason to think that improving this aspect of a person's functioning will play a part in optimising recovery. To fail to identify PoTS and focus exclusively on addressing the psychology, however, might arguably be doing a greater disservice to patients. Mood and anxiety often directly and rapidly benefit from receiving a diagnosis of PoTs; and PoTS symptoms in the majority of cases respond well to symptomatic management and treatment.

Interestingly in PoTS survey data, psychiatric misdiagnosis was markedly different according to gender, being reported by 75% of women, but only 25% of males [5]. It is clearly unacceptable that men presenting with symptoms of unexplained dizziness, fatigue and palpitations appear more likely to be taken seriously than women with a similar presentation. A recent large, cross-sectional online community-based survey reported that PoTS patients on average experience a 24 month delay and are evaluated by 7 physicians from initial presentation to diagnosis, and often experience misdiagnosis, again with findings more prominent in women compared with men [28]. It is hoped that these unfortunate diagnostic delays in PoTS will improve with ongoing physician education and awareness.

An unhelpful outgrowth of the conceptual separation of mind and body is an erroneous view that disorders involving psychological factors are somehow more of a person's choosing, or under their control, than those of the body. This in turn leads to prejudice, discrimination, and has implications for access to care. This seems to be especially the case in relation to fatigue. PoTS patients may be labelled as lazy, affiliated to outdated assumptions that PoTS is predominately caused by deconditioning associated with avoidance and secondary gain. In fact, survey data suggests that prior to the onset of PoTS, 66% of patients were engaged in regular physical exercise and were high functioning immediately before onset of PoTS symptoms [5]. At a time when there are international criteria, emerging biomarkers, and that many symptoms such as gastric disturbances, somatic anxiety and brain fog respond to treatment, it is surely time to move beyond debates about whether PoTS is real, psychosomatic or 'middle-class.' We should focus energy instead on identifying therapeutic targets and patient-specific multi-specialty coordinated care pathways.

Formulating the triggers for the onset of PoTs, might best be conceptualized, much as in other systemic and autoimmune chronic health conditions, as understanding the brewing of a perfect storm. Physical and psychological stressors such as trauma, loss, life change, concussion or viral illness are quietly accruing contributory factors against a climate of physiological predisposition, with the syndrome often triggered suddenly after one insult too many for the body to maintain equilibrium. Thereafter, challenging and unpredictable symptoms and life changes take their toll, and instinctive coping mechanisms such as rest and avoidance are often unhelpful. This reinforces the important role of maximising all other aspects of health, including mental health and social support, to begin the important process of reconstruction. Calling the crisis early, and making available rapid diagnosis and access to multidisciplinary medical care, including psychological care, is critical to this end.

Trauma Work

Anecdotally, many clinicians report that a disproportionate number of their patients seem to have experienced trauma or abuse. Again, this is an area with little research.

Intuitively one can hypothesize that previous emotional or physical trauma could lead to tendencies to dissociate in order to continue to function amongst emotional or physical pain. This could potentially become habitual, reducing attunement to the body's needs, and leaving a person more likely to plough on and miss physical cues to slow down, heal, restore and reduce stressors. We know that attentional biases, and tendencies towards both extreme hypervigilance and avoidant or dissociative coping strategies, are implicated in whether a traumatic event develops into post traumatic stress disorder (PTSD). Research is currently in progress investigating whether associated conditions such as hypermobility syndromes are more likely to experience adversity as trauma, or develop PTSD or dissociative coping patterns.

While numerous consultants have noticed that a prior trauma history is common in PoTS, we need to remain mindful to the sad reality that many young women, who are the predominant group, have an elevated background rate of exposure to a sexual or violent trauma. One in five women in England and Wales have experienced sexual violence or assult, which is five times the rate for men [29].

Patient Interactional and Cognitive Styles

It is important to acknowledge the view amongst some clinicians that PoTS patients are difficult, draining, overwhelming and even melodramatic or confrontational; the classic 'heart sink' patient. Certainly a PoTS patient's interactional skills may be compromised by 'brain fog' on presentation (40% of patients report this phenomenon, and for them it is often cited as the most troubling symptom) [5]. Patients report that while they still look, move, and sound the same, that they feel somehow removed from their personality and lack full access to their cognitive function. Patients can feel they are compromised in the very capacities which are central to their identity, including ability, creativity and sociability. This can result in a sense of loss of self, and insinuations of exaggerating severity or malingering. Normalising and empathizing with this type of thinking can be therapeutically validating and help a patient move forward by focusing on what they can change.

A patient struggling with the level of disability typically associated with PoTS for the typical seven-year delay between symptom onset and accurate diagnosis may well also be desperate and despondent [5]. Such a patient is likely to have a long list of complaints, overwhelming both for them and the clinician. Often, the complaints that are most distressing and emphasized by the patient (such as brain fog or fatigue) are nebulous and non-specific. They are likely to be so desperate to resolve them that may react very strongly or defensively if such concerns are not treated seriously or empathically. In contrast, they may have adapted to experiencing palpitations and light-headedness so that these are not initially emphasized, or may even be unaware of them given that dissociation from physical symptoms can emerge as a coping strategy. They are likely to be wary of doctors and misdiagnosis, and have thick files which raise a red flag in clinicians trained to be suspicious of a history of unexplained symptoms and referrals to multiple specialists. Such a presentation is more likely to be turned away by physical health professionals, labelled as functional or somatoform disorders or personality disorders, and the somatic aspects of PoTS explained away as a combination of anxiety and depression.

In terms of reaching a workable diagnosis and making sense of complex symptoms straddling the physiological/psychological interface, there is currently no short-cut to a detailed patient-centered history coupled with psychological measures which clearly separate cognitive and somatic hallmarks of depression and anxiety. After this, PoTS-associated compromised attentional and cognitive processes may be evident versus clinically significant 'pure' depression or anxiety. With regard to mood and sympathetic arousal processes, reactive minor depression and symptom-specific anxiety may typically be recognised as the culprits and therapeutic targets. This combination of time required and a rather intimidating interpersonal profile to work with may initially lack appeal to the aspiring clinician. However, these are fascinating presentations and patients often respond extremely well to appropriate intervention. Often offering understanding, a plan, and some hope, are catalysts for significant change with enormous rewards for all involved.

Therapy Evidence Base

Studies may not agree about the nature of processes involved in the mind/body interface in PoTS, but all concur that patients are likely to do better by addressing the psychological, attentional, and adjustment challenges associated with PoTS.

Stress-reduction techniques and CBT are typically advocated; however, there is a paucity of robust, high quality research for cognitive-behavioral interventions in PoTS. Much of the evidence for its recommendation stems from research on associated conditions with similar challenges. There is good evidence, for example, that patients with medical conditions generally benefit from psychotherapies. This is born out for example in COPD [30] which has a comparable impaired health-related QoL to PoTS [9]. CBT has good face validity for treatment of physical health conditions with distressing symptoms. It is centered on developing awareness of the interaction of physical responses with situations, thoughts, emotions, and actions, with the ultimate goal of identifying and changing unhelpful patterns. As an example, catastrophic thinking, a standard target for modification with CBT, has been associated with functional disability in PoTS [1].

Evidence is growing rapidly for variants of traditional CBT approaches based on mindfulness, such as Mindfulness-based cognitive therapy (MBCT). Mindfulness is defined as paying attention to what is happening in the present moment with acceptance, curiosity, and compassion [8]. A large systematic review and meta-analysis, demonstrated that mindfulness-based interventions significantly improved symptoms of depression, anxiety and stress, QoL, and physical functioning [31]. Mindfulness training has been shown to reduce heart rate and stress-related changes in blood pressure in healthy individuals, reduce hypervigilance for, and overly negative interpretations of, bodily sensations, and dampen vicious cycles of worry and physical manifestations of anxiety [32–35].

Practicing mindfulness on a regular basis supports enhanced awareness of experiences and actions, and better adaptations (e.g. responding more flexibly and skillfully to changing symptoms such as palpitations). This can help break cycles of unhelpful thoughts and actions (such as avoidance), which can otherwise increase distress, exacerbate symptoms, and limit functioning. The use of standardized mindfulness-based interventions has been shown to alleviate mental and physical symptoms in patients with cardiovascular disease, cancer, chronic pain, depression and anxiety disorders, as well as prevent symptoms in healthy populations [31] Mindfulness training has also been shown to improve autonomic responses to stress, [32, 35] and, relevantly, to reduce hypervigilance and catastrophic interpretations of symptoms [33, 34].

Some caution appears warranted by a study reporting different outcomes following specialist CBT for patients with chronic fatigue syndrome/ myalgic encephalomyelitis (CFS/ME) diagnosis according to whether they also had PoTS. The study reported a smaller improvement in fatigue, and even deterioration in some cases, in the comorbid PoTS-CFS/ME group [36]. There was a high attrition rate in this study, however, and fatigue was the only reported outcome measure. The authors do not elaborate on the specific CBT techniques used in the study, or on how and over what time period they were delivered, and there seems to have been an emphasis on increasing physical activity. It would be useful to understand the specific elements of the intervention that were perhaps more challenging for PoTS patients, and to explore mood, QoL, and psychosocial outcomes.

An interesting and unanticipated finding emerged from a recent small outcome study of a Mindfulness-Based Stress Reduction (MBSR) program adapted for teenagers with cardiac diagnoses (in which category the investigators included PoTS) [37]. That the comparison group, who received facilitated small group support via video, had outcomes equivalent to the treatment group suggests that group support is perhaps best understood as an intervention, not a non-treatment comparison. This is in line with accruing evidence of the pivotal role of reducing social exclusion and perceived helplessness for positive outcomes in chronic illness [38]. Indeed, reducing isolation may be a very significant factor in any therapeutic intervention. In a study examining adults with congenital heart disease, social adjustment was more predictive of health outcomes than medical variables [39]. Isolation may be a particularly significant factor for young bed-bound women with PoTS. Many patients describe living a life unfathomable to their peers and having been misbelieved and ostracized [5]. It is our opinion that clinicians who work with PoTS patients have an opportunity to engender hope and reduce isolation.

Similar psychosocial adjustment factors could arguably be implicated in the case study of successful CBT treatment in a member of the American military with PoTS [40]. Positive outcomes were recorded in self-assessment of functional symptoms, improved mental well-being, and return to work. As might be anticipated, significant emphasis was placed on the positive effects of challenging catastrophizing thoughts, reducing avoidance of symptom-triggering environments, and practicing tolerating frightening symptoms. While this is a case study, many key aspects of this intervention concur with our own clinical opinion of best practice psychological interventions for patients with PoTS.

ACT is another 'third-wave' outgrowth of CBT. It includes a component of mindfulness, but places greater emphasis on the principle that unpleasant thoughts and emotions are part of life, trying to avoid them is understandable but counterproductive, and a more useful aim is to live in accordance with our values [41]. This seems particularly relevant in the context of chronic medical conditions which might lead to frustration and anxiety. A large meta-analysis of randomised controlled trials demonstrated its efficacy in improving a variety of outcomes in the context of a range of physical and psychological health problems including, for example, blood glucose control in diabetes and seizure frequency in drug refractory epilepsy [42]. We hope that research exploring the efficacy of ACT in patients with PoTS will be forthcoming soon.

Psychiatry Best Practice Considerations in PoTS

As we have discussed, patients with PoTS commonly experience modestly elevated depressive and anxiety symptoms compared to the background population, and are at increased risk of insomnia and experiencing suicidal ideation. In clinical practice, PoTS patients are not immune to experiencing the typical mental health disorders one would expect in the young female adult population in general. This would include major depression, and anxiety disorders including phobias, generalized anxiety disorder, panic disorder and PTSD [43]. PoTS patients should be assessed for psychiatric disorders with a complete psychiatric history, paying particular attention to assessing suicidality. The treatment plan should be consistent with evidence-based mental health guidelines, with an appropriate psychotherapeutic treatment modality, psychotropic medications, or a combination of both.

There are very limited data available to guide choice of pharmacotherapy in patients with PoTS. Selective serotonin reuptake inhibitors (SSRIs), such as sertraline, are often used first line in the treatment of depression and anxiety disorders. A study of the acute effects of sertraline in patients with PoTS revealed a trend towards increased blood pressure, and PoTS symptoms were actually slightly worse in the sertraline group compared to placebo [44]. This study corresponds with our clinical experience in treating PoTS patients. We generally find that they exhibit variable tolerance of antidepressant medications, and may discontinue their medication if their PoTS symptoms are exacerbated. It is also our clinical experience that patients who tolerate their antidepressant medication are able to obtain similar psychiatric benefits to patients without PoTS; however, research is needed to verify this clinical impression.

Selective norepinephrine reuptake inhibitors (SNRIs), in addition to inhibiting the reuptake of serotonin (like SSRIs), also inhibit the reuptake of norepinephrine. They are often used second line for the treatment of depressive and anxiety disorders [45]. A study of the acute effects of atomoxetine, a norepinephrine reuptake inhibitor, in PoTS showed that it significantly increased standing heart rate and exacerbated all symptoms compared to placebo [46]. Due to the significant risk of increased symptom burden associated with SNRI use in PoTS, The Heart Rhythm Society Expert Consensus Statement considers the use of SNRIs in PoTS a class 3 recommendation, i.e. their use should be generally avoided [47]. In clinical practice, SNRIs and other non-SSRI antidepressants are commonly used second line in PoTS patients with a poor response or inability to tolerate an SSRI trial. It is our experience that SNRIs tend to be more poorly tolerated in patients than SSRIs due to their increased tendency to exacerbate PoTS symptoms. We find that those patients who do tolerate these medications, however, often experience good clinical benefit.

In general, we tend to avoid the use of tricyclic antidepressants (TCAs) and monoamine oxidase inhibitors (MAO-Is) due to their profile of high side effect burden, including orthostatic hypotension.

When to Refer

It would seem likely that patients would benefit from psychological support, either in its protective or therapeutic capacities. Referrals are especially recommended when mood is compromised, the patient has reduced activities, sleep is affected, and relationship or appetite changes have occurred. This is especially urgent where a patient is fearful of, and avoidant of triggering, the physiological symptoms that they are experiencing; or indeed even more so if there are any safety concerns around self-harm or suicidal ideation.

Clinical Red Flags Supporting Rapid Access to Mental Health Care in PoTS

- Safety concerns such as self-harm or suicide—never be afraid to ask a patient as this will not 'suggest' an action that they otherwise would not have undertaken
- Despondency and hopelessness
- Fear of physiological symptoms
- Withdrawal, sleep deprivation, dissociative episodes or significant weight change.

While professionals with experience with PoTS may be hard to find, patients will be most likely to benefit from a clinician with experience of the interface between physical and mental health in other LTCs. In addition to this chapter, there is information on the PoTS UK website (www.potsuk.org) that may be helpful for clinicians to know before working with patients with PoTS. In psychotherapy, expectancy, engagement, and creating a positive therapeutic connection, are critically important in maximizing outcome. In addition, feeling understood, accepted, hopeful, and able to take control of managing a complex medical condition are essential for optimal progress.

A physical health clinician actively involved in patient care is probably best placed to introduce patients to the idea of engaging in psychological support without being misconstrued as suggesting symptoms are "all in the head." Introducing this support early on is likely to be an important factor in preventing QoL deterioration and associated secondary factors such as reactive depression, avoidance, and physical deconditioning [5]. A clinical or health psychologist is then well positioned with sufficient contact time and specialist skills to formulate, develop, and implement the integrated psychological, physiological, and behavioral/lifestyle treatment approach required. Unfortunately, before being correctly diagnosed with PoTS, many patients have had their symptoms misdiagnosed, often hearing they are 'all in their head' (for example 48% of a recent UK sample of patients, [5] which is conservative in comparison to previous findings). As a consequence, a suggestion by a medical professional to seek psychological support can be misinterpreted by patients as a trivialization and misunderstanding of the physical nature of their illness, leaving them reluctant to access this important form of support. It can help to use a parallel with physiotherapy. Explaining that just as patients with illnesses that are not caused by deconditioning may require input from physiotherapy services to prevent future deterioration and adjust to the changes brought about by their illness (e.g. patients with Parkinson's disease), so too patients with illnesses not caused by psychological processes can benefit enormously from psychological support going forward.

A sensitively discussed stigma-free referral and ongoing collaboration can help patients confidently access this important part of their treatment package. To reap the full benefit of the CBT family of therapies generally requires a patient to be committed to engaging fully in sessions and tasks between sessions, to have some hope or confidence in the approach, and, they must have the cognitive capacity to gain insight into the consequences of their thinking styles and behavioural patterns (see Box 1). Ideally, it would be preferable to have an in-house therapy team working in collaboration with other specialties in a multidisciplinary approach. The creation of specialist centres, supporting patients towards optimal outcome in a person-centered integration of psychological and physiological care, seems ideal in the context of our understanding of this complex multi-system syndrome.

Socializing a patient to the treatment approach is standard best practice for CBT and essential for engagement and active collaboration. We know that patients actively involved in their health care do better. The rationale for psychological intervention, which can be helpful to share with patients, includes those specific to PoTS as well as those more broadly applicable to many chronic illnesses. It is worth emphasizing that we know that patients with many chronic illnesses do better with access to CBT. Factors common to many health conditions that can be usefully highlighted include:

a. What we know about the impact of chronic stress, isolation and compromised sleep on disease prognosis.
b. Help with adjustment to diagnosis, grief and fears for the future.
c. That psychotherapy can also help to enhance motivation to engage in appropriate lifestyle changes and adhere to pharmacological regimes more consistently.
d. Advice around appropriate pacing and engagement in the right activities for the right amount of time to live optimally.
e. That it is common to harbor frustration at past mistakes, misdiagnosis and failings amongst family and friends.
f. The rationale that if one aspect of our health or functioning is compromised it makes sense to optimize all other aspects of our health and functioning to compensate; including identifying and changing unhelpful assumptions and thinking styles.

In terms of factors more specific to PoTS, support can be targeted at:

a. Getting the delicate balance right of responding appropriately to, but not getting distressed or overwhelmed by, somatic symptoms.
b. Learning strategies to calm down the fight/flight response and preventing anxious thinking from escalating the 'anxiety-mimicking' somatic symptoms.
c. Presyncope specific strategies including counter-maneuvers and not continuing on and ignoring physiological cues.
d. Addressing unhelpful dissociative tendencies, which can arise as a coping strategy in the wake of distress and discomfort (which untreated can exacerbate a vicious cycle of deteriorating functioning).
e. Challenging the unhelpful idea that the body is scary, unpredictable, out of control and has let them down.

Our experience with co-morbid difficulties and common challenges reported by PoTS patients suggests some key therapeutic interventions, from both CBT and so-called 'third-wave' CBT approaches, which incorporate mindfulness, self-compassion, and acceptance principles. After socialisation to the model, and based on individual needs identified in case-formulation, these techniques should be considered for inclusion in treatment plans. They can be usefully adapted for individual or group interventions (please see Appendix Table A1 for a detailed suggested treatment approach for psychologists). Given the rather unpredictable response to treatment of this complex syndrome, however, we would advocate that further work is needed to begin to construct and assess the incremental benefits of various elements of manualized therapy protocols, in addition to standard medical care. It is worth noting that not all patients with PoTS need psychological therapies to manage their condition. Adjustment to this challenging disorder will depend on their unique symptom profile, history and severity, as well as factors including extrinsic supports and acquired or intrinsic psychological resilience. Arguably, however, all will benefit from a paradigm for systemic illness which moves beyond the

Table A1

Skill	Suggested techniques	Rationale
Core CBT skills for identifying and challenging unhelpful thinking	Thought records, coping cards (summary of coping statements to use when symptomatic), behavioral activation, behavioral experiments, data gathering	Understandable tendencies towards catastrophizing, minimizing achievements, black and white thinking, future related thoughts, and learnt helplessness
Acute anxiety skills	Psychoeducation, breathing skills, relaxation, visualization (including 'turning down the dial' of anxiety volume), defusing from emotions, refocusing/healthy distraction, self-soothing tool-kit. Treating any preexisting trauma which exacerbates difficulties	Mismatch between measurable physiology and self-reported experiences. Managing scary sensations including a racing heart, dizziness and brain-fog Preventing unhelpful responses e.g. avoidance or dissociation including conversion phenomena
Worry skills	Decision trees, delayed 'worry hours' (including health anxiety/planning), generating alternative explanations with probabilities, rating importance of worries, challenging perfectionism and control	It makes sense that the somatic symptoms of PoTS which mimic anxiety make emotion-congruent memories and worrisome thoughts more accessible. Compensatory over-control in another aspects of life can develop
Adjusting to unpredictability	Enhancing belief in capacity to cope with situations as they arise. Flexible planning, Acceptance and commitment based skills	Difficulty planning activities due to not knowing how symptoms can generate 'learned helplessness' and avoidance of making plans
Syncope and pre-syncope related skills	Skills in healthy body-scanning, counter-maneuvers, life-style changes and 'grounding' (mindfully staying present),	The tendency to feel out of control, vulnerable and distressed by symptoms can cause lack of attunement to physical cues
Improved sleep	Mindfulness for sleep strategies and sleep-hygiene	Patients report being 'tired but wired'. Poor sleep is implicated in mood, anxiety, suicidal ideation and brain-fog
Pain management	Mindfulness skills and behavioral activation	PoTS patients report pain from migraine, coat-hanger pain and chest pain. Comorbid disorders such as hEDs are associated with significant additional pain
Interpersonal skills	Appropriate assertiveness. Developing empathic awareness and compassion. Revising expectations of others. Role play and 'empty-chair' strategies	Illness places strains on interpersonal relationships. Preventing isolation is important for outcome. Socializing requires creative adaptions in lieu of fatigue and physical limitations
Managing grief and guilt	Psychoeducation, awareness and insight. Aim to 'banish guilt' and be compassionate of grief	Losses include of the anticipated future, passions, and trust in body. Guilt about effect of illness on others
Anger management	Reframing anger as a helpful 'flag' of issues to resolve or let go. Always valid, but needs to be harnessed usefully	Often develops during period before diagnosis relating to not being believed, being misdiagnosed or feeling unsupported
Mindfulness (presence in the moment with curiosity, compassion and acceptance)	Meditation, body scanning, adapted yoga or tai-chi	Associated with improved energy, heart-rate, blood pressure and blood-sugar levels, interpersonal skills, sleep and QoL
Consolidating advice and over-seeing behavior changes	Practical skills for usefully undertaking life-style and daily planning (water, nutrition, medication, activities), motivation, priority setting, initiating action, & problem solving	Actively coordinating own care plan improves engagement and outcome. Without being integrated, advice from multiple specialists can feel overwhelming and lead to inertia/helplessness

Continued

Table A1 Continued

Skill	Suggested techniques	Rationale
Activity pacing	Developing an appropriately flexible regime for slowly and appropriately escalating challenges, and self-reward. Listening to body rather than ploughing on to burn-out	Fatigue and limited energy make choosing the right activities to stay fit and to enjoy life without set-backs more challenging and more critical
Self-compassion, self-worth and self-care	Meditation skills, value-based living (rather than goal driven self-esteem), self-soothing	Capacity to be a good friend to oneself essential for making positive health choices and valuing oneself even when not able to meet previous goals or levels of productivity
Challenging illness identity	Keeping interests and activities rich, varied and in keeping with pre-illness self, limiting time on health-related matters, maintaining key relationships, recognizing and celebrating individuality and achievements	Managing appointments and health can begin to take up all time and energy, leaving patients feeling there is nothing else to them (further increasing isolation and despair)
Hope and positivity	Cognitive reframing, focusing on positives, life-planning and prioritizing, and the therapeutic alliance itself (in generating hope)	The idea that when energy is compromised what really matters is brought sharply into focus, we potentially bring new appreciation and priorities to the fore in our day to day lives, which adds to and enriches pre-diagnostic lived experience

unjustifiable separation of somatic and psychological phenomena, and tailors treatment to the whole person in their wider social context.

Box 1: Common Themes in CBT for PoTS

- Coping with scary physiological sensations
- Adjusting to unpredictability (Acceptance)
- Identifying and changing unhelpful assumption and thinking styles
- Strategies for switching off fight/flight mode/dial turning
- Grief associated with loss of health and life changes
- Activity pacing
- Sleep difficulties
- Relationship difficulties
- Self-esteem, identity (values work) and self-compassion and self-care
- Mindfulness—appropriate body scanning and emotional awareness.

Appendix

Summary of Mental Health Recommendations in PoTS

Patients with PoTS are at risk of experiencing at least modest depressive and anxiety symptoms, and are at significantly increased risk of experiencing insomnia and suicidal ideation. They warrant and should have access to mental health assessment, treatment and support. We would advocate that:

- Given the likelihood of patients being referred to mental health professionals, they and allied disciplines should be educated about PoTS and how to refer appropriately if they suspect it.
- Most patients with long-term conditions would benefit from, and all should have ready access on request, to psychological support.

- Introducing this support as early as possible is likely to be a very important factor in preventing QoL deterioration and associated secondary factors such as reactive depression, avoidance and physical deconditioning.
- Uptake and engagement is likely to be increased if therapeutic support is offered as part of standard treatment and is seen as endorsed by a medical consultant active in the patient's care.
- CBT has a good evidence base in LTCs assuming a patient is motivated and has cognitive capacity.
- Evidence supporting the value of Mindfulness-based CBT and ACT in the context of chronic illness is increasing.
- These 'third wave' CBT approaches are likely to be helpful in appropriately modifying vigilance to somatic changes, and tolerating the frustrations that come with ill-health, while continuing to engage in manageable activities which enhance QoL.
- Therapists with a good understanding of supporting patients with chronic health issues, and experience with formulating and treatment in the context of multiple co-morbidities, are most likely to benefit patients.
- It can be very challenging making all the necessary life adaptations to live with PoTS. It can help patients to know that after the hard work of adjusting to what they cannot do and prioritizing and appreciating what they can do, many patients with PoTS report enjoying happy and fulfilling lives.

References

1. Benrud-Larson LM, Dewar MS, Sandroni P, Rummans TA, Haythornthwaite JA, Low PA. Quality of life in patients with postural tachycardia syndrome. Mayo Clin Proc. 2002;77(6):531–7.
2. McDonald C, Koshi S, Busner L, Kavi L, Newton JL. Postural tachycardia syndrome is associated with significant symptoms and functional impairment predominantly affecting young women: a UK perspective. BMJ Open. 2014;4(6):e004127.
3. Moon J, Kim DY, Byun JI, Sunwoo JS, Lim JA, Kim TJ, et al. Orthostatic intolerance symptoms are associated with depression and diminished quality of life in patients with postural tachycardia syndrome. Health Qual Life Outcomes. 2016;14(1):144.
4. Pederson CL, Brook JB. Health-related quality of life and suicide risk in postural tachycardia syndrome. Clin Auton Res. 2017;27(2):75–81.
5. Kavi LN M, Low DA, Opie M, Nicholson LM, Caldow E, Newton JL. A profile of patients with postural tachycardia syndrome and their experience of healthcare in the UK. Br J Cardiol. 2016;23:33.
6. Pederson CL, Blettner BJ. Sleep disturbance linked to suicidal ideation in postural orthostatic tachycardia syndrome. Nat Sci Sleep. 2017;9:109–15.
7. Anderson JW, Lambert EA, Sari CI, Dawood T, Esler MD, Vaddadi G, et al. Cognitive function, health-related quality of life, and symptoms of depression and anxiety sensitivity are impaired in patients with the postural orthostatic tachycardia syndrome (POTS). Front Physiol. 2014;5:230.
8. Mindfulness All-Party Parliamentary Group. Mindful Nation UK. 2015; Available from: https://themindfulnessinitiative.org.uk/images/reports/Mindfulness-APPG-Report_Mindful-Nation-UK_Oct2015.pdf.
9. Grubb BP. Postural tachycardia syndrome. Circulation. 2008;117(21):2814–7.
10. Department of Health. Psychological assessment and treatment for medically unexplained symptoms and long-term conditions. 2009; Available from: https://arms.evidence.nhs.uk/resources/qipp/29417/attachment.
11. McGrady A, Kern-Buell C, Bush E, Khuder S, Grubb BP. Psychological and physiological factors associated with tilt table testing for neurally mediated syncopal syndromes. Pacing Clin Electrophysiol. 2001;24(3):296–301.
12. Raj V, Haman KL, Raj SR, Byrne D, Blakely RD, Biaggioni I, et al. Psychiatric profile and attention deficits in postural tachycardia syndrome. J Neurol Neurosurg Psychiatry. 2009;80(3):339–44.
13. Khurana RK. Experimental induction of panic-like symptoms in patients with postural tachycardia syndrome. Clin Auton Res. 2006;16(6):371–7.
14. Masuki S, Eisenach JH, Johnson CP, Dietz NM, Benrud-Larson LM, Schrage WG, et al. Excessive heart rate response to orthostatic stress in postural tachycardia syndrome is not caused by anxiety. J Appl Physiol (1985). 2007; 102(3):896–903.
15. Ross AJ, Medow MS, Rowe PC, Stewart JM. What is brain fog? An evaluation of the symptom in postural tachycardia syndrome. Clin Auton Res. 2013;23(6):305–11.
16. Arnold AC, Haman K, Garland EM, Raj V, Dupont WD, Biaggioni I, et al. Cognitive dysfunction in postural tachycardia syndrome. Clin Sci (Lond). 2015;128(1):39–45.
17. Ocon AJ, Messer ZR, Medow MS, Stewart JM. Increasing orthostatic stress impairs neurocognitive functioning in chronic fatigue syndrome with postural tachycardia syndrome. Clin Sci (Lond). 2012;122(5):227–38.

18. Stewart JM, Medow MS, Messer ZR, Baugham IL, Terilli C, Ocon AJ. Postural neurocognitive and neuronal activated cerebral blood flow deficits in young chronic fatigue syndrome patients with postural tachycardia syndrome. Am J Physiol Heart Circ Physiol. 2012;302(5):H1185–94.
19. Stewart JM, Del Pozzi AT, Pandey A, Messer ZR, Terilli C, Medow MS. Oscillatory cerebral blood flow is associated with impaired neurocognition and functional hyperemia in postural tachycardia syndrome during graded tilt. Hypertension. 2015;65(3):636–43.
20. Raj V, Opie M, Arnold AC. Cognitive and psychological issues in postural tachycardia syndrome. Auton Neurosci. 2018;215:46–55.
21. Moriarty O, McGuire BE, Finn DP. The effect of pain on cognitive function: a review of clinical and preclinical research. Prog Neurobiol. 2011;93(3):385–404.
22. Dubey DH S, Vernino S. M1 and M2 muscarinic receptor antibodies among patients with postural orthostatic tachycardia syndrome: potential disease biomarker. J Clin Neuromuscul Dis. 2016; 17(3):179.
23. Fadgyas-Stanculete M, Buga AM, Popa-Wagner A, Dumitrascu DL. The relationship between irritable bowel syndrome and psychiatric disorders: from molecular changes to clinical manifestations. J Mol Psychiatry. 2014;2(1):4.
24. Baeza-Velasco C, Bourdon C, Polanco-Carrasco R, de Jouvencel M, Gely-Nargeot MC, Gompel A, et al. Cognitive impairment in women with joint hypermobility syndrome/Ehlers-Danlos syndrome hypermobility type. Rheumatol Int. 2017;37(6):937–9.
25. Bagai K, Song Y, Ling JF, Malow B, Black BK, Biaggioni I, et al. Sleep disturbances and diminished quality of life in postural tachycardia syndrome. J Clin Sleep Med . 2011;7(2):204–10.
26. Mallien J, Isenmann S, Mrazek A, Haensch CA. Sleep disturbances and autonomic dysfunction in patients with postural orthostatic tachycardia syndrome. Front Neurol. 2014;5:118.
27. Miglis MG, Barwick F. Sleep disorders in patients with postural tachycardia syndrome: A review of the literature and guide for clinicians. Auton Neurosci. 2018;215:62–9.
28. Shaw BH, Stiles LE, Bourne K, Green EA, Shibao CA, Okamoto LE, et al. The face of postural tachycardia syndrome—insights from a large cross-sectional online community-based survey. J Intern Med. 2019.
29. Office of National Statistics. Crime in England and Wales. 2016; Available from: https://www.ons.gov.uk/peoplepopulationandcommunity/crimeandjustice/bulletins/crimeinenglandandwales/yearendingmar2016.
30. Smith SM, Sonego S, Ketcheson L, Larson JL. A review of the effectiveness of psychological interventions used for anxiety and depression in chronic obstructive pulmonary disease. BMJ Open Respir Res. 2014;1(1):e000042.
31. Gotink RA, Chu P, Busschbach JJ, Benson H, Fricchione GL, Hunink MG. Standardised mindfulness-based interventions in healthcare: an overview of systematic reviews and meta-analyses of RCTs. PLoS ONE. 2015;10(4):e0124344.
32. Zeidan F, Johnson SK, Gordon NS, Goolkasian P. Effects of brief and sham mindfulness meditation on mood and cardiovascular variables. J Altern Complement Med. 2010;16(8):867–73.
33. Garland EL, Gaylord SA, Palsson O, Faurot K, Douglas Mann J, Whitehead WE. Therapeutic mechanisms of a mindfulness-based treatment for IBS: effects on visceral sensitivity, catastrophizing, and affective processing of pain sensations. J Behav Med. 2012;35(6):591–602.
34. Vujanovic AA, Zvolensky MJ, Bernstein A, Feldner MT, McLeish AC. A test of the interactive effects of anxiety sensitivity and mindfulness in the prediction of anxious arousal, agoraphobic cognitions, and body vigilance. Behav Res Ther. 2007;45(6):1393–400.
35. Nyklicek I, Mommersteeg PM, Van Beugen S, Ramakers C, Van Boxtel GJ. Mindfulness-based stress reduction and physiological activity during acute stress: a randomized controlled trial. Health Psychol. 2013;32(10):1110–3.
36. Roerink ME, Lenders JW, Schmits IC, Pistorius AM, Smit JW, Knoop H, et al. Postural orthostatic tachycardia is not a useful diagnostic marker for chronic fatigue syndrome. J Intern Med. 2017;281(2):179–88.
37. Freedenberg VA, Hinds PS, Friedmann E. Mindfulness-based stress reduction and group support decrease stress in adolescents with cardiac diagnoses: a randomized two-group study. Pediatr Cardiol. 2017.
38. Hawton A, Green C, Dickens AP, Richards SH, Taylor RS, Edwards R, et al. The impact of social isolation on the health status and health-related quality of life of older people. Qual Life Res. 2011;20(1):57–67.
39. Kovacs AH, Saidi AS, Kuhl EA, Sears SF, Silversides C, Harrison JL, et al. Depression and anxiety in adult congenital heart disease: predictors and prevalence. Int J Cardiol. 2009;137(2):158–64.
40. Ralston TE, Kanzler KE. Symptom discrimination and habituation: a case study of behavioral treatment for Postural Orthostatic Tachycardia Syndrome (POTS). Behav Med. 2016;42(1):57–62.
41. Harris R. ACT made simple: an easy-to-read primer on acceptance and commitment therapy Oakland. CA: New Harbinger; 2009.
42. JG AT, Davis ML, Morina N, Powers MB, Smits JA, Emmelkamp PM. A meta-analysis of the efficacy of acceptance and commitment therapy for clinically relevant mental and physical health problems. Psychother Psychosom. 2015;84(1):30–6.

43. Kessler RC, Chiu WT, Demler O, Merikangas KR, Walters EE. Prevalence, severity, and comorbidity of 12-month DSM-IV disorders in the s. Arch Gen Psychiatry. 2005;62(6):617–27.
44. Mar PL, Raj V, Black BK, Biaggioni I, Shibao CA, Paranjape SY, et al. Acute hemodynamic effects of a selective serotonin reuptake inhibitor in postural tachycardia syndrome: a randomized, crossover trial. J Psychopharmacol. 2014;28(2):155–61.
45. Blier P. Neurobiology of depression and mechanism of action of depression treatments. J Clin Psychiatry. 2016;77(3):e319.
46. Green EA, Raj V, Shibao CA, Biaggioni I, Black BK, Dupont WD, et al. Effects of norepinephrine reuptake inhibition on postural tachycardia syndrome. J Am Heart Assoc. 2013;2(5):e000395.
47. Sheldon RS, Grubb BP 2nd, Olshansky B, Shen WK, Calkins H, Brignole M, et al. 2015 heart rhythm society expert consensus statement on the diagnosis and treatment of postural tachycardia syndrome, inappropriate sinus tachycardia, and vasovagal syncope. Heart Rhythm. 2015;12(6):e41-63.

Service Models

PoTS in Primary Care

Lesley Kavi

Introduction

Disorders of the autonomic system can be difficult to diagnose in primary care as symptoms are often non-specific, wide-ranging and subtle. Patients frequently present to the primary care clinician with undifferentiated conditions and a high index of suspicion is required. In dysautonomia, an increased or reduced/absent change between lying and standing heart rate or blood pressure can be the only examination findings. However, such orthostatic recordings may not be recorded at all (especially in younger people) or recorded over an inadequate duration of time, and consequently, these conditions can be easily overlooked.

PoTS was named and formally described in 1993 and is not yet included in most medical school or GP training curricula. Informal polls of GPs around the UK conducted by the author at GP educational events revealed in 2014 that only 10–15% had heard of PoTS. This combination of lack of awareness and non-specific symptoms make it unsurprising that patients experience difficulty in obtaining a diagnosis (a mean of almost 4 years [1] from presentation to diagnosis and 7 years from symptom onset to diagnosis [2]). In only 7% of patients did the GP suggest that PoTS might be the cause of patients' symptoms and in one fifth, the patient suggested their diagnosis to their healthcare professional [1]. In the UK, half of patients are initially given a psychological or psychiatric diagnosis such as anxiety, panic disorder, depression or hypochondriasis to explain their symptoms. This misdiagnosis occurs in a much higher proportion of female patients (75%) than male (25%) [1].

Investigation and management of PoTS has not been studied in the primary care setting and there are no current recognised care pathways.

When to Suspect PoTS

The more common symptoms of PoTS are a triad of lightheadedness, fatigue and palpitations [1, 3]. However, patients may experience a long list of non-specific symptoms similar to those listed as common 'medically unexplained symptoms' [4].

There should be a high index of suspicion in chronic fatigue syndrome; in one UK study 27% of CFS patients had PoTS [5]. PoTS is common in hypermobile Ehlers-Danlos syndrome and hypermobility spectrum disorder (previously known as joint hypermobility syndrome (JHS)) [6] and conversely, over 50% of patients with

L. Kavi (✉)
Solihull Healthcare Partnership, 3 Grove Road, Solihull B91 2AG, West Midlands, UK
e-mail: lesley@potsuk.org

N. Gall et al. (eds.), *Postural Tachycardia Syndrome*, https://doi.org/10.1007/978-3-030-54165-1_41

PoTS have JHS [1] with some centres suggesting that this percentage is higher.

Testing for PoTS in a Primary Care Setting

If PoTS is suspected, it may be necessary to exclude other conditions with similar symptoms such as anaemia, thyroid disorders, phaeochromocytoma, Addison's disease and other conditions associated with orthostatic hypotension.

It can be helpful to undertake an active stand test in the consulting room. After taking a history that might suggest PoTS, it may be more practical to ask the patient to attend on a different day with a longer appointment, and to suggest that they do not plan to drive home as they may feel a little unwell if the stand test is positive.

It is only possible to accurately record around a maximum of 4 blood pressure recordings within one minute and ideally beat-to-beat monitoring of heart rate and blood pressure during a stand test would detect short-lived changes such as drops in blood pressure or periods of asystole. Such monitors are expensive to buy and maintain and it is unlikely that they will be available in the primary care setting. Furthermore, a GP is likely to be single-handed when undertaking such testing and it can be difficult to continue to operate a manual or battery-operated sphygmomanometer whilst a patient experiences presyncope or syncope. Therefore, if the stand test is inconclusive or it has been difficult to obtain reliable results and symptoms are strongly suggestive of PoTS, referral for tilt table testing in secondary care is recommended.

Organising blood tests, ECG and echocardiogram (if appropriate) can help to ensure appropriate referral.

Referral to Secondary Care

Referral to a secondary care physician with little or no knowledge of PoTS can be a frustrating experience for the patient. In the UK the majority of hospital consultants who have expertise in diagnosing and managing PoTS are cardiologists (often specifically heart rhythm specialists (electrophysiologists)), often working within a syncope or blackouts clinic. There are also medicine for the elderly consultants, neurologists and paediatricians with an interest in PoTS.

There is a list of consultants with an interest in PoTS on the PoTS UK website www.potsuk.org/specialists.

In many localities there is no service for patients with PoTS; this is especially problematic for those who live in Scotland and Wales, and also for children and adolescents. Some consultants will accept 'out of area' patients, although patients often experience problems in achieving such referrals.

Managing PoTS in Primary Care

It is important to review current medication and consider stopping any drugs that may cause or contribute to symptoms. Culprits can include medication that raises heart rate or lowers blood pressure.

Self-management measures:

- Advise increased fluids and salt to increase blood volume (where there are no contraindications such as renal, cardiac or hypertensive disease) [7].
- Compression tights may be prescribed or purchased.
- Cautious resistance training and graduated supine exercise such as swimming, rowing or recumbent exercise cycling can be recommended for some patients [7].

If physiological therapies fail to sufficiently improve symptoms, medication may be initiated. There are no drugs that are licensed for use in PoTS although some are familiar to GPs from their use in other conditions. Medications used in PoTS include low dose beta blockers, ivabradine, fludrocortisone, midodrine, pyridostigmine and clonidine. Modafinil may improve fatigue and cognitive dysfunction, but has the potential to worsen tachycardia [7]. GPs may be willing to initiate or continue to prescribe drugs after recommendation from secondary care. Some trusts operate shared care agreements for the less familiar drugs.

Hospital clinicians are sometimes not aware of medication that the patient is taking as prescribed in primary care. If a new drug is initiated in secondary care, it is in the patient's interests to check interactions in primary care using in-house consulting room software (e.g. by adding it to the patient's record as a 'hospital issued drug') and report any significant issues to the consultant. Some drugs, such as ivabradine, have the potential for teratogenicity and provision of reliable contraception and preconception counselling may be necessary.

Patients with PoTS often have symptoms affecting many bodily systems and may also have associated conditions such as hypermobile Ehlers-Danlos syndrome/hypermobility spectrum disorder (see Chapter "Rheumatology and Postural Tachycardia Syndrome"), mast cell activation syndrome (see Chapter "Mast Cell Activation Syndrome (MCAS)") or auto-immune conditions (see Chapters "Rheumatology and Postural Tachycardia Syndrome" and "Is PoTS an Autoimmune Condition?") [7, 8]. As multidisciplinary teams to manage such conditions are not yet the norm in secondary care, the GP can have an important role in co-ordinating and rationalising services for and with their patient.

Such consultations can be complex and prolonged and, especially in the early stages of diagnosis and management, the provision of appointments that are longer than the traditional 10 minutes may ease frustration for both doctor and patient.

Future Priorities

Research

The prevalence of PoTS is unknown. It has been estimated at 0.2% of the US population [7] and 1 in 100 teenagers. Work needs to be undertaken to determine how common PoTS is in the UK population and a national registry may help to clarify prevalence, identify phenotypes and provide a basis for multicentre clinical research.

There are many unanswered questions in PoTS which include:

- Why there is a preponderance of PoTS in females, and why people aged 15–50 appear to be most affected
- The physiological mechanism(s) underlying PoTS, and in particular, one of the most disabling symptoms, cognitive impairment
- The relationship between associated conditions including CFS, vasovagal syncope, orthostatic hypotension and likely triggers which include viral illness, trauma, surgery and pregnancy
- The most effective physiological and pharmaceutical treatments for PoTS.

Research aimed at answering such questions, could assist the GP in identifying and managing affected patients.

Education

With limited knowledge of PoTS in primary care there is a need for inclusion of this subject in medical school and GP training curricula.

References

1. Kavi L, Nuttall N, Low PA, Opie M, Nicholson L, Caldow E, et al. A profile of patients with postural tachycardia syndrome and their experience of healthcare in the UK. Br J Cardiol. 2016;23(33).
2. McDonald C, Koshi S, Busner L, Kavi L, Newton JL. Postural tachycardia syndrome is associated with significant symptoms and functional impairment predominantly affecting young women: a UK perspective. BMJ Open. 2014;4(6):e004127.
3. Thieben MJ, Sandroni P, Sletten DM, Benrud-Larson LM, Fealey RD, Vernino S, et al. Postural orthostatic tachycardia syndrome: the Mayo clinic experience. Mayo Clin Proc. 2007;82(3):308–13.

4. Psychiatrists RCO. https://www.rcpsych.ac.uk/healthadvice/problemsanddisorders/medicallyunexplainedsymptoms.aspx.
5. Hoad A, Spickett G, Elliott J, Newton J. Postural orthostatic tachycardia syndrome is an under-recognized condition in chronic fatigue syndrome. QJM. 2008;101(12):961–5.
6. Gazit Y, Nahir AM, Grahame R, Jacob G. Dysautonomia in the joint hypermobility syndrome. Am J Med. 2003;115(1):33–40.
7. Sheldon RS, Grubb BP 2nd, Olshansky B, Shen WK, Calkins H, Brignole M, et al. 2015 heart rhythm society expert consensus statement on the diagnosis and treatment of postural tachycardia syndrome, inappropriate sinus tachycardia, and vasovagal syncope. Heart Rhythm. 2015;12(6):e41–63.
8. Hoffman-Snyder C, Lewis J, Harris L, Dhawan P, Goodman B. Evidence of mast cell activation disorder in postural tachycardia syndrome. Neurology. 2015;84(14):P1.277.

Nurse-Led PoTS Clinics: A Framework

Melloney Ferrar and Helen Eftekhari

Introduction

The focus of this chapter is on the importance of the role nurses play in the delivery of care for people with PoTS within nurse led clinics, for example in a cardiology setting. Anecdotally, cardiology has historically been a specialist area with extensive experience of nurse-led clinics in the UK. The rationale for the transferability of nursing skills from these clinics to the care of people with PoTS is explored and the competencies required for delivering a nurse-led PoTS clinic are outlined. The main principles outlined could potentially be transferable to any speciality wanting to establish nurse-led care for people with PoTS.

In cardiology there are two main areas where specialist nursing has made significant contributions to improving patient care and clinical pathways: nurse-led clinics, patient education with supportive self-management. Nursing has an important contribution to make in improving the care, support and management of people with PoTS. Nurse-led clinics are discussed in the context of advanced nursing practice, in line with current developments in the United Kingdom. We have used the framework for advancing nursing practice, combined with clinical nursing experience of working with people with PoTS, to propose nursing competencies for delivering a nurse-led PoTS clinic.

Background

For the past two decades cardiology has led the way in developing nurse-led clinics for rapid access chest pain [1, 2], heart failure [3–5], palpitations [6] and atrial fibrillation. Studies confirm the positive impact on care that these clinics have had. In nurse-led rapid access chest pain, a retrospective 6 year study found that the clinic offered enhanced prevention focus with outcomes comparative to international studies [1]. Nurse-led heart failure clinics improve medication management and adherence, and patient outcomes, whilst reducing the overall health care burden [3–5, 7, 8]. In atrial fibrillation management, arrhythmia nurse-led clinics have improved adherence to anticoagulation, reduced risk factors and improved quality of life associated with AF, whilst being cost effective [9–13].

As with all research in PoTS, there is limited literature available on nurse-led PoTS clinics. The only study relating to nurse-led clinics

M. Ferrar (✉)
Syncope and PoTS Nurse Specialist, Sheffield Teaching Hospitals Foundation Trust, Sheffield, UK
e-mail: melloney.ferrar@nhs.net

H. Eftekhari
Arrhythmia and Syncope Nurse Specialist, University Hospitals Coventry Warwickshire, Coventry, UK

N. Gall et al. (eds.), *Postural Tachycardia Syndrome*, https://doi.org/10.1007/978-3-030-54165-1_42

and PoTS highlights the important contribution arrhythmia nurse-led clinics can make to increasing PoTS diagnostic rates. This can be achieved by recognising the symptoms and screening for PoTS through the simple active stand test. One study of a nurse-led palpitations clinic found 5% of diagnoses made were of PoTS [14]. On average in the UK, it takes 7 years to be diagnosed with PoTS [15] and experts agree upon the need for increased awareness and diagnostic rates [16]. Arrhythmia nurses need to have an awareness of PoTS and be part of improving the diagnostic rates through screening within their general arrhythmia clinics.

Increasingly, hospitals in the UK are supporting and commissioning two specific arrhythmia nurse-led clinics, the rapid access palpitations clinic [6] and the syncope clinic. By embedding the active stand test in the clinical assessment, both clinics ensure the arrhythmia nurse-led clinic is contributing to improving diagnostic rates of PoTS and the PoTS pathway, whilst reducing the length of time to diagnosis. It is essential when running any general arrhythmia clinic to ensure there is robust screening in place for PoTS. Nursing assessment and support intensifies therapeutic interventions and surveillance in the most complex patients.

Supportive Self-Management

Self-management programs have supported people with long-term conditions since the 1980s [17]. Many of these have been studied in patients with cardiac and respiratory conditions, arthritis and diabetes [18]. Self-management is collaborative working between health-care services and people who are managing and living with a long-term condition. Supportive self-management refers to the interventions delivered by the health-care services to support these people [19].

The NIHR (National Institute for Health Research) commissioned a systematic review and meta-analysis of self-management interventions. This research found overall cardiac conditions had the highest number of published studies in self-management (29%). Out of all of the self-management programmes, the cardiac interventions had the highest impact on improving quality of life, whilst reducing health care utilisation [18]. The components and formats of self-management support interventions vary considerably, even across similar cardiac patient groups [20, 21].

To clarify what supportive self-management should comprise of, one study (PRISM) developed a taxonomy [19] of 14 core components for supported self-management. This included information and education on the condition, resources, monitoring, support in adherence to treatments, regular review, access to advice and support, including lifestyle support and support with psychological strategies. The cornerstone of PoTS management is lifestyle changes, including good hydration and diet (Chapter "Non-pharmacological Management (Hydration, Diet and Compression)"), exercise (Chapter "Exercise Guidelines for Postural Tachycardia Syndrome") management of fatigue (Chapter "Chronic Fatigue Syndrome") and psychological well-being (Chapter "Psychological and Psychiatric Support; When, Why and What to do"). Nurses dealing with long term health conditions, especially the cardiac conditions, often have the skills and are in an ideal position to support people with PoTS with self-management interventions.

Evidence supports the positive impact of cardiac nurse-led clinics in cardiac conditions and self-management support. A PoTS nurse-led clinic can improve clinical care and management. The key to further support and develop the role of a PoTS nurse-led clinic is to improve the evidence base in this area through gathering and publishing outcomes.

Historically, cardiac nurse-led clinics are led by clinical nurse specialists. There is ongoing work in the UK and other countries on expanding nursing roles, including developing clinical nurse specialists as advanced nurse practitioners [22–24]. In 2018 the Department of Health,

Social Services and Public Safety published the UK National Advanced Nursing Practice Framework [25]. The document defines the four pillars of advanced nursing practice, benchmarking the same pillars with the clinical nurse specialist role. The core distinction between a clinical nurse specialist or advanced nurse practitioner, in essence, is how autonomous the nurse's practice is [25].

The four pillars of practice are:

- direct clinical practice
- education and learning
- leadership and collaborative practice
- research and evidence-based practice.

The following components of a nurse-led PoTS clinic have been developed from the competencies in the advanced nursing practice framework [25] and draw from the authors' clinical experience.

Nurse-Led PoTS Clinic: Service Specifications

To provide a clinic-based service in which patients would be efficiently assessed and managed requires:

- A lead consultant to provide a service overview for clinical governance purposes and lead the medico-legal dimensions of the service.
- Agreed pathway, protocols and referral criteria for nurse specialist assessment.
- Clinical supervision arrangements agreed with designated consultant.
- Consultation duration agreed locally. We would suggest 45 minutes to 1 hour for new appointments and 20 minutes for follow up appointments.
- The appointment letter will outline the purpose and duration of the consultation, so that the patient is aware of the time required for assessment. (Morning appointments can be problematic for some patients, although not all nurse led PoTS services find this. Telephone clinics can help to resolve this problem).
- Appropriate nursing expertise for symptom assessment and risk stratification to develop a care plan according to symptoms and patient's preferences.
- Effective IT and administrative support for timely communication with referring clinician and general practitioner.
- New referrals require an ECG and 10-minute active stand test, ideally conducted by a qualified technician and ideally phlebotomy for baseline, locally agreed, blood tests.
- Access to tilt table testing with a beat-to-beat blood pressure assessment system.
- Ensure pathways, job descriptions and protocols revised regularly and kept up to date.

Direct Clinical Practice

A benefit to the structured approach detailed below is the co-ordination of appropriate referrals to other specialist services in a timely manner with demonstrable inter-professional communication of agreed patient clinical outcomes.

History Taking and Risk Stratification to Include the Following:

- Transient loss of consciousness (T- LOC)/ pre-syncope / palpitations/chest pain/shortness of breath
- Identify when symptoms began and symptom triggers
- Other symptoms: sleep pattern/fatigue/ headaches/sweating/temperature regulation/ bowels/ bladder problems/rashes and other symptoms of Mast Cell Activation Syndrome (MCAS)
- Past medical history
- History of sudden adult death (unexplained sudden death under the age of 40) within the immediate family and other family history

- Full medication history to include over the counter/herbal/recreational drugs—assessing the effect of drug therapies
- Allergies including drugs
- Dietary assessment (alcohol/meals/allergies/intolerances/fluid and salt intake)
- Exercise—amount and type
- Occupational health, college/university, DVLA
- Assessment of mood following NICE Clinical guideline [CG90] Depression in adults: recognition and management https://www.nice.org.uk/guidance/cg90
- Assessment of quality of life.

Physical Examination to Include

- Active stand test
- Assessment of venous pooling
- Assessment of joints using Beighton hypermobility score/EDS diagnostic criteria.

Supportive self-management to deliver therapeutic interventions (for more details on specific interventions see relevant chapters of this book).

Lifestyle Management

- Fluids and salt—ensure consistency at every appointment
- Wearing of compression tights/stockings/sports leggings
- Exercise advice
- Instruction in physical counter-pressure manoeuvres to avoid syncope/increase orthostatic tolerance
- Dietary advice
- Joint management (see Chapter "Rheumatology and Postural Tachycardia Syndrome").

Strategies to Recognise/Avoid Potential Triggers Including

- Managing the effects of gravity, heat, menstruation
- Preventing venous pooling
- Daily activities—eating, exercise
- Pain
- Anxiety.

Referral for Delivery of Specific Therapeutic Interventions Delivered by Other Health Care Professionals

- Physiotherapy
- Occupational therapy
- Clinical Psychology
- Dietetics
- Orthotics.

Psycho/Social/Educational Information Support to Patients and Families

- Recommended information literature (PoTS UK, STARS, EDS Support UK) and telephone support
- Support a self-management strategy with the transition from passive recipient to active participant
- Provide parental support where appropriate
- Discuss the benefits and pitfalls of using social media forums as a source of reliable information for PoTS management.

Medication Compliance

The nurse can play a significant role in helping patients with PoTS manage their medicines carefully. Consideration needs to be made as to which aspect of managing medicines would best suit the patient. Compliance can be achieved using the following strategies:

- Initiation and education on how to take, mode of action, timings, side effects
- Contraception/pregnancy avoidance advice in relation to the medication used
- At follow up: adjusting medicines to suit patient's needs
- Identify side effects, intolerances and allergies
- Monitoring safety of medications—appropriate checks on long term therapies (such as Midodrine, Octreotide, Ivabradine, Fludrocortisone) with 24-hour Holter and 24-hour blood pressure monitoring and relevant blood tests as needed.
- Management of medicines can be achieved, for example, through patient group directions (PGDs) to supplementary and independent prescribing.
- Liaising with primary care physicians on the long-term prescribing of medication to improve local access to therapeutic medication.

Education and Learning

In a nurse-led PoTS clinic there are two areas to address in education and learning: the individual nurse education and education of other health care professionals on PoTS diagnosis and management. The nurse has a responsibility to increase awareness of and improve the management of PoTS either through opportunistic teaching or formal teaching sessions.

Individual Recommended Skills

- Health Assessment Course
- Teaching qualification
- Interpretation skills in ECG/ active stand test/ tilt table test/24-hour holter and blood pressure monitoring/blood tests
- Non-medical prescribing
- Counselling
- IT and audit skills.

There is currently a climate within the UK to expand the role of the nurse to advanced nurse practitioner level. The PoTS specialist nurse ideally suits this model due to the wide area of responsibility and expertise required to fulfil this role.

Centres are strongly advised to invest and support nurses running PoTS clinics to undertake Masters level courses and work towards advanced practitioner level.

Leadership and Collaborative Work

The key to a successful nurse-led clinic is a strong collaborative working relationship with a clinician who has an interest in PoTS. This collaborative working can then move forward towards a service providing expert consultation for medical and other staff, development of robust pathways, guidelines and protocols, the establishment of a formal MDT, and establishing effective methods for shared expertise and skills transference. This includes working with the primary care team to improve communication between specialist centres, improving support for people with PoTS, and improving awareness of PoTS. Collaborative working also feeds into the national picture, with PoTS services supporting each other, working to improve the evidence base in PoTS, sharing workload and contributing towards development of guidelines.

Research and Evidence-Based Practice

Earlier in this chapter, the rationale behind a PoTS nurse-led clinic was discussed; however, the actual evidence base for a nurse-led PoTS clinic is limited and further information need to be gathered to validate and refine this.

Audit is key to ensuring that patients' needs are met, and that standards of care improve.

This begins with monitoring activities, outcomes and quality of care through ongoing data collection and acquiring additional retrospective data that may be retrieved through information technology (IT) departments. Consider exploring demand and capacity figures. Measuring active stand measurements over a period of time, adherence to medication, effectiveness of prescribing practices and quality of life measurements may be helpful.

Important tools for subjective measurements should include a validated quality of life tool and a patient satisfaction survey. In PoTS research studies, the most commonly used validated quality of life measures include generic quality of life tools like the short-form 36 (SF36), EQ5D or the autonomic nervous system questionnaire (ANSQ). Although not PoTS specific, the ANSQ tool has been validated and used in PoTS research [26–30]. Through audit and collection of objective and subjective measurements, the evidence base for PoTS and nurse-led clinics can be better established.

The 2015 Heart Rhythm Society guidelines on vasovagal syncope, inappropriate sinus tachycardia and PoTS includes management recommendations [31]. One IIB recommendation is that "Patients with PoTS might be best managed with a multidisciplinary approach." While aspirational, there currently is insufficient evidence to support this as a higher recommendation. Nurse-led clinics and supportive self-management within the cardiology setting in other cardiac conditions have anecdotally been shown to be effective. Therefore, centres implementing a nurse-led clinic for managing people with PoTS need to gather evidence on the effectiveness and cost effectiveness of this service delivery model.

References

1. McLachlan A, Aldridge C, Lee M, Harper C, Kerr A. The development and first six years of a nurse-led chest pain clinic. N Z Med J. 2019;132(1489):39–47.
2. Pottle A. A nurse-led rapid access chest pain clinic–experience from the first 3 years. Eur J Cardiovasc Nurs. 2005;4(3):227–33.
3. Cheng HY, Chair SY, Wang Q, Sit JW, Wong EM, Tang SW. Effects of a nurse-led heart failure clinic on hospital readmission and mortality in Hong Kong. J Geriatr Cardiol. 2016;13(5):415–9.
4. Stewart S, Chan YK, Wong C, Jennings G, Scuffham P, Esterman A, et al. Impact of a nurse-led home and clinic-based secondary prevention programme to prevent progressive cardiac dysfunction in high-risk individuals: the Nurse-led Intervention for Less Chronic Heart Failure (NIL-CHF) randomized controlled study. Eur J Heart Fail. 2015;17(6):620–30.
5. Smith CE, Piamjariyakul U, Dalton KM, Russell C, Wick J, Ellerbeck EF. Nurse-led multidisciplinary heart failure group clinic appointments: methods, materials, and outcomes used in the clinical trial. J Cardiovasc Nurs. 2015;30(4 Suppl 1):S25–34.
6. Scott PA, Appleford P, Farrell TG, Andrews NP. A nurse-led palpitations clinic: a 2-year experience. Postgrad Med J. 2010;86(1011):3–7.
7. Driscoll A, Srivastava P, Toia D, Gibcus J, Hare DL. A nurse-led up-titration clinic improves chronic heart failure optimization of beta-adrenergic receptor blocking therapy–a randomized controlled trial. BMC Res Notes. 2014;7:668.
8. Thompson DR, Roebuck A, Stewart S. Effects of a nurse-led, clinic and home-based intervention on recurrent hospital use in chronic heart failure. Eur J Heart Fail. 2005;7(3):377–84.
9. Yaeger A, Cash NR, Parham T, Frankel DS, Deo R, Schaller RD, et al. A nurse-led limited risk factor modification program to address obesity and obstructive sleep Apnea in atrial fibrillation patients. J Am Heart Assoc. 2018;7(23):e010414.
10. Bowyer JL, Tully PJ, Ganesan AN, Chahadi FK, Singleton CB, McGavigan AD. A randomised controlled trial on the effect of nurse-led educational intervention at the time of catheter ablation for atrial fibrillation on quality of life, symptom severity and rehospitalisation. Heart Lung Circ. 2017;26(1):73–81.
11. Qvist I, Hendriks JM, Moller DS, Albertsen AE, Mogensen HM, Oddershede GD, et al. Effectiveness of structured, hospital-based, nurse-led atrial fibrillation clinics: a comparison between a real-world population and a clinical trial population. Open Heart. 2016;3(1):e000335.
12. Hendriks JM, Vrijhoef HJ, Crijns HJ, Brunner-La Rocca HP. The effect of a nurse-led integrated chronic care approach on quality of life in patients with atrial fibrillation. Europace: Eur Pacing, Arrhythmias, and Cardiac Electrophysiol: J Working Groups on Cardiac Pacing, Arrhythmias, and Cardiac Cellular Electrophysiol Eur Soc Cardiol. 2014;16(4):491–9.
13. Hendriks J, Tomini F, van Asselt T, Crijns H, Vrijhoef H. Cost-effectiveness of a specialized atrial fibrillation clinic vs. usual care in patients with atrial fibrillation. Europace: Eur Pacing, Arrhythmias, and Cardiac Electrophysiol: J Working Groups on Cardiac Pacing, Arrhythmias, and Cardiac Cellular Electrophysiol Eur Soc Cardiol. 2013;15(8):1128–35.

14. Said A, Bloo R. Outcomes of fast-track outpatient clinic for rhythm and conduction disorders: focus on Postural Tachycardia Syndrome and literature review. Asian J Cardiol Res. 2018;1(1):1–22.
15. Kavi L. A profile of patients with postural tachycardia syndrome and their experience of healthcare in the UK. Br J Cardiol. 2016.
16. Brinth L, Pors K, Spahic JM, Sutton R, Fedorowski A, Mehlsen J. Postural Orthostatic Tachycardia Syndrome (POTS) in Denmark: increasingly recognized or new epidemic? Auton Neurosci: Basic Clin. 2018.
17. Clark N, Becker M, Janz N, Lorig K, Rakowski W, Anderson L. Self-management of chronic disease by older adults. J Aging Health. 1991;3(1):3–27.
18. Panagiot M, Richardson G, Murray E, Rogers A, Kennedy A, Mewman S, et al. Reducing care utilisation through self-management interventions (RECURSIVE): a systematic review and meta-analysis. In: Research NIfH, editor. National Institute for Health Research;2014.
19. Pearce G, Parke H, Pinnock H, Epiphaniouu E, Bourne C, Sheikh A, et al. The PRISMS taxonomy of self-management support: derivation of a novel taxonomy and initial testing of its utility. J Health Serv Res Policy [Internet]. 2015;0(0).
20. Buck H, Stromberg A, Chung M, Donovan K, Harkness K, Howad A, et al. A systematic review of heart failure dyadic self-care interventions focusing on intervention components, contexts and outcomes. Int J Nurs Stud. 2018;77:232–42.
21. Jonkman N, Westland H, Groenwold R, Agren S, Anguita M, Blue L, et al. What are effective programm characteristics of self-management interventions in patients with heart failure? An individual patient data meta-analysis. J Cardiac Fail. 2016;22(11):861–71.
22. Mayo AM, Ray MM, Chamblee TB, Urden LD, Moody R. The advanced practice clinical nurse specialist. Nurs Adm Q. 2017;41(1):70–6.
23. Suller S. The advanced practice nurse in the emergency department. J Emerg Nurs. 2017;43(6):504–5.
24. Pearce C, Breen B. Advanced clinical practice and nurse-led clinics: a time to progress. Br J Nurs. 2018;27(8):444–8.
25. Midwifery NIPaECfN. Advanced Nursing Practice Framework: Supporting Advanced Nursing Practice in Health and Social Care Trusts. In: Department of Health SSaPS, editor. Belfast2018.
26. Ashangari C, Suleman A. A comprehensive study on postural orthostatic tachycardia syndrome (POTS) symptoms. Auton Neurosci: Basic Clin. 2015;192:123.
27. Iodice V. The postural tachycardia syndrome: a multi-system condition: clinical features, pathophysiology, genetics and novel treatment [10297995]. Ann Arbor: Imperial College London (United Kingdom); 2013.
28. Ives CT, Kimpinski K. Higher heart rate increments on head-up tilt in control subjects are not associated with autonomic dysfunction. Clin Neurophysiol: Official J Int Fed Clin Neurophysiol. 2014;125(10):2109–14.
29. Kimpinski K, Figueroa JJ, Singer W, Sletten DM, Iodice V, Sandroni P, et al. A prospective, 1-year follow-up study of postural tachycardia syndrome. Mayo Clin Proc. 2012;87(8):746–52.
30. Sletten DM, Suarez GA, Low PA, Mandrekar J, Singer W. COMPASS 31: a refined and abbreviated Composite Autonomic Symptom Score. Mayo Clin Proc. 2012;87(12):1196–201.
31. Sheldon RS, Grubb BP 2nd, Olshansky B, Shen WK, Calkins H, Brignole M, et al. 2015 heart rhythm society expert consensus statement on the diagnosis and treatment of postural tachycardia syndrome, inappropriate sinus tachycardia, and vasovagal syncope. Heart Rhythm. 2015;12(6):e41–63.

A Tertiary Referral Centre for PoTS: The Autonomic Unit at the National Hospital for Neurology and Neurosurgery Experience

Valeria Iodice and Christopher J. Mathias

Abbreviations

Non-Pharma	Non pharmacological measures
HUT	Head up tilt
EDS	Ehlers-Danlos Syndrome
Fludro	Fludrocortisone
PoTS	Postural tachycardia syndrome
MDT	Multi-disciplinary team

Introduction

The postural tachycardia syndrome (PoTS) is an autonomic condition that may cause significant morbidity and impairment of quality of life. It often is associated with multi-system involvement and multiple co-morbidities [1, 2]. The pathophysiological basis can include the interrelationship between autonomic, biochemical, genetic and environmental factors. This can result in different subgroups with important and at times subtle clinical differences with divergent responses to treatment. Contributory factors in PoTS could include neural involvement (with a limited autonomic neuropathy possibly of autoimmune basis), physical deconditioning, chronic hypovolemia, hyperadrenergic tone, impaired cerebral autoregulation and genetic mutations [1].

The complexity of multi-system conditions such as PoTS requires an accurate approach to evaluate the aetiology and pathophysiology (which often is heterogeneous), and depending on the contributory issues the need for holistic management [1, 3].

Detailed autonomic assessment in PoTS, including the evaluation of haemodynamic autonomic responses to daily stimuli is important in establishing definitive diagnostic criteria (Fig. 1). Management, in addition to non-pharmacological measures may need a multi-step pharmacological approach and especially in severe cases specific targeting, including medication such as Octreotide to reduce post prandial exacerbation of postural tachycardia and orthostatic intolerance [1] (Fig. 2).

The differences in pathophysiology and multi-systemic involvement can affect all stages of care, and at the Autonomic Unit at the National Hospital for Neurology and

V. Iodice (✉) · C. J. Mathias
Queen Square Institute of Neurology, University College London, London, UK
e-mail: v.iodice@ucl.ac.uk; Valeria.iodice@nhs.net

V. Iodice
Autonomic UnitNational Hospital for Neurology and Neurosurgery, Queen Square, UCLH Trust, London, UK

V. Iodice · C. J. Mathias
Hospital of St. John and St. Elizabeth, Autonomic and Neurovascular Medicine Centre, London, UK

C. J. Mathias
Lindo Wing, St. Mary's Hospital, Imperial College Healthcare Trust, London, UK

N. Gall et al. (eds.), *Postural Tachycardia Syndrome*, https://doi.org/10.1007/978-3-030-54165-1_43

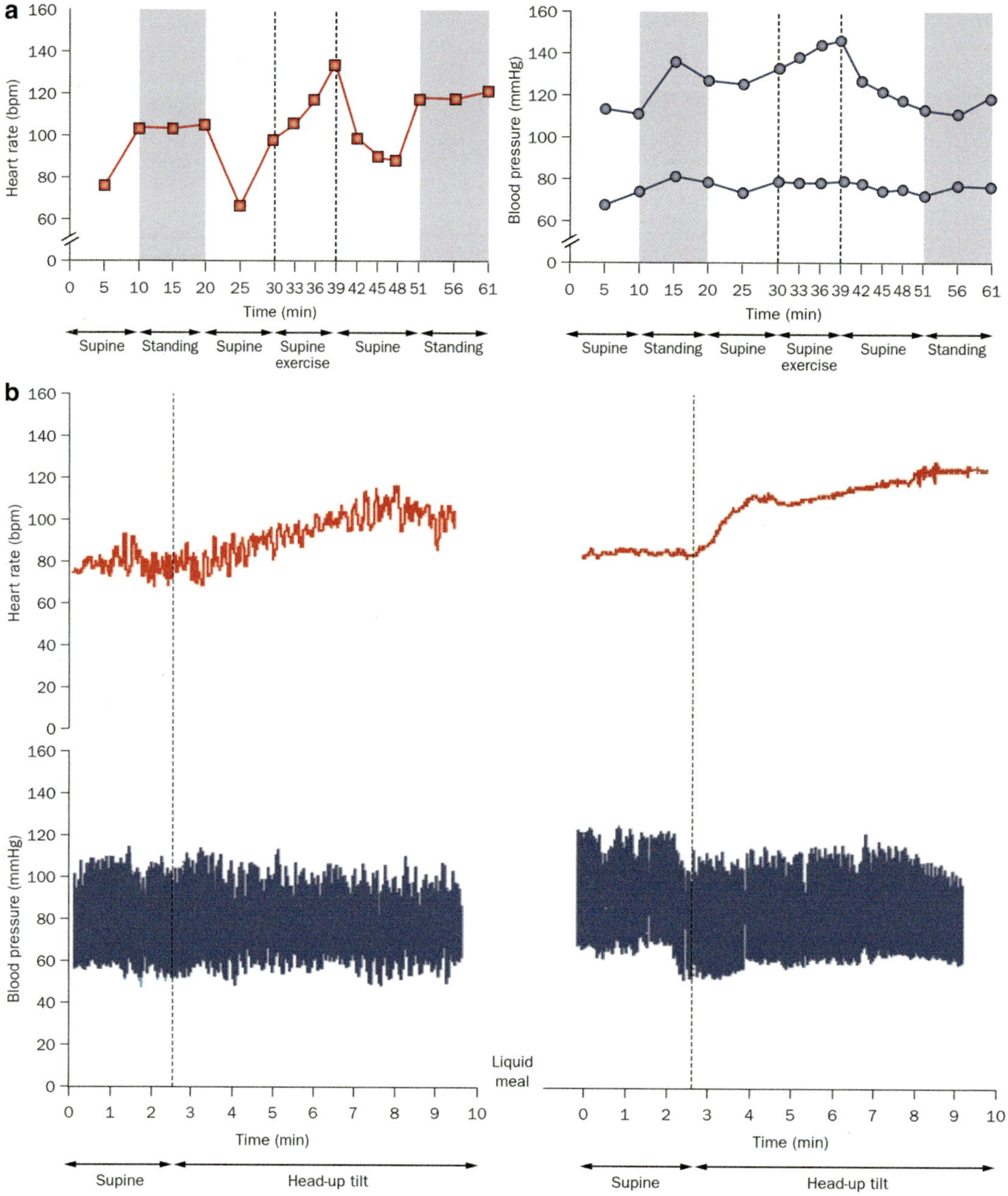

Fig. 1 Changes in heart rate and blood pressure associated with various stimuli in a patient with PoTS. **a** Changes observed during standing, as well as before and after a graded supine cycling exercise. **b** Changes observed while supine and during head-up tilt, before and after ingestion of a balanced liquid meal. The patient's blood pressure (top line, systolic blood pressure; bottom line, diastolic blood pressure) and heart rate responses to exercise are preserved, but while standing after exercise (even 10–15 min later) the heart rate remains elevated and above the rate measured before exercise. A greater rise in the heart rate is observed on head-up tilt after ingestion of the meal, compared with the rate during head-up tilt before the meal. *Abbreviation* PoTS, postural tachycardia syndrome [5]

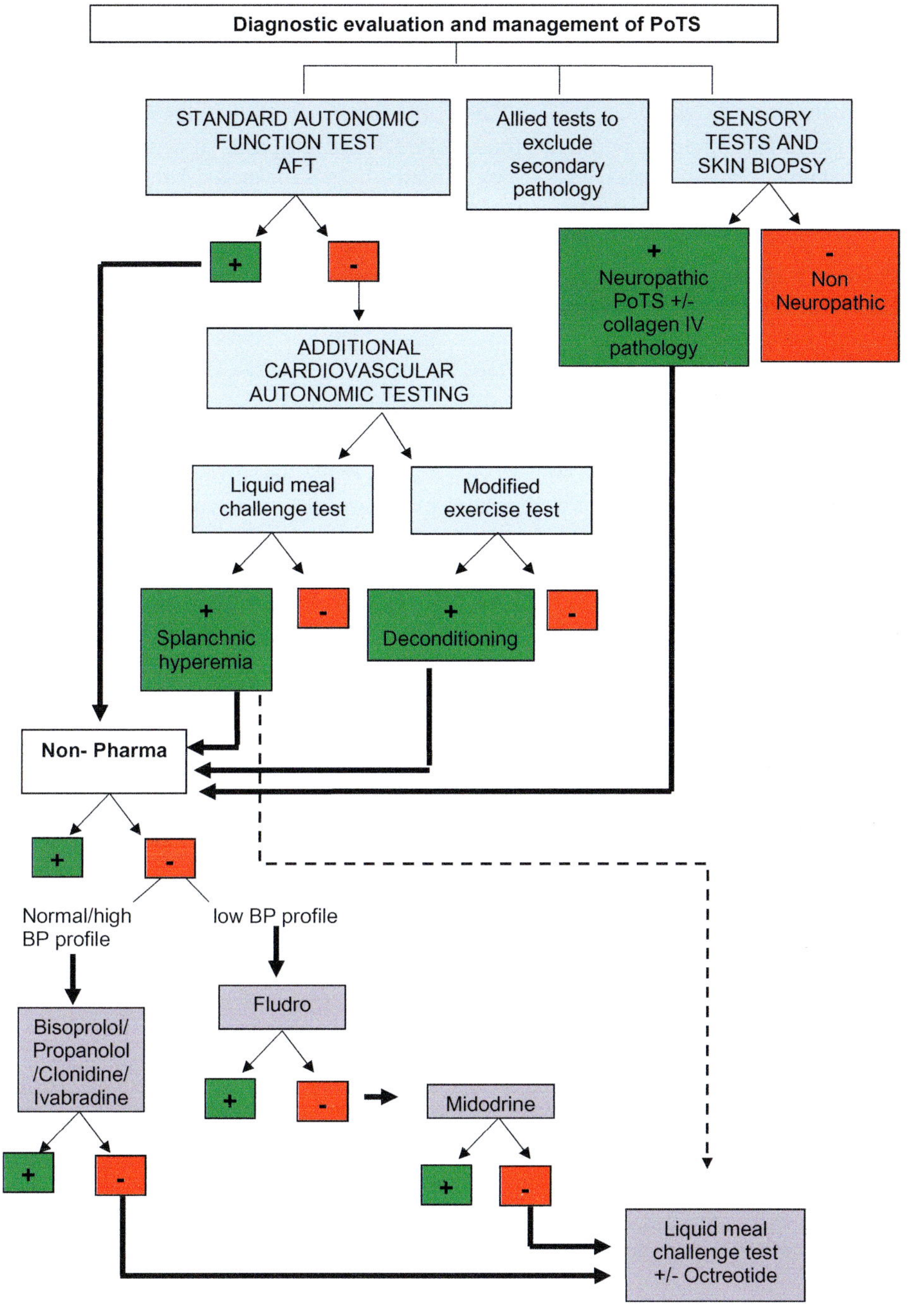

Fig. 2 Diagnostic evaluation and management of PoTS including the standard autonomic evaluation (Head up tilt and standing tests), allied investigation to exclude secondary pathology [5], and skin biopsy to define the Neuropathic phenotype and the collagen pathology [7]. Patients who are negative on standard autonomic investigation are investigated with liquid meal and exercise challenge tests, which are also informative in terms of pathophysiology, indicating predominant splanchnic hyperemia and pooling in the muscle vascular beds after exercise. The autonomic cardiovascular investigation is crucial in tailoring the patients management. Patients who do not response to first and second line treatment and with evidence of splanchnic hyperemia (liquid meal challenge test with and without octreotide) can benefit from octreotide

Neurosurgery we have adopted a multi-disciplinary team (MDT) approach, with an established care pathway for patients with different autonomic disorders that includes PoTS. This is especially so in PoTS and in particular those with multi systemic involvement.

Patient Care Pathways for PoTS: The MDT Approach

In our tertiary referral centre patients with autonomic disorders are seen by consultants with an extensive and broad experience in different types of autonomic disorders. In addition there are specially trained clinical autonomic scientists who are essential for precise and individualised investigation. There are experienced specialist nurses to ensure streamlined care.

The patient pathway in the Autonomic unit at National Hospital for Neurology and Neurosurgery (NHNN) includes an initial consultation with an autonomic consultant, to determine if there is multi-domain autonomic involvement (cardiovascular, sudomotor, bladder and GI tract, amongst others), to focus on appropriate autonomic evaluation followed by targeted treatment [1].

Patients are assessed with a range of autonomic cardiovascular tests and sudomotor assessment, both in the laboratory and also in the home [3]. This quantifies the degree of autonomic dysfunction, determines if there are factors which can overlap and affect autonomic dysfunction, and helps to establish phenotypes of PoTS in relation to probable pathophysiology (Fig. 2).

Details of the different autonomic investigations have been described in detail. The initial focus of investigation should be on cardiovascular autonomic function, and in particular to exclude disorders that cause autonomic failure, some from a fixed and irreversible lesion.

The cardiovascular responses to head up tilt (HUT) and standing are key diagnostic tests to identify PoTS, and contributors to orthostatic tolerance at our centre. A number of factors can exacerbate orthostatic intolerance, and are of particular importance in those who initially do not meet the PoTS criteria on HUT or standing, but in whom the diagnosis is likely. In them PoTS features can be worsened by stimuli in daily life, such as food ingestion, exertion and heat. Assessing the haemodynamic responses to these daily life stimuli is of importance in the diagnosis of PoTS and determining which factors are of relevance (Fig. 1), especially with management.

24-hr autonomic profiles using ambulatory monitoring of blood pressure and heart rate using the protocol devised in our department, with a diary that details the times of prescribed exercises and manoeuvres, ascertains valuable information in the daily life of patients with PoTS and other autonomic conditions (Fig. 3).

In subgroups, nonautonomic investigations and evaluations may be indicated to exclude secondary pathology. These may include echocardiography in suspected mitral valve prolapse, neuroimaging of cranio-cervical junction to exclude Chiari malformation, thermal threshold studies in possible smallfibre neuropathy, and psychological assessment. Depending on the patient's clinical features, urinary bladder, gastro-intestinal and pelvic investigations may also be needed [1].

Each case is reviewed by the MDT which consists of autonomic consultants, clinical autonomic scientists and autonomic specialist nurses, resulting in a comprehensive evaluation of each PoTS patient from different points of view tailored to the needs of the individual.

Following MDT evaluation, if a diagnosis of PoTS is confirmed, patients are invited to a management clinic led by a specialist nurse. These are group clinics aimed at providing the patients with an educational session exploring non-pharmacological strategies that include exercise management.

Once non-pharmacological approaches are established, if needed drug treatment is tailored to each patient, guided by symptomatology, phenotype and the cardiovascular autonomic profile [1, 4] (Fig. 2).

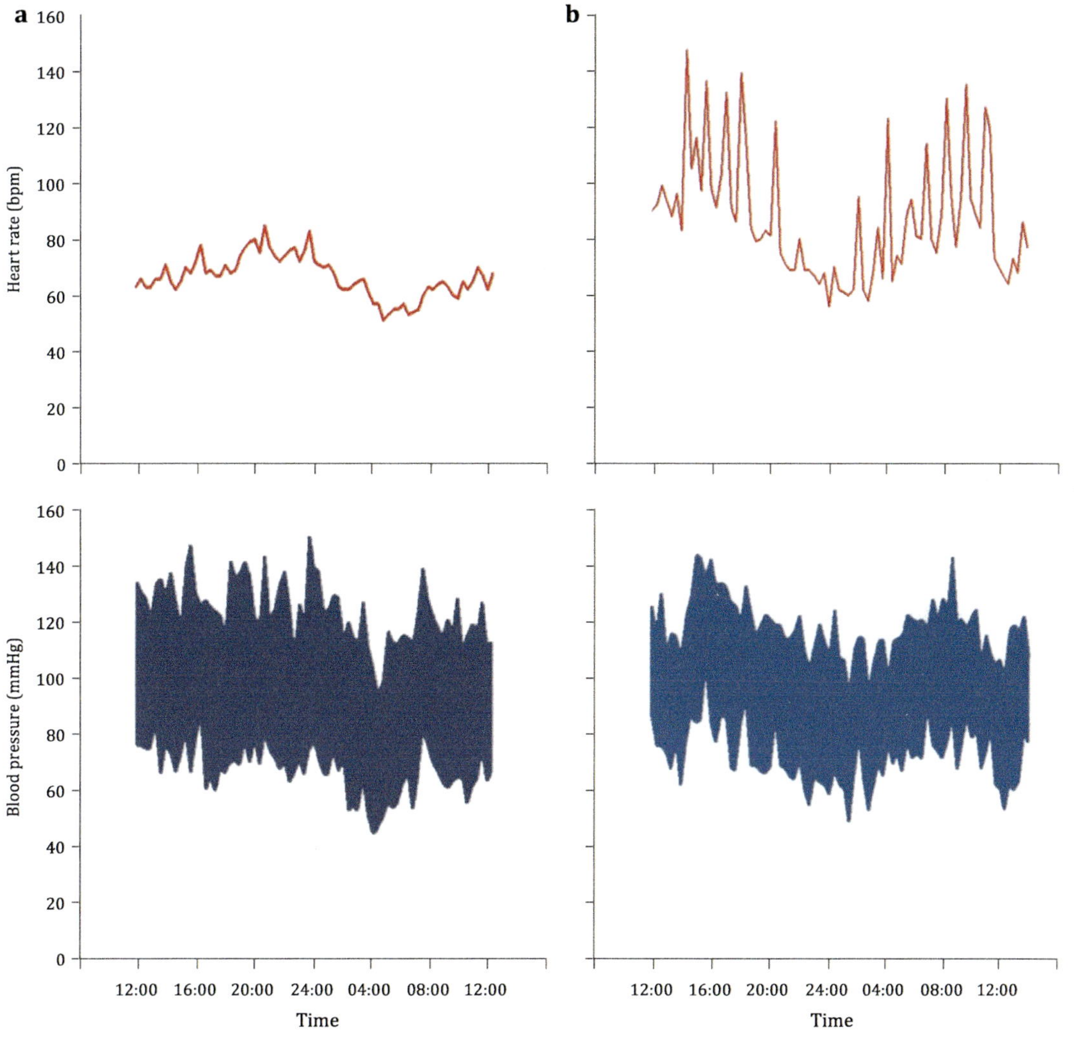

Fig. 3 Blood pressure and heart rate profiles during 24-h ambulatory monitoring using the London Autonomic Units protocol. **a** Profile from a healthy individual. **b** Profile from a patient with PoTS. The elevations in heart rate observed in the patient with PoTS were mainly related to periods of being upright. Abbreviation: PoTS, postural tachycardia syndrome [6]

Multi-Systemic Disorder

Given the considerable variability in both pathophysiology, patient characteristics, and the associated condition the joint hypermobile form of Ehlers-Danlos syndrome (EDS), we recognise that although an autonomic physician manages key aspects of PoTS, co-ordination with specialists offering differing expertise is often are required. This could include a gastroenterologist, uro-neurologist, sleep specialist, psychologist and rheumatologist, and ideally in those with previous experience in dealing with autonomic conditions.

At University College London Hospital (UCLH) and at the Autonomic Unit at the NHNN, clinicians with different specialisations and expertise are part of a network that address patient needs on different aspect of their care.

The Impact of a MDT Approach in Diagnosis and Management of PoTS

MDT evaluation at a tertiary referral centre such as ours has resulted in phenotyping of PoTS patients with a quantitative assessment of the autonomic nervous system, and this aids development of a targeted treatment plan.

Patients return for at least 2 follow up consultations, depending on their response to treatment and to refine management strategy if needed. The MDT approach, in addition to beneficial patient outcomes after optimisation of therapy should be associated with reduced healthcare costs, both primary and secondary.

When to Refer to a Tertiary Referral Centre?

1. To confirm the diagnosis of PoTS and determine associated features that influence symptoms.
2. To establish the phenotype in PoTS.
3. To improve management in PoTS not responsive to non-pharmacological approaches.
4. For PoTS patients in whom orthostatic tachycardia and symptoms are likely to be worse after daily stimuli such as food ingestion, exertion and heat, and to aid different treatment schedules and strategies.
5. For PoTS patients with severe or debilitating symptoms not responding to standard treatment and who may need autonomic inpatient rehabilitation. This enables objectively quantifying exercise tolerance and closely monitoring response during rehabilitation.

Concluding Remarks

The evaluation and accurate diagnosis of autonomic dysfunction continues to be challenging, particularly in PoTS patients, many of which in the past have been considered to have "medically unexplained symptoms". More knowledge is needed to better define the varying PoTS phenotype, to dissect genetic components, and link these with differing therapeutic strategies, especially in complex and resistant cases. Our experience in a tertiary referral centre over the last 2 decades confirms that the MDT approach to PoTS, results in an earlier and definitive diagnosis and in individualised management with positive patient outcomes.

References

1. Mathias CJ, Low DA, Iodice V, Owens AP, Kirbis M, Grahame R. Postural tachycardia syndrome–current experience and concepts. Nat Rev Neurol. 2011;8(1):22–34.
2. Mathias CJ, Ingle G. Autonomic aspects of neurology. In: Clarke C, Howard R, Rossor M, Shorvon S, editors. Wiley-Blackwell; 2016.
3. Kimpinski K, Figueroa JJ, Singer W, Sletten DM, Iodice V, Sandroni P, et al. A prospective, 1-year follow-up study of postural tachycardia syndrome. Mayo Clin Proc. 2012;87(8):746–52.
4. Mathias CJ, Low D, Iodice V, Bannister R. Investigation of autonomic disorders. Mathias CJ, Bannister R, editors. Oxford University Press, Oxford; 2013.
5. Wells R, Elliott AD, Mahajan R, Page A, Iodice V, Sanders P, et al. Efficacy of therapies for postural tachycardia syndrome: a systematic review and meta-analysis. Mayo Clin Proc. 2018;93(8):1043–53.
6. Mathias CJ, Low DA, Iodice V, Owens AP, Kirbis M, Grahame R. Postural tachycardia syndrome–current experience and concepts. Nat Rev Neurol. 2012;8(1):22–34.
7. Jacob G, Costa F, Shannon JR, Robertson RM, Wathen M, Stein M, et al. The neuropathic postural tachycardia syndrome. The New England J Med. 2000;343(14):1008–14.

The Management of PoTS in a District General Hospital, A Personal View

Diane Bruce

Introduction

Most individuals with autonomic dysfunction suffer with symptoms which may have a potential cardiac cause. In an audit of patients attending my specialist secondary care cardiac clinic, the top three most frequently presenting complaints were rhythm disturbance, syncope/presyncope and fatigue/exercise intolerance. This finding was independent of the referral source and included patients referred from the emergency department (ED).

The Role of the Cardiologist

A cardiologist is very well-placed to see and manage this group for a number of reasons. They are experienced in rhythm management, its investigation and treatment. We also manage disorders of blood pressure on a daily basis. The exclusion of sinister causes of such symptoms is very important. For example, in our clinic cohort we have three patients who were found to have both PoTS and Long QT Syndrome (LQTS), previously unrecognised. Referral to clinical genetics confirmed evidence of familial LQTS and hypermobile EDS. Occasionally patients may have a co-existing cardiac diagnosis such as a re-entry tachycardia requiring a referral to electrophysiology.

Cardiologists have access to imaging and physiological tests such as exercise testing and cardio-pulmonary exercise testing. It is an interesting point however that within the large cohort of patients seen in our service, no significant echocardiographic abnormalities have been found other than mild mitral valve prolapse and/or mild dilatation of the aortic root. Very occasionally a slightly low left ventricular ejection fraction (LVEF) has been noted, although no significant findings on subsequent cardiac MRI have been found and often with improvement on serial echos. It may be that a rapid resting rate will confound measures of LVEF.

Ideally, in view of the wide array of systems affected by autonomic dysfunction, it is preferable to have experience in general medicine.

The "goal" for the doctor is to help the patient back to a normal life for them, using both non-pharmacological and pharmacological treatments [2]. They can be managed as out-patients in most circumstances. In our cohort, patients have never required admission.

Very rarely, a patient may require a more invasive approach, such as the need for an implantable loop recorder (ILR), to facilitate the diagnosis of syncope for instance, or an

D. Bruce (✉)
Consultant Cardiologist, The Royal Bournemouth Hospital, Castle Lane East, Bournemouth BH7 7DW, United Kingdom
e-mail: dianebruce@me.com

N. Gall et al. (eds.), *Postural Tachycardia Syndrome*, https://doi.org/10.1007/978-3-030-54165-1_44

electrophysiological study to investigate an SVT; an ILR was implanted in less than 0.2% of patients in our cohort.

So far in our cohort, two patients have proceeded to pacing for significant pauses (>10 s) associated with a syncopal episode. However, both were counselled to the effect that the cause of syncopal events in dysautonomia is often multifactorial, with both bradycardia and hypotension, and that pacing would not necessarily be a "cure". Both patients continue to have episodes unfortunately.

The running of a PoTS service lends itself to doctors and other practitioners working part-time; indeed, by not having duties associated with ward rounds and on-call, the clinician can focus more on the expansive needs of this patient group.

Developing a PoTS Service

In persuading colleagues and managers that a specialist PoTS service is not only desirable but necessary, one needs evidence that these patients exist within the provider group, but also that investment of the clinical time and effort will produce results, reducing unplanned attendances, admissions and repeated investigations. One patient seen in our department had attended the ED over a hundred times before reaching a diagnosis of autonomic dysfunction. Subsequently, after diagnosis, he has only attended twice in the last six months.

It is appropriate to highlight to managers and commissioners that these individuals are already in the system within the hospital and often are referred back multiple times due to persistently unexplained symptoms. General practitioners often struggle to know which sort of specialist to approach next. By initiating a specialist clinic, one is simply "streamlining" and facilitating a more holistic approach for these patients. Patient choice and "cost-neutral" can be useful terms to include in any proposals. Examples of other specialist services such as Atrial Fibrillation or Syncope Clinics may be used as an illustration. Admission avoidance is a top priority for most healthcare organisations.

Referral Sources

Patients may be referred from a variety of sources; initially our referrals came from cardiology colleagues who had failed to find a cardiac explanation for their patient's symptoms. However, with spreading knowledge, general practitioners, ED consultants and other internal medicine colleagues began to refer patients because of 'medically unexplained symptoms". After interacting with social media and support groups, patients began to request a referral from their GP. The key to identifying more patients where an autonomic problem is underlying was through the education of colleagues, particularly those working in "frontline" areas. Our team of advanced cardiology nurse practitioners have quickly become adept at recognising patients in ED or on cardiology ward rounds.

Going Live with the Service

Our service was facilitated by changes to our general cardiology outpatients' service. Patients with autonomic problems such as inappropriate sinus tachycardia, PoTS or syncope/presyncope were diverted into one of two four hour clinics run by a single consultant with ad hoc support from the team of cardiology specialist nurses. The investigations required for this group were all located within cardiology. We no longer have tilt table and autonomic function testing on site, but we refer to a nearby hospital, as required.

Currently our service accepts referrals from Dorset, (population 425,000), Hampshire (population 1.37 million) and Wiltshire (population 480,000). At times, referrals are accepted from 'out of area' but this can prove difficult with arranging investigations and can affect waiting times for local patients. This sometimes led to closing to referrals out of area until the waiting times for appointments improved.

Arranging both a morning and an afternoon clinic is desirable as some patients find it easier to travel and attend at certain times of day, especially if they are unable to drive. Contacting patients by telephone 48 hours beforehand reduced non-attendance rates. Ideally any necessary investigations are carried out prior to the consultation, so that results are available at the first consultation. All our new patients have a 12 Lead ECG and seven-day ECG monitoring to assess the burden of arrhythmia, a 24 hour ambulatory BP monitor and a transthoracic echocardiogram. If these have been carried out within the last 12 months by other practitioners, there is no need for them to be repeated unless there has been a significant change in symptoms.

Allowing adequate time to take a full and detailed history cannot be over-emphasised; we allow one hour per patient. Our patients have usually had years, if not decades, of problems, that have been unexplained [3] and understandably many feel angry, dissatisfied and disillusioned. We emphasize that there may still be much to discuss and further outstanding information can be obtained at subsequent appointments. We hope they feel valued with this approach. We encourage patients to bring a partner or relative; it helps with obtaining a family history and the details of syncopal episodes, for example.

History Taking

Patients with autonomic problems have numerous symptoms which can be very variable; we concentrate on their "Top Three" symptoms, to focus the dialogue in the "here and now" before going on to a more extensive medical history. Early life medical history can offer useful clues to any underlying pre-disposition to dysautonomia. Finding out about prolonged periods of school/college absence is vital. "Trigger" factors, physical, mental or emotional, should be sought; many patients will not raise these issues unless specifically asked. We often ask "When do YOU feel that you were last well"; this is often pertinent as many patients cannot recall ever having felt well!

It is not uncommon for patients to have had dissociative episodes. Many are reluctant to divulge information about these unless probed but feel very relieved when it is covered. A full dietary history can provide valuable insight and again needs a sensitive approach. Sleep and any disruption of sleep pattern is also important.

Physical Examination

The physical examination should include the identification of possible joint hypermobility examining the skin for "extensibility", stretch marks and abnormal scars. Flushing and urticaria may also be relevant. Acrocyanosis of the hands and feet should be documented.

In addition to the standard cardiovascular examination, we also measure heart rate and blood pressure supine and after five and ten minutes of upright posture. Asking the patient to place their hands on the back of a chair for support can be useful to maintain safety. Encourage them to report any light headedness or the need to sit or lie down.

Patients often have lots of questions they feel need answering and it is worth having a selection of useful patient leaflets available (such as those from PoTS UK, STARS, EDS UK and Mast Cell Action). One needs to highlight that Classical or Vascular-Type EDS are rare and almost never found.

Making a clear plan for follow-up is vital. The trend to try to keep outpatient follow up to a minimum is difficult to apply to this group of patients.

Autonomic dysfunction is not a "quick-fix" and a range of treatment modalities may be used over time. Ideally the next appointment should be within three months and the patients encouraged to monitor changes in their symptoms with treatments, including lifestyle measures and pharmacological therapy. It cannot be over-emphasised that the investment of time in this first consultation reaps benefits by allowing time to educate the patient and their family about their condition and how best to manage it.

Our clinic is designed such that it has no more than two new patient consultations in any one session with up to four follow ups. We see a further two new PoTS referrals from the ED most weeks in a separate service (ambulatory cardiac clinic). Our clinic at the Royal Bournemouth Hospital has been running for almost five years now with around 300 new and 500 follow up patients each year.

The specialist nurses support the doctor working within the clinic, sitting in on clinics providing a part-time support role seeing patients for follow-up. They also provide telephone review and will answer patient emails. It is vital that the time spent dealing with patients by phone or email is documented so that it can be included in job planning. There is a significant workload in terms of administrative duties which must be recognised such as replying to phone calls, and writing letters of support for schools, colleges, and welfare assessments.

Children and Adolescents with Dysautonomia

This group of patients is currently not well-provided for in the UK for a variety of reasons, yet PoTS/vasovagal syncope does occur in children and adolescents; puberty may often "kick start" the disorder. On a positive note, with appropriate support, PoTS may be a less chronic, more self-limiting disorder in this age group [4]. Our service sees patients from 13 years and older, usually referred by paediatricians.

Training in Safeguarding and Paediatric Life Support Training are vital. Patients under 16 requiring cardiac investigations are referred on to another local trust.

We recommend, when possible, arranging a multidisciplinary meeting with the referring paediatrician to discuss the patients and to formulate a treatment plan.

It is important to allow more time for consultations involving young people as it can take time to encourage them to discuss their symptoms and to listen to their "version" which may differ from their parents! More often than not, several family members may have similar symptoms, perhaps related to hypermobility. There is a distinct lack of local support groups for people of this age group. Many are inappropriately referred to adolescent mental health services waiting months for assessment.

The Role of Other Practitioners

Cardiologists working with PoTS patients soon need to diversify and call on wider general medical knowledge. Many have issues affecting their gastrointestinal and urological systems and may also have skin/allergy problems. Building up a team of interested and sympathetic colleagues is important. Multidisciplinary meetings with neurology and the ED are particularly useful. Presenting case studies at wider meetings can be useful in making other specialties aware of this group of conditions.

Exercise is an important part of the treatment plan and one must explore the services available locally. A scheme called "Move to Improve" exists in our local Rheumatology Department and has had fantastic results for our patients. Our Cardiac Rehabilitation service also has a "Keep Well" scheme with exercise prescription and healthy lifestyle advice which is also proving beneficial.

Caring for the Carers

Working in this type of service is extremely rewarding but also challenging. Even colleagues within the department may appear disinterested because of the multiple symptoms and co-morbidities. Often these patients are thought of as "difficult". My personal view is that the cardiologist should only work part-time in this field and also have another role within the department. Delegating uncomplicated patients back to the original referrer or a specialist nurse helps to keep the service open to new referrals.

Many patients are reluctant to be discharged but that is important, as is having an "open door policy". In our service, a registered patient can "self-refer" back within six months. We refer to tertiary centres for advice and guidance if a patient is not progressing as one expects.

Occasionally one may see patients who have many features of PoTS but something is "not quite right". We had three patients who clinically had PoTS but inflammatory markers were high and they did not seem to improve as quickly as expected on initial therapy. All three developed lymphomas within weeks of their initial review despite there being no obvious signs of a haematological malignancy at presentation. One must always be alert to the threat of misdiagnosis.

There are usually very few other specialists in this field in any one region. By attending clinical meetings with other specialist colleagues, one gets reassurance about one's own practice. Holiday cover for the service and "succession planning" must be discussed once the service is established. Obviously not all patients with dysautonomia can be seen by a single practitioner, and it can be helpful to educate colleagues at every possible opportunity. PoTS and other dysautonomias are not uncommon and remain eminently treatable; the lives of these patients and their families can be improved, sometimes by even the most basic of therapies, and this is surely a worthy message to disseminate.

Summary

There is increasing acceptance of the need to manage chronic conditions such as PoTS and related disorders of autonomic function in the world of health care. This can only improve the lives of the patients who struggle with autonomic symptoms but also empower the specialist teams looking after them.

The provision of a local service in every district hospital, which accepts the reality of PoTS and associated disorders and provides care and hope for everyone facing the life-changing scenario of autonomic symptoms, must truly be the vision of all of us working in this field.

References

1. Cornwall DJ. Invisible illness-how to sustain hope. Huffington Post July 11 2014.
2. Boris JR. The role of the cardiologist in the evaluation of dysautonomia. Cardiol. Young. 2010;133–9.
3. Freeman K, Goldstein DS, Thompson CK. The dysautonomia project. USA: Bardolf and Company;2015.
4. Kizilbash SJ, Ahrens SP, Bhatia R, Killian JM, Kimmes SA, Knoebel EE, Muppa P, Weaver AL, Fischer PR. Long-term outcomes of adolescent-onset postural orthostatic tachycardia syndrome. Clin Auton Res. October 2013. In: Abstract presented at the 24th international symposium on the autonomic nervous system.

A Tertiary Hospital Cardiology Model of Care

Nicholas Gall

Previous chapters in this textbook have detailed the complexity of PoTS in view of its relatively recent discovery and indeed its definition which describes a significant aspect of the physiology although whether that remains the sole and major driver to the condition remains uncertain. Details relating to the complexity of the pathophysiology, differing presentations and widespread effects have also been discussed. It is clear that, in understanding the management of this condition both in the UK and with colleagues around the world, there is no single, successful model for the assessment and management of this group of patients. As the condition seems to associate with a number of other conditions it may be managed in many different settings. It seems likely to have an autonomic neurological basis but presents significantly with cardiovascular symptoms and therefore it may present to cardiologists or to autonomic neurologists in most part. Provision of autonomic neurology in the UK certainly is limited and therefore in most part it will tend to present to cardiologists. Much of the symptomatology relates to palpitation, presyncope and syncope and in association with the sinus tachycardia, it often presents to cardiac electrophysiologists with questions relating to whether there may be an underlying arrhythmic problem leading to syncope associated with a risk of sudden cardiac death; alternatively palpitations with a possibility that a supraventricular tachycardia may be relevant are also raised.

It was on this basis that the PoTS unit based at King's College Hospital developed. While a number of the patients presenting described frequent ectopic beat-related palpitation, much of the presentation seemed to relate to tachycardia and therefore the question of an SVT was paramount. Patients were therefore seen in the clinical electrophysiology clinics. It became increasingly clear that the presentation, while occasionally highlighting frequent ectopy or SVT, mostly related to the findings of an inappropriately fast sinus tachycardia. We took a particularly cardiological view to investigate the symptoms, undertaking an echocardiogram to exclude structural heart disease, several days of Holter monitoring to investigate the tachycardia profile and in an attempt to exclude significant arrhythmia, a cardiopulmonary exercise test in view of the presentation with chest pain, breathlessness and fatigue and the tilt test/active stand to investigate the autonomic orthostatic haemodynamics. We have the advantage of in-house autonomic neurology so that more complex symptoms could be investigated with more formalised autonomic function tests to investigate more significant autonomic neuropathic

N. Gall (✉)
Department of Cardiology, King's College Hospital, London SE5 9RS, UK
e-mail: nickgall@doctors.org.uk

N. Gall et al. (eds.), *Postural Tachycardia Syndrome*, https://doi.org/10.1007/978-3-030-54165-1_45

processes. While there remains uncertainty as to which investigations to undertake in any individual patient, these investigations became our standard and allowed us to focus on a number of individual symptomatic aspects of our patients leading on to therapeutic options for the low and variable BP, the sinus tachycardia and dysfunctional breathing, as detailed in other areas of this textbook.

The investigations undertaken are mostly available in any hospital via cardiology although tilt provision is not available in all hospitals and cardiopulmonary exercise testing may only be available in certain tertiary centres. They are not critical to the diagnosis but certainly have proven beneficial to assist in our understanding of the condition and have driven therapeutic benefits.

The main challenge has focused on the increasing numbers of referrals and fitting those into a busy tertiary centre practice where there is a focus on the ablation of arrhythmia and both simple and complex device work. The management of patients revolves around standard non-pharmacological approaches and advice is offered with specialist arrhythmia nurses available to discuss further management and provide advice during more symptomatic episodes. We use a number of medications particularly focusing on the more cardiovascular-acting medications, as we have become familiar with their use. We often give patients the first dose of midodrine or ivabradine to ensure that there are no adverse haemodynamic consequences and indeed that is now enshrined in local South-East London guidelines. In general, the assessment of patients taking their first dose of medication tends not to highlight any significant adverse cardiovascular consequences but provides reassurance particularly for patients and primary care physicians who are not familiar with these medications.

We have taken a multidisciplinary approach to the management of our patients, as while they may present predominantly with cardiovascular symptoms, as is obvious from the chapters in this book, there do seem to be many associated conditions and symptoms. Patients are often particularly symptomatic in multiple territories and merely focusing on the haemodynamic changes does not necessarily lead to enormous symptomatic benefit. In that regard, therefore, we have developed links with a number of specialists both in our hospital and in others, in an effort to deal with these more widespread symptoms. There do seem to be very characteristic symptomatic conditions in a number of organ systems and we have developed links with like-minded physicians who can provide support with those individual symptoms although the overall care of the patients has remained with our unit. The model therefore is one of the management of the cardiovascular symptoms in an arrhythmia clinic with support from specialist arrhythmia nursing while maintaining an interest in the more widespread symptoms and enlisting the assistance of associated specialties.

Patient Considerations

PoTS from a Patient's Perspective

Lesley Kavi and Lorna Nicholson

Awareness of PoTS

Lack of awareness amongst medical professionals remains problematic for patients. PoTS was recognised, named, and defined in 1993, and is not a prescribed part of medical school curricula or specialist training in the UK. Anecdotally, many healthcare professionals have not heard of the condition.

The word 'syndrome' is derived from a Greek word meaning 'running together' or 'concurrence'. It is recognised that PoTS is **not** a diagnosis in its own right, with one single underlying pathophysiology or disease entity. Rather, it is a syndrome consisting of a collection of similar symptoms and signs. An analogy may be drawn with heart failure which is also a syndrome, with similar symptoms and signs, yet multiple disparate mechanisms, underlying diseases and treatments (e.g. rheumatic valve disease, inherited cardiomyopathy, amyloidosis, ischaemic heart disease). However, there are clinicians who do not believe that PoTS exists as a syndrome, or that there are no treatment options if a patient meets the diagnostic criteria for PoTS.

L. Kavi (✉)
Solihull Healthcare Partnership, 3 Grove Road, Solihull B91 2AG, West Midlands, UK
e-mail: lesley@potsuk.org

L. Nicholson
PoTS UK, Sheffield, UK

Obtaining a Diagnosis

The first challenge for patients is to obtain an accurate diagnosis, which for many can take several years. The mean time from first consulting a healthcare professional in the UK with symptoms to obtaining a diagnosis was almost 4 years [1] and from symptom onset to diagnosis is 7 years [2] with a number taking over 20 years before obtaining an explanation for their symptoms.

Patients often describe a prolonged battle with the health service, having experienced a number of specialist referrals over a period of years. In one UK study, almost half of affected people were initially given a psychiatric diagnosis such as anxiety, depression, panic disorder or hypochondriasis as an explanation for their physical symptoms; this occurs more commonly in female patients (75%) compared to males (25%) [1]. Consequently, mistrust of doctors and other healthcare professionals is common.

In our experience, it is common for patients to suggest that they have PoTS to their healthcare professional after learning about it from family or friends or following research on the internet. In the UK it is most common for a cardiologist to suggest the diagnosis, followed by the patient [1]. The commonest symptoms of PoTS are light-headedness, fatigue and palpitations. These are non-specific symptoms found in many conditions, and it needs a high index of suspicion to

N. Gall et al. (eds.), *Postural Tachycardia Syndrome*, https://doi.org/10.1007/978-3-030-54165-1_46

detect PoTS in people who present with these symptoms (especially younger women).

During their diagnostic journey, patients often undergo multiple investigations. Due to lack of communication, the same test may be repeated several times. When patients undergo tests such as prolonged ECG monitoring or event recorders, recurrent tachycardias that may suggest PoTS are interpreted as due to anxiety.

Patients are often visibly relieved to receive a diagnosis and to have their symptoms validated by a healthcare professional.

For patients who do receive a 'diagnosis' of PoTS, there is often no attempt to identify any co-morbidities such as connective tissue or autoimmune disorders.

Referrals

Patients in the UK are often referred to cardiology when they present with palpitations or chest pain. Many, but not all the cardiologists who are experienced at managing PoTS are cardiac electrophysiologists. Referral to syncope or blackout clinics may occur when fainting is a presenting complaint. Patients may also be seen by neurologists, autonomic specialists, general physicians or paediatricians. Some elderly medicine specialists who have access to the tilt table as a diagnostic tool will also see and manage younger patients with PoTS.

Many patients report difficulties in obtaining referrals to knowledgeable specialists. Problems include:

- GPs can be unwilling to refer to a specialist.
- Waiting times to see a specialist can be lengthy; this can be up to one year.
- Due to lack of understanding of symptoms, multiple referrals are often made to multiple specialities.
- In some areas there are few or no clinicians with an interest in PoTS. This is especially problematic in Scotland and Wales and for children throughout the UK.
- Where no local specialist with training and experience in managing PoTS patients exists, patients experience difficulty in obtaining out of area referrals.
- Some specialist PoTS centres have been overwhelmed with referrals resulting in a number no longer accepting out of area patients.

Management

Management is inconsistent throughout the UK. Sometimes when a diagnosis is made, patients are discharged from the service with little information on how to manage their condition. 43% of patients reported that their healthcare advisors admitted that they did not know what advice to give their patient [1].

Patients often have symptoms involving multiple systems, and therefore specialists in a variety of clinical areas may be involved in their care. This can lead to communication difficulties between healthcare professionals and repetition of investigations. It can be helpful if a nominated healthcare professional takes on the lead role of co-ordinating care with the patient.

There is limited evidence for PoTS treatments. Much of what is recommended is based on consensus and clinician experience [3]. Management by a multidisciplinary team is often recommended [3], but no such service is known to exist in the UK at the time of writing.

Disability

PoTS can be a life-changing illness. Functional limitations of PoTS patients have been compared with, and found to be equivalent to those of patients with chronic obstructive airways disease and congestive heart failure [4].

PoTS often (although not exclusively) has a predilection for people during their formative or most productive years. It affects young people who could otherwise be in education, the workforce or raising a family, and interferes with their ability to participate in education, or to support themselves or their families financially. Affected people can struggle to participate in normal family life or interact with their peers. Social isolation is a common challenge.

A survey of over 1000 PoTS patients in 2016 [1] revealed that:

- 84% described a reduction in their quality of life
- 5% were bedbound
- 23% were wheelchair users
- 37% had to stop working due to their PoTS symptoms.

PoTS has been described as an invisible illness; patients may appear well yet experience substantial disability. Consequently, they often have had difficulty obtaining relevant health, disability and employment benefits.

Lack of understanding by employers is a common reason for patients to seek help from the national charity, PoTS UK. Patients often experience fluctuations in their health, and small numbers of separate days of sick leave can trigger tools (e.g. the Bradford Factor Calculator [5]) which penalise people who have several short-term absences over those who have the same number of days off work in a single or fewer blocks.

Family and Friends

Patients seem to do best when they are empowered to be coordinators of their own care and with a good support team that involves friends and family to prevent all of the problems associated with isolation. Just as for the patient, the unpredictability of symptoms can be difficult for family and friends to manage, but having a support team that is patient and believes in them can make all the difference in weathering flares in symptoms, and not sinking a into mental health crisis in addition to the physical health burden. For patients and their supporters alike there can be a fine line between encouraging activity and being compassionate when activities are not possible, but seeing this as a team's problem rather than an individual's problem can make a big difference in overall outcome and functioning.

What Would Help Patients

- Obtaining a prompt diagnosis
- Better identification of PoTS in primary care
- Where necessary, prompt referral for a definitive diagnosis to a secondary care specialist with knowledge in this area
- Greater awareness and management at a local level
- Specialist centres throughout the country for those who are more complex—with appropriate funding to take out of area patients
- Clear, accessible out of area referral pathways
- Greater consistency in diagnosis and management throughout the UK
- Management to be multidisciplinary involving support from medical, psychological, dietetic/nutritional, exercise physiology, and physiotherapy services, all tailored to the individual's needs. Most importantly, help to manage lifestyle changes
- Multicentre research into aetiology and best management.

What Are the Charities Doing to Help?

- Providing evidence-based information in the form of websites and patient information leaflets
- Raising awareness amongst the general public and health professionals
- Providing information and support through social media platforms
- Offering an email enquiry service and telephone helpline
- Writing for peer reviewed medical journals
- Organising educational events for patients and healthcare professionals
- Speaking at other medical conferences
- Campaigning for improved services including a multidisciplinary approach to care and shorter waiting times for hospital services.

Negotiating for specialised commissioning for PoTS

- Working towards developing an international patient registry and research network
- Coordinating national guidelines
- Supporting research projects.

We would like to thank the PoTS UK trustees and the members of PoTS UK for their contributions to this article.

References

1. Kavi L, Nuttall N, Low PA, Opie M, Nicholson L, Caldow E, et al. A profile of patients with postural tachycardia syndrome and their experience of healthcare in the UK. Br J Cardiol. 2016;23(33).
2. McDonald C, Koshi S, Busner L, Kavi L, Newton JL. Postural tachycardia syndrome is associated with significant symptoms and functional impairment predominantly affecting young women: a UK perspective. BMJ Open. 2014;4(6):e004127.
3. Sheldon RS, Grubb BP 2nd, Olshansky B, Shen WK, Calkins H, Brignole M, et al. 2015 heart rhythm society expert consensus statement on the diagnosis and treatment of postural tachycardia syndrome, inappropriate sinus tachycardia, and vasovagal syncope. Heart Rhythm. 2015;12(6):e41–63.
4. Benrud-Larson LM, Dewar MS, Sandroni P, Rummans TA, Haythornthwaite JA, Low PA. Quality of life in patients with postural tachycardia syndrome. Mayo Clin Proc. 2002;77(6):531–7.
5. The Bradford Factor Calculator. 2013. https://www.bradfordfactorcalculator.com/.

Living with the Ehlers-Danlos Syndromes (EDS)—The Patients' Perspective

Kay Julier

Introduction

Increased knowledge about the molecular basis for the majority of the Ehlers-Danlos syndromes is not yet impacting the time to diagnosis for the majority of patients. The pathway to diagnosis and correct management is often long and challenging, with multiple misdiagnoses along the way. Families with children who show signs and symptoms face additional challenges. While living positively with the conditions requires active self-management, access to knowledgeable healthcare professionals to provide initial, accurate information and advice is extremely limited. Patients can experience significant disability without the correct diagnosis and management advice. The current reality for most patients is discussed along with the role of patient organisations in providing information, support and shaping service provision.

Getting a Diagnosis

As with PoTS, the key challenge for the majority of patients with Ehlers-Danlos syndrome (EDS) is getting an accurate diagnosis. The increased understanding of the molecular basis for most of the Ehlers-Danlos syndromes now means diagnosis of 12 of the sub-types can be confirmed genetically [1]. However, even in these cases, getting to the point of testing can be a challenge and can take several years. The situation for those with hypermobile EDS (hEDS) or the related hypermobility spectrum disorder (HSD) [2] is particularly bleak. In the UK, the average time from first consulting a healthcare professional with symptoms to obtaining a diagnosis is 10 years [3]. In a survey of Ehlers-Danlos Support UK members in Scotland in 2017, the average time between first seeing a GP about symptoms and being given a diagnosis of EDS was 19 years (based on 316 respondents).

The majority of patients who engage with patient organisations describe 'fighting' to be taken seriously over years, sometimes decades. They experience multiple primary care appointments and specialist referrals with no clear outcomes, commonly being told that symptoms have a psychological cause. Common misdiagnoses include fibromyalgia, chronic pain syndromes, chronic fatigue syndrome or myalgic encephalomyelitis (ME), anxiety, irritable bowel syndrome and functional dyspepsia, medically unexplained symptoms and Munchausen's syndrome.

There continues to be a widespread belief that the symptoms of the Ehlers-Danlos syndromes are musculoskeletal and dermatological,

K. Julier (✉)
The Ehlers-Danlos Support UK, Devonshire House, Manor Way, Borehamwood, Hertfordshire WD6 1QQ, United Kingdom
e-mail: kay@ehlers-danlos.org

N. Gall et al. (eds.), *Postural Tachycardia Syndrome*, https://doi.org/10.1007/978-3-030-54165-1_47

apart from those of vascular EDS, where the involvement of the vasculature is more easily recognised once the diagnosis has been made. The majority of patients interacting with patient organisations report symptoms beyond their joints and skin; mainly gastrointestinal, autonomic, gynaecological and allergy-like problems.

Parents who see signs and symptoms in their children often face an additional battle. Due to the difficulty diagnosing some types of EDS in children and the understandable reluctance of paediatric specialists to label children with a chronic condition early in life, it is almost impossible at the time of writing to get a diagnosis of hEDS for a child in the UK via the National Health Service. At Ehlers-Danlos Support UK, we advise parents not to pursue a diagnosis but instead to seek help to manage their child's symptoms, whatever cause they have been attributed to. Sadly, even this course of action increasingly backfires. With the widespread lack of awareness of the Ehlers-Danlos syndromes and their impact, parents are given little information and guidance. As the child's symptoms get worse, further medical appointments are sought and school hours may be increasingly missed. An increasingly common scenario then is the involvement of child protection services and the investigation of the family for potentially fabricating an illness in the child, which is a form of abuse [4, 5]. (Talem Law, 2018; BBC 5 Live Investigates, 2019).

The Ehlers-Danlos Support UK runs a helpline (as do other organisations supporting this patient group), currently handling around 1,500 telephone and email enquiries per year, with many more attempts to access the service. Over the past three years, finding information about getting a diagnosis has remained the main reason for calling (29%). The next most common calls are about accessing a specialist (23%) and managing symptoms (19%). Callers report that the information they seek is not readily available elsewhere. Figure 1 shows the breakdown of all call types over the period 1 April 2017 to 31 March 2019.

Patients report an improved sense of well-being by having a diagnosis even if treatment options are sparse or uncertain. Especially where lifestyle factors can influence the progression of symptoms, a diagnosis can also encourage people to make positive changes to help manage their condition.

There is sufficient evidence and knowledge about the management of EDS symptoms [6–9], alongside the impact of not having a clear diagnosis [10, 11] to warrant urgent efforts towards faster, more accurate diagnosis and that is what we must all work towards.

Referrals

Patients are usually referred to rheumatology in the first instance due to widespread joint pain and/or frequent unexplained dislocations in the most common types of EDS. However, in primary care, EDS patients may present initially with non-musculoskeletal symptoms such as chronic fatigue, IBS-like symptoms or prolapses [12]. It is expected that the majority of EDS and HSD cases could be managed in primary care but there is an urgent need for increased awareness and understanding first. A primary care multidisciplinary team approach, including physiotherapy, occupational therapy, nurse specialists, possibly psychology and dietetics (as required) would be ideal.

Lack of awareness amongst rheumatologists of the association with multisystemic symptoms means questions are not routinely asked about problems not directly related to the musculoskeletal system or else these are dismissed as being irrelevant if mentioned by the patient. This often results in a refusal to refer on to other specialities (e.g. gastroenterology, urology, gynaecology). As already stated, a multidisciplinary team approach is ideal but is unfortunately very rare at present.

The very small number of EDS specialists with the knowledge and capacity to manage more complex cases leads to long waiting times. As with PoTS, the few specialist centres which

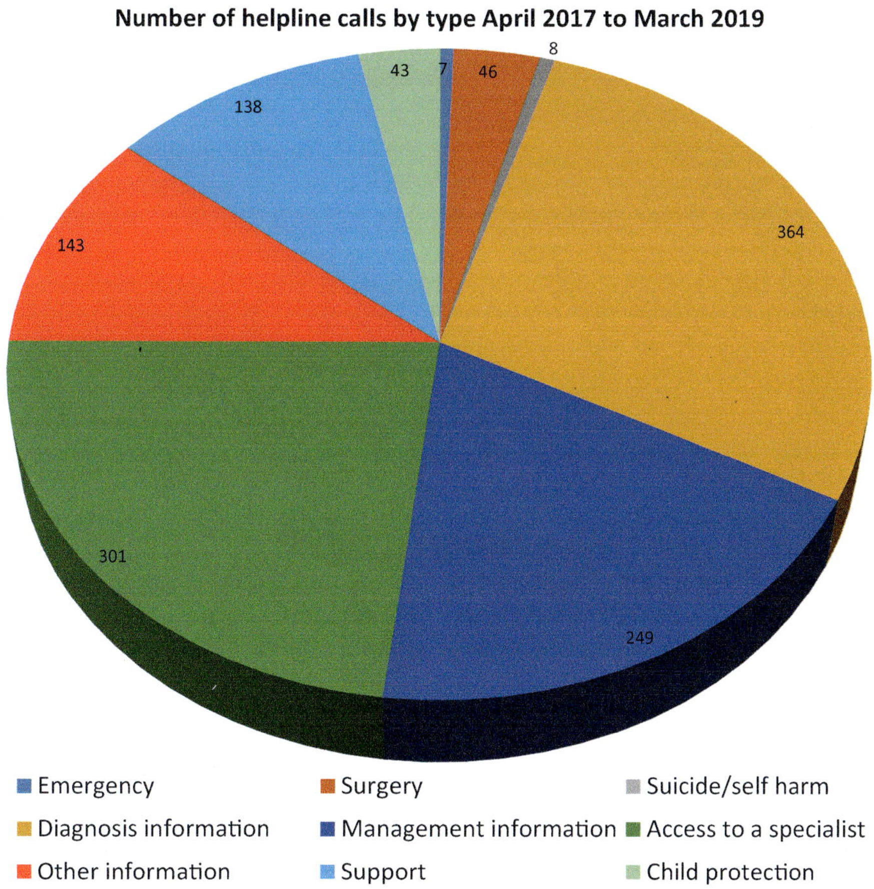

Fig. 1 All call types April 2017 to March 2019

exist are regularly overwhelmed with referrals and frequently have to close to out of area patients. The lack of specialist centres means patients often have to travel very long distances which can be extremely challenging and expensive for those with restricted mobility. In the UK (at the time of writing), there are no formally commissioned services for people with hEDS or HSD, therefore centres seeing these patients, especially the more complex cases, are doing so in the absence of funding and only due to the interest and compassion of the consultants involved.

Again, from a UK perspective, there are slightly more EDS specialists who exclusively see patients through private practice. Many people feel pushed into private healthcare out of sheer frustration, at least to obtain a diagnosis, only to then find that their diagnosis may be questioned as it has been obtained through a private route. Similarly, faced with a diagnosis obtained privately, at present few local services have the knowledge to manage or advise these patients, leading to the majority feeling abandoned unless they can afford to continue seeking advice privately.

There seems to be an increasing number of referrals to local genetics services, possibly as a result of expansion of genomic medicine initiatives such as the 100,000 Genomes Project but this may also be due to increased awareness of the rarer types of EDS, such as vascular EDS, through media exposure. Patient organisations can play an education role here, both in emphasising to patients the rarity of the majority of EDS subtypes (and so providing reassurance) and in helping to explain the lack of genetic tests for hEDS, HSD and related conditions.

Management

Often a diagnosis is made and patients are sent on their way with little advice as to how to manage day to day living with their condition(s). Some clinicians are open about their reluctance to give a diagnosis due to the incorrect belief that there is no treatment or management which can help so 'what's the point?'.

EDS and conditions often associated with it, like PoTS, largely depend on self-management by the patient, and patient organisations play a key role here in offering evidence-based information, advice, encouragement and support. The mainstays of treatment and management are covered elsewhere in this book and these are reinforced by patient groups, who are often in a position to develop engaging materials and use a variety of media and methods to widely share the information.

For patients who are diagnosed late and especially for those who have deconditioned, there can be a period of grieving for the life they had planned or for the activities and events they have missed out on. However, with the right support and advice, this can be worked through and both physical and mental health improved.

With the correct management advice which recognises related multisystemic problems, the majority of patients can self-manage their conditions (with support provided by patient groups), seeking medical appointments only when symptoms flare and the usual strategies no longer work. An improved understanding of the management of these conditions in primary and secondary care has the potential to free up resources and reduce costs.

From an economic perspective, improved management also has the potential to reduce the amount of school missed by young people affected by the conditions and to give adults more options for paid work. Advice on pacing, as one example, helps people to do more, not less.

The Role of Patient Organisations

Condition-specific patient organisations are often the only expert source of holistic advice and support for people living with lesser known conditions. They have a particularly important role in conditions like EDS and PoTS where self-management is central to controlling symptoms and preventing deconditioning. They are able to reinforce information from medical professionals and provide the emotional support and practical advice often not available elsewhere due to resource constraints. This includes providing information to help with access to benefits and education support and signposting to tailored support to help people get into or stay in work while also managing their condition.

The charities in the UK supporting people with EDS, PoTS and related conditions work closely with medical and allied healthcare professionals either in a formal advisory capacity or as a part of the charities' governance structures. In this way, they are generally up to date with the latest research and clinical opinion around the conditions they are supporting and can provide information to patients based on this. There are some excellent examples of collaborations between patient organisations and the medical community, for example educational masterclasses for medical professionals organised by patient organisations, symposia where experts discuss their research and form new international collaborations which advance knowledge of the condition and the development of an online toolkit aimed at primary care.

Wider collaboration between patient organisations and healthcare and other professionals has the potential to reduce the burden of these conditions on health services. Services provided by patient organisations complement treatment and care by providing support for self-management but there seems to be a reluctance to engage in some areas. This may be due to a misunderstanding of the messages the charities are providing to their beneficiaries. However, through the advent of social prescribing [13] we are starting to see small changes in the right direction.

Patient organisations like Ehlers-Danlos Support UK also bring people together through support groups, workshops and other events which encourage peer-to-peer support and reduce isolation. In a 2019 survey about the impact of the charity's services, 86% of 900 respondents said our services reduced feelings of isolation, 88% said the information provided had improved their understanding of managing their health through gentle exercise and healthy eating and 90% said the information and support had positively impacted how they manage their health needs.

When canvassed in 2018, Ehlers-Danlos Support UK members' top three requests for additional services from the charity were increased availability of the helpline, more local support and steps to ensure there are more EDS-trained medical professionals across the UK. The charity has developed a five year plan to address these priorities.

Patient organisations can also play a key role in funding, supporting and shaping essential research. The research priorities of patients may be different to those of clinicians or academics and funding by patient organisations ensures research which is most relevant to patients happens. Patient groups generally have access to a large number of people experiencing the condition(s) in question and can therefore play a pivotal role in recruitment to research studies.

In summary, patient organisations for people affected by EDS, PoTS and related conditions manage the human fall-out from gaps in clinical and social care for these complex conditions on a daily basis. We are also taking a more long-term view by trying to address the lack of awareness and understanding in the medical community through education and influencing commissioners and service providers using real-world data demonstrating the widespread impact of the conditions.

References

1. Malfait F, Francomano C, Byers P, Belmont J, Berglund B, Black J, et al. The 2017 international classification of the Ehlers–Danlos syndromes. Am J Med Gen Part C Semin Med Genet. 2017;**175C**:8–26. https://doi.org/10.1002/ajmg.c.31552.
2. Castori M, Tinkle B, Levy H, Grahame R, Malfait F, Hakim A. A framework for the classification of joint hypermobility and related conditions. Am J Med Genet Part C Semin Med Genet. 2017;175C:148–57. https://doi.org/10.1002/ajmg.c.31539.
3. Hakim A. Hypermobility, overmedicalised? J Rheumatol. 2012;51(suppl_3):iii2 (I11) (Abstract).
4. Talem Law. Fabricated and Induced Illness—Cases on the Rise, Apparently. 19 March 2018. http://talemlaw.co.uk/fabricated-induced-illness-cases-rise-apparently/.
5. BBC 5 Live Investigates. Parents accused of exaggerating illness in children. Broadcast 5 May 2019. https://www.bbc.co.uk/sounds/play/m00050jw. Accessed 7 May 2019.
6. Castori M, Camerota F, Celletti C, Grammatico P, Padua L. Quality of life in the classic and hypermobility types of Ehlers-Danlos syndrome. Ann Neuro. 2010;67:145–6.
7. Bowen JM, Sobey GJ, Burrows NP, Colombi M, Lavallee ME, Malfait F, Francomano CA. Ehlers-Danlos syndrome, classical type. Am J Med Genet Part C Semin Med Genet. 2017;175C:27–39. https://doi.org/10.1002/ajmg.c.31548.
8. Byers PH, Belmont J, Black J, De Backer J, Frank M, Jeunemaitre X, Johnson D, Pepin M, Robert L, Sanders L, Wheeldon N. Diagnosis, natural history, and management in vascular Ehlers-Danlos syndrome. Am J Med Genet Part C Semin Med Genet. 2017;175C:40–7. https://doi.org/10.1002/ajmg.c.31553.
9. Engelbert RH, Juul-Kristensen B, Pacey V, de Wandele I, Smeenk S, Woinarosky N, Sabo S, Scheper MC, Russek L, Simmonds JV. The evidence-based rationale for physical therapy treatment of children, adolescents, and adults diagnosed with joint hypermobility syndrome/hypermobile Ehlers Danlos syndrome. Am J Med Genet Part C Semin Med Genet. 2017;175C:158–67. https://doi.org/10.1002/ajmg.c.31545.
10. Smith GR, Monson RA, Ray DC. Patients with multiple unexplained symptoms: their characteristics, functional health, and health care utilization. Arch Intern Med. 1986;146:69–72.
11. Hiller W, Fichter M, Reif W. A controlled treatment study of somatoform disorders including analysis of healthcare utilisation and cost-effectiveness. J Psychosom Res. 2003;54:369–80.
12. Royal College of General Practitioners. The Ehlers-Danlos Syndromes Toolkit. 2018. https://www.rcgp.org.uk/eds. Accessed 6 May 2019.
13. Frostick C, Bertotti M. Social prescribing in general practice. Br J Gen Pract. 2019;69(688):538–539. https://bjgp.org/content/69/688/538.

Index

N. Gall et al. (eds.), *Postural Tachycardia Syndrome*, https://doi.org/10.1007/978-3-030-54165-1